MW00527308

THE HANDBOOK OF SANDPLAY THERAPY

Barbara A. Turner, Ph.D.

TEMENOS PRESS®

The Handbook of Sandplay Therapy

Published by

TEMENOS PRESS®
Box 305
Cloverdale, California 95425
USA
www.temenospress.com

3 4 5 6 7 8 9 10

ISBN 0-9728517-3-9

Cover and book design by Charlotte M. Turner, Ph.D.
Printed in the United States of America

Library of Congress Cataloging-in-Publication Data

Turner, Barbara A.
The handbook of sandplay therapy / Barbara A. Turner.
p.cm.
Includes bibliographical references and index.
LCCN 2004090235
ISBN 097285173-9

Sandplay Therapy—Psychology—Depth Psychology—
Symbolism—Child Psychology—Jungian Psychology—
Mental Health Treatment—Handbooks, manuals.
I. Title.
RC489.S25T87 2004 616.89'1653

For Dora Kalff

Acknowledgements

My deepest appreciation to,

My Sandplay Clients, who generously agreed to share their intimate journeys in order that other people might be relieved of pain and suffering and that others might know the joys of their unique inner light. I have an abiding love and respect for each of you. Moreover, I am humbled by the profound lessons each of you taught me along the way. Bless you.

Thomas Armstrong, my husband, for his inspiring demonstration of writing as a vocation.

Charlotte Turner, my sister, for the precision and clarity of her intelligence and her dedication to what has been very hard work and a lot of fun.

Pam Starr, my friend, for her wisdom, caution, unfailing generous support, and tireless fun.

My Vision Sisters, our women's group that has met for over a decade now, who held me during this project and simply assumed that I could do it. Thanks Jan, Penel, Lucia and Pam.

Linda Dean, my theory consultant, for her deep understanding and tenacious dedication to precision in the finer points of Jungian psychology.

My Content Editors, who dared to be brutally honest, Paula Hall, Robin Anderson, Thomas and Pam.

Ralph Metzner, who awakened in me the mysteries of the Yggdrasil.

Dora Kalff, who, in her no-nonsense manner, sternly set me on this path many years ago. Thank you, for showing me that to be truly seen by another is all that is necessary.

TABLE OF CONTENTS

PART TWO — Process Concepts: Healing and Transformation In Sandplay Therapy

Section I
Developmental Considerations in Sandplay

Section II
Themes in Sandplay Therapy

Section III
Understanding Sandplay Therapy

PART THREE — Procedural Concepts: Implementing Sandplay in the Practice

Section I
Before the Sandplay Session

Section II
During the Sandplay Session

Section III
After the Sandplay Session

PART FOUR — Client Case Examples

The Handbook of
Sandplay Therapy

THE HANDBOOK OF SANDPLAY THERAPY

Introduction

Overview of Sandplay Therapy

Sandplay therapy is a psychotherapeutic tool that has its roots in early twentieth century Europe. Sandplay stems from the work of British physician, Margaret Lowenfeld (1939), who developed the "World Technique" as a means of communicating non-verbally with children in treatment. For a history of the development of sandplay and similar miniature world therapies, please refer to Appendix B, "The History and Development of Sandplay Therapy."

The late Jungian therapist, Dora M. Kalff (1980/2003), of Switzerland developed what she termed *sandplay* for use in Jungian therapy. Our investigation of sandplay therapy builds upon the pioneering work of Dora Kalff, and is specifically a Jungian approach to the material. The reason for this is that the Jungian approach to the work allows for the deepest order of psychic transformation. This will become clearer as we progress through our consideration of the subtleties of sandplay therapy. For now, as an overview, the sandplay method consists of the psychotherapy client's creation of a three-dimensional picture with miniature figures in a tray of sand in the protective presence of a trained practitioner.

The sand tray is 28-1/2 inches long by 19-1/2 inches wide and 3 inches deep. The sides and bottom of the inside of the sand tray are colored light blue. By moving the sand aside, the blue coloration can be used to represent areas of water in the sandy landscape. Real water can be added to the sand to make it adaptable for shaping and sculpting. Miniature figures representing all aspects of life and fantasy are arranged on shelves near the sand tray. A wide variety of building materials out of which the client can fashion needed items is also available.

The therapist encourages the client to make whatever he or she likes in the sand tray and gives no further instructions. As the client works in the sand tray, the therapist sits nearby making note of what figures the client uses and what the client says, or does, if anything. The therapist sketches, or *maps* a diagram of the sand tray for future reference and takes photographs when the sand tray is completed. The actual completion of a sand tray is thus deceptively simple. It is the profound psychological and spiritual process that underlies this simple creation of a picture in the sand that will concern us in our examination of sandplay. The understanding and containment of sandplay is anything but simple. There is a quality of unsullied elegance in a sandplay that embodies a psychic process so complete as to defy all attempts to comprehend its fullness.

The theoretical foundation of sandplay therapy is based on the Jungian concept that the psyche has an autonomous disposition to heal itself and to grow toward fullness (Jung, 1960/1981). Given the proper conditions, this natural tendency is activated. The act of creating a series of three-dimensional sandplays facilitates healing and transformation by bringing up conflicts from the unconscious in symbolic form and by allowing a healthy re-ordering of psychological contents. Through the transformative nature of what is known as the *transcendent function*, the symbolic process of sandplay involves a re-ordering of the conscious ego to the Self, which is considered the central archetype in Jungian psychology.

Symbols appear in sandplay as individual figures, clusters of figures or whole sand trays, and in the series of sand trays, which is referred to as a *process*. The sandplay method facilitates the healing of psychic wounds and taps latent developmental potentials. Sandplay permits the client to align his or her identity and experiences with this inner core of the Self. Through the course of the sandplay process the client comes to know that who he or she "*is*" is anchored in the deepest inner truth—in something divine.

Within the safety of the therapeutic relationship between therapist and client, sandplay allows the client to go beyond the limits of the conscious mind, to stimulate psychic development, and to access channels to fuller, more creative living. Sandplay therapy is used in treatment of both adults and children. No analysis or interpretation is made to the client until after the process is completed and sufficient time has passed to allow for the integration of the work undergone.

Although no interpretation is made with the client at the time the sand tray is produced, it is very important that the therapist develops an understanding of what is transpiring in the client's sandplay process. This understanding plays a critical role in the *containment*, or *holding*, of the client's emerging unconscious material (Turner, 1994). The therapist's more conscious awareness of the symbolic process, which is yet largely unconscious to the client, acts as a stabilizing factor to the often uncertain and tumultuous qualities of the emergence and integration of unconscious material for the client. The capacity of the therapist to safely hold the client's emerging unconscious content works cooperatively with the client's ability to integrate and make conscious this symbolic material. It is thus essential that the sandplay therapist continually refines and cultivates the ability to hold and have a degree of conscious awareness about the symbolic contents of the sandplay process. It is not necessary, nor is it possible, to understand everything that transpires in sandplay. The nature of symbolic process is that it always leads beyond itself and is not reductive. However, Dora Kalff (1988) stated that, in order to provide adequate containment for the process, it is necessary that the sandplay therapist be continually engaged in the process of becoming conscious of what is transpiring.

Several noted sandplay scholars pay particular attention to the therapist's involvement in the sandplay process. Martin Kalff (1993), noted sandplay teacher and Tibetan Buddhist scholar, emphasized that the verbal analysis of sandplay cannot fully represent the contents of the symbolic images and is only successful when the analysis points beyond itself. Interpreting sandplay involves the thinking process, but it should also include the functions of intuition, feeling, and sensation. Martin Kalff emphasized that the analysis of the sandplay is secondary to the capacity to understand and participate in the client's process on a preverbal level. Observing that these activities work together, M. Kalff noted that the refined ability to interpret sandplay cultivates deeper respect for the healing and transformational process. Bradway and McCoard (1997) emphasized the responsibility of the therapist to become familiar with the cultural and archetypal dimensions of the content of the sand trays. Like M. Kalff, they also stressed the importance of understanding the sandplay through both thinking and feeling. Estelle Weinrib (1983/2004) observed that the therapist must empathetically "enter" the sandplay process with the client.

> The silent capacity to enter into the creation of his world with the patient can, in itself, help repair the feeling of isolation with which so many people are afflicted (2004, p.33).

THE HANDBOOK OF SANDPLAY THERAPY

In the pages ahead we will take a close look at the varied aspects of sandplay therapy. The material is divided into four primary parts:

I. Theoretical Concepts
II. Process Concepts
III. Procedural Concepts
IV. Case Illustrations.

Our exploration of sandplay necessarily entails some repetition and overlapping discussion. What follows stems from the challenging task of attempting to describe in language that which is a non-verbal process. As the author, it is my hope to do this appropriately and with reverence for the mysteries of this ineffable psycho-spiritual engagement. My intent is always to share my experiences and understanding of sandplay from the loving spirit of healing and transformation. Perhaps in this way the restorative and regenerative spirit of sandplay that has been so generously shared with me by my teachers can be further passed along to more therapists. And perhaps in some small way this can work to facilitate the healing of our individual and communal souls that is so urgently needed. This book is addressed to the psychotherapist, but it might be found interesting by non-professionals curious to know more about sandplay therapy.

I ask that you undertake the reading of this material with a spirit of compassion. Nothing that is said here is either a "rule" or "right." Neither the psyche nor sandplay lend themselves to the confines of such dualistic limitations. As a sandplay therapist, you must find your own way with the work. This emerges ultimately from the truth of knowing your Self. Following black and white rules is far easier than the rigors of this engagement. However, nothing is as fulfilling as coming to understand and live your own truth. Furthermore, nothing is as healing to our clients as witnessing them from this place of center. Ultimately, the re-ordering of our cultural and global ills begins with such a re-ordering of our selves. This is what sandplay is about. Throughout this journey into sandplay the reader is continually reminded to listen deeply to the callings of his or her inner truth and to always honor it.

I hope that you will enjoy what lies ahead, and that this material will challenge your body, mind and spirit. Perhaps you will find that you have responses to the material ranging somewhere between disinterest, deep inspiration, and strong dislike. Sandplay has the capacity to touch the deepest layers of the psyche and can evoke very strong emotions. Should you feel greatly inspired by what you read, please use this to move deeper within your Self personally and professionally. And should you find that you strongly resist or clash against something you come across, be assured that something deep within you has also been touched. Sandplay can engage us at such fundamental levels as to make us feel that our very existence is threatened. When this occurs we can be certain that we have definitely entered into the process of sandplay. Holding these inner struggles within ourselves and allowing them to move and transform us can be some of the most difficult challenges we face. Throughout this work, it is my hope that whatever places are tapped within ourselves, we welcome them as evidence that we are deeply involved in the sandplay process. It is my deepest hope that we will be able to hold them and allow them to transform us, to carry us beyond the limits of our known selves, to realize the possibilities innate in each of us, and to become more of who we have the potential to be.

Barbara Turner, PhD
Cloverdale, CA 2005
bturn@sonic.net

PART ONE

Theoretical Concepts: How Sandplay Therapy Works

PART ONE

Theoretical Concepts: How Sandplay Therapy Works

Introduction

Jungian sandplay therapy is distinguished from other methods of work in the sand tray by what is known as the *transcendent function*, the agent or faculty of the deepest order of psychic change. In order come into relationship with the unconscious and to allow a place for the transcendent function in our therapeutic work, we must have a conceptual framework of the psyche and its functioning. The psyche is, of course, beyond words and description. Jung (1960/1981) said that attempting to describe the psyche is like trying to describe the world. Where do we start, and through what lens do we look? As sandplay therapists we use a Jungian lens as a way of engaging with the client's work in the sand tray. The reason for this is that Jung's theoretical model of the psyche intentionally makes space for the deepest order of transformation and the fullest development of human potential.

In any theoretical description of the psyche, what we are describing is the map, not the territory. The definitions of the various psychic structures and dynamics that we will be discussing build upon themselves and are defined by their own terms. These concepts can be difficult to grasp and require frequent review on our part as therapists in order to deepen our working relationship to them. This requires that we be patient with ourselves.

The examples used in this Handbook to illustrate the various concepts have been abstracted from case material and are not reflective of overall process. The case illustrations are alphabetized by pseudonym in PART FOUR and are used with the kind permission of the clients. Each image is provided in an attempt to illustrate a particular theoretical concept or process. Some of these examples may work better for you than others. At all times it is important to keep in mind that you may never see examples like these in your own clinical work. The nature of sandplay is so diverse and unique that there is no limit to the ways the psyche might manifest in your own case material. The examples are furnished only to lend the flavor of the particular psychic construct

In Chapter One, we review the elements of the *structure* of the psyche. Chapter Two looks at the *dynamics*, or interactions, of these elements. Chapter Three examines symbolic process and how symbols work to heal and transform. Finally, Chapter Four explores the critical *role of the therapist* in sandplay therapy.

Chapter 1

The Structure of the Psyche

Jung (1956/1976) observed that there appear to be two types of thinking: directed and undirected. In his observations of people, he noticed that directed thinking attempts to establish order. Directed thinking is characterized by speech, is linear, sequential, and rational. Jung noticed however, that this directed form of thinking appeared to emerge out of another form of thought. He observed that the underlying mental process was altogether different from what we know as conventional, rational thinking. What he discerned was an undirected type of thought, which was characterized by image. Jung perceived that undirected thinking was not at all random; rather, it appeared to be a meaningful product of underlying mental processes. From these observations, Jung developed his concepts of the *unconscious* and the *conscious* mind.

The Unconscious

The unconscious is essentially that of which we are inseparably constituted yet remain largely unaware. The unconscious consists of two primary components, the *personal* and the *collective* (Jung, 1953/1977).

> **Personal Unconscious:** The personal unconscious is created essentially by repression. We become conscious of something, but forget it, find it unacceptable or intolerable, and "tuck it away" back in the unconscious (Jung, 1953/1977).
>
> **Collective Unconscious:** The collective unconscious is made up of instincts and archetypes. Jung (1960/1981) postulated that,
>
> > The collective unconscious contains the whole spiritual heritage of mankind's evolution, born anew in the brain structure of every individual (p.158).

The collective unconscious might be likened to the entirety of humankind's potential and history, which crosses all limits of culture and time. Myths and fairy tales are projections of the contents of the collective unconscious. The personal and collective psyches are not as clearly divided as their definitions might seem to indicate.

Images and symbols are the language of the unconscious. Jung (1959/1980; 1960/1981) saw the unconscious as creative potential and as functioning to support the developmental possibility of individuals and of humankind.

Consciousness and Being Conscious

Consciousness and being conscious are two of the most important concepts in understanding Jungian psychology. Because the two terms are frequently confused and used interchangeably, we must first distinguish between the *domain of consciousness* and the *activity of being conscious.*

Consciousness is basically that of which we *can be* aware. Consciousness rises out of the unconscious. In its essence, consciousness is a province of the psyche and is neither awareness nor the process of thought. Jung defined the domain of consciousness as consisting of what he called *the four functions,* or styles of processing inner and outer world information.

The ego reflects upon, illuminates, elements that are in the domain of consciousness, thus bringing them into *conscious awareness.* To become conscious is an essential element in the process of *individuation,* which concerns the relationship of the ego to the contents of the psyche. As the organ of consciousness, the ego, which we will discuss more in detail later, has the ability to access some of the hidden contents of the psyche, thus making them conscious. The larger body of the psychic contents not reflected by the ego remains unconscious and nothing can be conscious without an ego to which it refers.

The Conscious and Unconscious in Sandplay

Sandplay creations involve components of the boundary between what is conscious and what is unconscious. As they are three-dimensional, there are clearly elements of the sand tray that are conscious to the client. If the client places a cow in the sand tray saying, "This is certainly a cute cow!" he or she is conscious that that is a cow. What, why, and how other elements of the tray might be in relationship to that cow may be far less conscious, however.

Portions of the sandplay content may move to greater levels of conscious awareness as the client reflects on his or her sand tray. For the large part however, the sandplay production is not rational to the client at the time of its creation. It might be best thought of as *in advance of* the client's conscious awareness. By virtue of its creation in a three-dimensional, concrete form in the presence of a witness, the sandplay content is intentionally set in position to effect potential changes in the conscious awareness of the two participants. The sandplay therapist never amplifies the symbolic content, as may occur in dream work or traditional analysis. Rather, he or she holds the client's work in silence and allows its potentials to develop in their own time.

The sandplay tradition articulates two modes of psychic process. Martin Kalff (1993) referred to the work of Erich Neumann (1953/1973, 1972/1955) and distinguished between what he called *lunar* and *solar* forms of consciousness. M. Kalff observed that sandplay is characterized by the lunar form of awareness. Lunar consciousness is not unconscious, but it is to be distinguished from the rational, verbal characteristics of solar consciousness. Thus, what appears in the sand tray is a form of conscious awareness, but it has not risen to a fully conscious level. We might say that what appears in sandplay is on the crest of the wave of the unconscious, but it is conscious enough to be material and three-dimensional.

In her explanations of the world technique, Margaret Lowenfeld also spoke of an early less defined form of consciousness she called a *protosystem* (1993/1979). Lowenfeld observed that this was characteristic of the child's mental experience prior to the development of more advanced linear reasoning and verbal capacities. In the consciousness of the protosystem, the temporal passage of time does not exist. All that transpires does so "at once." Lowenfeld observed that world creations, for the most part, take place in this state of timelessness.

Lowenfeld's early observations provide a valuable tool for helping the therapist hold and understand what happens in sandplay. What appears in the sand tray does make a visible appearance, yet it is not so conscious as to be rationally understood or verbally articulated. Although what takes place in the sand tray may reflect historical or time-ordered conditions, what we see in the sand tray is the psyche's experience of the material occurring at the same time. It is outside of time.

LENAE Examples of the movement of consciousness and the unconscious in sandplay are seen in the work of **Lenae**, age eight, who entered treatment to deal with issues regarding her parents' divorce, her mother's suspicions of sexual abuse by the father, and her father's alcoholism.

The unconscious dynamics in the family system are evident in **Lenae's Tray 1**. The family of nesting dolls, a mother, father and two children, the same family configuration as the client's, are seen laying down on the shore of the body of water. Books covering the faces of the two children further suggest the unconscious condition. A bottle is half-buried, half-exposed on the left. While much is unconscious in this first sandplay, hopeful indicators include a pelican, representative of a profound form of nurture. A tiny pine tree, the beginnings of growth, is also present.

Later in **Lenae's** work, **Tray 6**, greater levels of conscious awareness surface as a family of whales emerges from the central spiral shell. Whales frequently represent a journey in the depths. Their surfacing here is a likely sign that they bring new awareness collected in their underworld journey. The progressively larger chambers of the spiraled nautilus shell also indicate a progressive form of growth or movement. The central presentation of the family of whales in this sand tray seems to indicate the emergence of something from the depths—a coming to conscious awareness in this family, or something about this family dynamic.

The Ego

The ego is an active complex and is the executive organ of consciousness. The ego complex reflects material that is in the domain of consciousness. The ego builds upon awareness and the retention of psychic contents through a discerning reflection regarding the relationship of these contents to what we have already learned. Building conscious awareness is a process of organizing the meanings of perceptions and their application to the individual's life. The ego's function is to both recognize and assimilate the external and internal realms, and to translate the world we experience into a manageable, coherent reality.

The ego discriminates among the contents of the psyche. It functions to control instincts and to facilitate adaptation to cultural norms. In the process of so doing it can become unbalanced and out of touch with the darker elements of the psyche. Jung (1956/1976) felt that it was essential that the ego reflect the presence and power of unconscious psychic contents, lest serious unconscious eruptions occur. This is a process that takes place on an individual as well as a collective, or cultural level. In fact, Jung (1954/1981) asserted that many of the ills of Western culture result from its one-sided valuation of rationalism and its avoidance of the less conscious, mysterious components of psychic life. Jung's observations, made in the earlier part of the twentieth century, anticipated the urgent warnings of today's philosophers and deep ecologists, who assail the global dangers of this unbalance in Western rationalism (Glendenning, 1994; Harman, 1988; Allen, 2007). If we do not, as individuals and as cultures, heed the unseen mysteries in ourselves and in our earth, many predict that our world cannot survive. The ego complex is a critically valuable psychic component, but what is needed to restore individual and global vitality is a healthy, balanced relationship between *ego-consciousness*, the activity of being conscious, and the deeper levels of the unconscious. As products of modern Western culture, we are painfully bereft of the means and knowledge of how to go about repairing this vital relationship between our conscious awareness and the greater mystery which surrounds and supports us, and of which we are an inseparable part. It is primarily for this reason that sandplay therapy is of such profound benefit. To enter the sand is to consent to the conscious engagement with the wonder of the unconscious, to acknowledge the vastness of its presence, and to allow it to inform us as to where we are wanting.

Frequently the ego is likened to a flashlight in a dark room. It can only focus on, or reflect, what is in its beam and does not see the big picture. The ego complex constructs *reality* out of bits, by illuminating mere pieces of the greater totality of the Self (Jung, 1971/1977).

For the sake of discussion let us borrow from the Eastern philosophies and assume that the entire universe (known as the Self in Jungian psychology) is unbounded energy, a unified wholeness, as described in several traditions (Eliade, 1958/1996). In order to function and make sense out of this totality, as human beings we must impose boundaries and limitations on what we perceive. Not to do so would result in our being overwhelmed. The ego is thus the psychic complex that functions to limit and to attempt to make sense of what we perceive in conscious awareness.

The ego complex is the center of consciousness. Jung described the ego as the subjective self of consciousness. He distinguished this characteristic of the ego from the Self, which he described as the subject of the entire psyche. Jung described the ego in this way,

> By ego I understand a complex of ideas which constitutes the center of my field of consciousness and appears to possess a high degree of continuity and identity (1971/1977, p.425).

To return to our flashlight analogy, the ego has the capacity to adjust and direct the beam of the flashlight. The ego is not the psychic content upon which its light shines. The sense of who we are, the subjective self, is formed as the ego illuminates and defines the parameters of ourselves in this world. As the central organizing point of conscious awareness, a reality is fashioned in the ego complex based on what is illuminated. Once this picture of reality is highlighted, the ego holds onto it tightly. In order to function as human beings, we need a sense of what is, or what is predictable. Without this we lapse into psychic chaos. Thus, the ego, is the psychic organ through which our realities and identities are defined and maintained.

This is a significant consideration when we extend this definition beyond our own individual perceptions of reality to broader social and cultural constructs. It is important to remember that what we take for granted as real, personally and as social groups, is nothing more than individual, or collective ego constructs. It is a reality assembled from bits and pieces of perceptions.

Another vital feature of the ego is that it has a drive to Self-actualize. Back to the flashlight analogy, while the ego only lights what is in its beam, at the same time, it has an intrinsic motivation to become whole. It wants to see more, to see the bigger picture. An inherent tension is implied here. As the organ of consciousness, the ego is quite limited in its purview, yet it creates the subjective awareness that the reality that it reflects is all that there is. However, it is concurrently discontented with its own limitations and is driven to become more. To become more requires that what it is, or its current limitations, be changed. In order for the individual to develop and to reflect more into conscious awareness, the ego must submit to its own partial destruction. In the process of growth and transformation, the ego structure must be sufficiently sturdy to withstand the assaults of the unconscious. It must be simultaneously strong enough to maintain a semblance of itself, while being flexible enough to undergo alteration. The beam and clarity of the flashlight need to be progressively increased without destroying the flashlight itself.

Because sandplay therapy probes the depths of being, the ego of the sand player must be sufficiently sturdy to withstand these rough undergoings. This can be a treacherous process. The presence of the sandplay therapist has the potential to provide added stability to the reconfiguration of the client's ego structure. Until such time as the client is able to do this for him or herself, the therapist's presence may bring the needed ego strength to the healing arena during this process. In addition to functioning to strengthen a fragile ego, sandplay may also work to soften an overly rigid ego. The therapist's presence has the potential to *contain* the client's process and *hold* the process, as he or she takes risks to release an overly rigid ego.

The sandplays in the following examples have been selected to evidence various qualities of ego functioning. As we look at these illustrations, let's remember that there is far more to each of these sand trays than we are currently taking into consideration. For the moment, we are directing our focus toward ego structure.

AARON Nine-year-old **Aaron's Tray 1** provides a good example of stable ego structure. **Aaron** entered treatment to deal with issues of anger regarding his absent, alcoholic father and his parents' divorce. As his sandplay process progressed, he did a lot of work on issues of his own masculinity. This sand tray indicates a stable, age-appropriate ego function. There is a great deal going on in the sand tray, but the ego strength is evident in that both its content and structure are organized, relational, and well defined. This sand tray seems to indicate that this child's ego structure is sufficiently intact to undergo the deep work that lies ahead of him.

ROSA Twelve year-old **Rosa's Tray 1** presents an entirely different picture. It is clearly evident that this child's ego stability and level of differentiation is gravely precarious, at best. The structure, organization, clarity, fluidity and relational qualities of our first example are absent in this tray. At first view, the sand tray does not appear to be the work of a twelve year-old child. Although she stood touching the sand for some time, her affect during the construction of the sandplay was fearful. When I quietly asked her if it was too scary, she looked relieved and bobbed her head up and down. I assured her that she did not have to do any more sand trays. This child's ego structure was so weak, she was not able to discern whether or not she even wanted to do a sandplay. It saddens me that I put her in the position of doing something so frightening.

TARA **Tara's Tray 1** is the first sandplay of a woman in her 30's, who entered therapy to address issues of childhood sexual molest and relationship difficulties. This sand tray appears to indicate a shaky ego structure. There is some organization and structure, particularly in the configuration of the sand, which assumes the form of a female torso. The neck and shoulder area is to the left, with the hip and pelvis to the right. The area of the breasts, the primary target of her abuse, is given particular attention. The landform is choppy, as if done nervously. The content and placement of the figures is random and there appears to be little or no relationship between the figures.

Tara's Tray 20 shows that the ego structure has been greatly strengthened, as is evidenced in the appearance of the spiral shell on the central mound. The significance of this manifestation is further highlighted by its intentional reflection in the round mirror. So many years later, I still smile warmly as I recall this client's delight when she adjusted the round mirror just so it would perfectly reflect this beautiful spiral.

LEO Eight-year-old **Leo's Trays 1, 4 and 6** are a wonderful example of the psyche's movement to establish a sturdy ego structure. The first tray indicates a chaotic circumstance and poor ego structure. **Tray 4** evidences ego establishment with the firm planting of a flag on top of a large central mountain. Subsequent to the establishment of the ego, **Tray 6** shows how he began to mobilize his forces. Although **Leo's** therapy ended abruptly at this point, he did make substantial progress in his abilities to initiate action and draw upon his inner resources for healing.

The Four Functions

From his experience, Jung identified four distinct styles, or types, of psychic activity, which constitute ways of perceiving and processing information from both the inner and outer world. The four functions constitute the domain of consciousness by being the modes whereby inner and outer experiences become potentially conscious.

Jung noticed that the psychic experience of people could be described by two rational, and by two irrational, modes of processing. He characterized these as *thinking* and *feeling*, and *sensation* and *intuition*. The *four functions*, as they are known, are present in varying combinations in each individual. Typically one or two predominate, while one or two are less developed. The less-developed functions are referred to numerically as *third* and *fourth* and are known as the *inferior function(s).* Jung introduced the four functions in *Psychological Types.*

> The conscious psyche is an apparatus for adaptation and orientation, and consists of a number of different psychic functions. Among these we can distinguish four basic ones: *sensation, thinking, feeling, intuition.* Under sensation I include all perceptions by means of the sense organs; by thinking I mean the function of intellectual cognition and the forming of logical conclusions; feeling is a function of subjective valuation; intuition I take as perception by way of the unconscious, or perception of unconscious contents (Jung, 1971/1977, p. 518).

Jung concluded that the individual must develop the inferior function or functions in order to grow and transform.

Another concept that has bearing on the perceptual faculties of the four functions is that of *extraversion* and *introversion*, the two primary styles of subjective perception. Jung biographer Deirdre Bair provided an excellent definition of extraversion and introversion in relationship to the four functions:

> ...the introvert sees the world in terms of his own situation within it, whereas the extravert defines himself in terms of what is happening in the world around him. To these two basic ways of perceiving the world, Jung added four basic functions that can be found in differing combinations within both types: thinking, feeling, sensation and intuition. He added a further division within the four functions, the rational pair of thinking and feeling, and the irrational pair of sensation and intuition. Such divisions and pairings gave Jung the model for how an individual both situated and adjusted himself or herself toward both the inner self and the external world (2003, pp. 255-6).

A rich body of literature has been written about the four functions, which extends beyond the scope of this inquiry. What is important to our understanding of sandplay is the role of the four functions as the constituents of consciousness.

The Persona

Persona is the Latin word for person. It refers to the mask an individual puts on in order to face the outer world in a particular role (Jung, 1971/1977). Each of us wears different faces in our various capacities as family members, professionals, etc. An individual may have several personae. These different faces may change, or evolve, over time. Further, a person can simultaneously employ a combination of two or more of these masks.

The persona is a necessary psychic element, and is not inherently pathological. The persona serves as our connection to the outer world and it is appropriate that each of us draws upon different personae to fulfill our various functions in the outer world. Pathology develops when we become overly identified with the persona, because the deeper callings of the Self are not addressed. If, for example, someone cannot see beyond the limits of a career role, it is clear to see how he or she is disregarding the greater part of his or her human potential. In the case of such a rigid fixation to the persona, the ego's drive to Self-actualize will create a pressure upon the fixed orientation, resulting in eruptions of compensatory unconscious material or energy.

In a more fundamental way, the persona consists of a set of skills and defenses that are developed for self-preservation and gratification (Jung, 1953/1977; 1971/1977). In the course of creating our realities we learn what works, how to go about relating to different people, and so on. Some of the adaptive tools we learn are healthier than others, but all initially serve a role in our survival. The persona is generally considered the adaptive personality, or *face,* that an individual presents or uses to adapt to a particular social role.

The persona is what we learned about *what is acceptable* from environmental feedback. *Who we are* is the job of the ego. The healthy ego interacts with the Self in the inner world. The persona facilitates our relationship with the external world. It weaves the survival skills, the ways it learns to get along, into an identity. However, sometimes the ego becomes identified with the persona. This refers back to the tension we spoke of in connection with the ego's move to Self-actualize. The ego's drive to Self-actualize frequently collides with the limitations of the persona. The persona can either support the relationship between the ego and the Self—or be a hindrance if too much over-identification occurs. In the course of healthy development we want to learn what is appropriate and what works in the outer world, and who we are in our inner truth. Most importantly, we want to know the difference between the two.

Developmentally, the parents are the primary instruments of persona formation. Through countless experiences of feedback and mirroring, the parents influence the growing child's sense of identity. To the child, the parents hold the projection of gods. In their secure presence, the child experiences a certain invulnerability, which allows him or her to take risks and to move into the unknown (Wickes, 1927/1966). It is thus that the child is able to learn and grow.

The safety needed to be psychically vulnerable breaks down when the parental images are flawed or when that safety is impaired. When the child's primary caregivers are not able to provide the physical and psychic security required by the child to proceed with growth and development, the child's fundamental need for self-preservation takes precedence. In place of growing into a greater sense of Self, the child's agenda becomes that of learning what tools to use to adapt and survive in the unsafe environment. Instead of relating to the Self, the ego becomes identified with the persona. The persona or set of skills developed by this child will be very different from the potential identity developed in a safe environment. In a healthy and secure setting the same child would be free to explore who he or she really is while concurrently addressing the demands of the environment. The responsibility of good parents is to acknowledge and accept the child's Self as they parent. The parents must ideally honor this unique Self in the child, while instilling their own values and directions as adult guides and protectors.

Needless to say, each of us marches forward with a persona developed out of these early childhood experiences, whether or not it works or fits with the demands of our new environment. The survival skills learned in a particular environment, especially if it was a dysfunctional and unsafe place, will not necessarily translate into safe and healthy ways of living. Who we learned to be, and how we learned to get along in the flawed environment, allowed us to survive that situation. However, these learned skills impose severe limitations in other settings. In such cases, the skills we learned to survive the original dysfunctional circumstances are not applicable or appropriate in other settings. In fact, in attempting to carry this persona forward, we will continually run into pain and problems. This is, of course, the reason many people enter psychotherapy. What we keep doing and how we see ourselves fails us. When the ego is not properly ordered to the Self and is identified with the persona, our energies are continually misdirected.

When there is an over identification with the persona, psychic growth and development requires that the limited ego identity risk an intrapsychic confrontation of the parents, as the original authorities. In such circumstances, it is inevitable that the archetypal images of these original gods must be met head-on and defied. To re-order the ego to the Self, we must stand singularly in the truth of who we are and face the false selves that were held and mirrored by the original caregivers. There is a great intrapsychic risk in doing so, as we must stand radically alone and defy the very people and things that have defined who we are. In the process of surrendering the disordered personae, we confront the need to find our own path. This often requires behaving in ways that were very unsafe in our original environments.

In traditional analysis it is the dissolution of the misconstrued persona that is often the first step toward individuation (Stein, 1982). In sandplay therapy the false persona may appear early in a process as the more conscious images of the sandplay client, or it may be bypassed as the sandplayer moves more immediately into less conscious levels of the work.

The Shadow

The shadow consists of features of the personality that we strive to hide or have never known. The aspects of the shadow that are closer to the realm of consciousness are referred to as the *personal unconscious*. This shadow consists of material that has been experienced by consciousness, but is incompatible with the ego and is repressed (Jung, 1959/1978; 1959/1980). The shadow also consists of the contents of the deeper collective unconscious. This aspect of the shadow is archetypal in nature and consists of all possible qualities potential to human experience that remain in the domain of the unconscious. The shadow includes our weakness, inferiority, and primitive qualities that are unacceptable and or unknown to ourselves or to the collective. Material from both the personal unconscious and the archetypal shadow is present in the sandplay process.

Just as the persona serves as our connection to the outer world, the personal shadow serves as a connection to the collective unconscious. As the shadow is more integrated into consciousness the personal unconscious diminishes, thus making the contents of the deeper collective unconscious more accessible.

Everyone has a shadow, and it is never fully eliminated. Everything in the light of the ego casts a shadow. When the shadow is secluded from consciousness, it is likely to erupt unexpectedly. An essential aspect of growth and psychological maturity is to come to terms with the shadow, to acknowledge its presence, and to develop a working relationship with this aspect of our nature. One of the tasks of analysis or of sandplay is to make the barriers between consciousness and the shadow more penetrable in order to become more conscious of its presence.

In traditional analysis, the shadow is one of the first psychic components dealt with as the persona breaks down (Stein, 1982). There is a flood of inferiority, failure, and weakness that the individual learns to deal with and ultimately to embrace. This course of events is not necessarily as orderly in sandplay, but the principle is the same. A part of the healing and transformative power of sandplay is that the shadow makes its appearance frequently and rather directly. This is facilitated by the *free and protected space* spoken of by Dora Kalff (1980/2003). The availability of the wide range of figures freely allows the shadow to emerge in the sand tray while the physical boundaries of the tray and the added security of the therapist's containment of the process help make its appearance tolerable to the client.

NORMAN Norman's Tray 1 illustrates the appearance of the shadow during the process of constructing the first sand tray through the removal and replacement of prominent figures. This is the work of a man in his 40's, who entered treatment to address erectile and relationship difficulties. The first figure shows Tray 1 in its completed form, while the second figure has been reconstructed to show the process Norman underwent during its construction.

Norman's process first includes a prominent pair of skeletons and a large gold skull. At the time of its construction, this felt like a nakedly authentic presentation of this part of his psychic process. Norman nervously examined this horrifying feature of the sandplay, quickly removed the death figures, and replaced them with a large, armored knight. The final presentation of the tray shows the powerful knight in the place of the more haunting specters that preceded him. Although they made their appearance, the shadowy qualities were once again consigned to an unconscious position.

Norman's Tray 5 illustrates substantial development, along with lurking shadow material. By this time in therapy there was significant improvement in the erectile dysfunction, perhaps evidenced by the large, extended stick in the hands of the unarmored person. However, the shadow of the issues remaining to be addressed makes a dramatic appearance as a threatening dragon directly behind the central figure.

Archetypes & The Self

The archetypes are the crystallized essence, or seeds, of psychic experience. They are the inherited component of the psyche that structure the cardinal forms for psychological experience. The archetypes are the essential patterns of psychic experience and should be distinguished from the images that are attached to them (Jung, 1960/1981). For example, the Venus of Willendorf, the Virgin Mary, and our favorite grandmothers are images attached to the lighter side of the archetype of the Great Mother, but do not constitute the underlying archetype itself.

Archetypes are points in the psyche that both attract and exert energy. They function to structure and organize the psyche. It might be said that the archetypes are the spiritual guides for the material instincts (Jung, 1960/1981; 1971/1977). As the instincts work to direct and organize material existence, so the archetypes function to structure the psyche. There is only an artificial, intellectual distinction between archetypes and instincts. They are two sides of the same coin. There are countless archetypes. Even our attempts to name them limits the fullness of their underlying energetic potentials. Archetypes that function to organize common experiences of life are mother, father, child, wise man, crone, and so on.

The Self is the central archetype, which includes in itself all other archetypes. The Self thus structures all experience—past, present, and future. The Self encompasses the full range of possibility. It is both the source and the goal of all life and manifestation. Archetypes are *patterns of potential* or possibility. Archetypes may manifest, or be active in, the psyche of an individual, or in a group or collective psyche. Mythological themes are the manifestation of archetypes. How they manifest is characterized by the individual or group personality as well as by cultural influences and variants. This accounts for the appearance of similar underlying themes or patterns occurring in a variety of ways in many of the religions and mythologies across cultures (Eliade, 1952/1991; 1958/1996; Wickes, 1927/1966).

It is my observation that what Jung attempts to describe with archetypes is essentially how manifest being configures itself out of the unmanifest. Looking to the Eastern philosophies, the *I Ching, or Book of Changes*, from the Chinese tradition describes this same process by saying,

> ...phenomena take form in the heavens. ...shapes come into being on earth (*I Ching* 1950/1971, p.283).

Jung commented that,

> ...the archetypes have, when they appear, a distinctly numinous character, which can only be described as 'spiritual,' if 'magical' is too strong a word (1960/1981, p. 205).

That is to say that they exert a compelling energy, or force. Archetypes provoke great feeling and have the capacity to overcome an individual or a group when not addressed consciously.

Traditional analysis and sandplay thus entail a deepening appreciation of the archetypal dimension of life. Cultivating the ability to interact consciously with the archetypal dimensions of being opens the individual to the deeper, collective roots of existence and to the essential connectedness of all of manifest being.

The archetypal accessibility afforded by the sandplay process holds tremendous potential for both individual and global healing. As we increase our awareness of our underlying connection to each other and to all things, our capacity to do violence to others or to our world is greatly diminished.

ADRIENNE **Adrienne's Trays 10, 11 and 12** tap a deep source of spirit and energy in this client. A woman in her 30's, she entered therapy to deal with a long-term depression and family of origin issues. Virtually neglected by her narcissistic mother and her weak father, who died of cancer when she was a teenager, this woman was left to grow up on her own. Suffering a lifetime of self-doubt and confusion, her sandplay allowed her to access archetypal sources of meaning and empowerment. In **Tray 10**, **Adrienne's** psyche arrives at the cruxes, or meeting point between her divine nature and the trials of her earthly journey. The meaning of her struggles in terms of her innate wholeness comes together as the archetypal holy mother, the angels and the weary wanderer worship together at the cross.

Having thus meaningfully anchored her passage in the Self, **Adrienne's** psyche is prepared to consciously face the tragedy of her earthly mothering. **Adrienne's Tray 11** pictures her life as a car crash, which kills a mother and leaves a little baby girl unattended.

This resolution of her own abandonment releases a surge of archetypal energy. **Adrienne's Tray 12** shows a thundering herd of sure-footed heavenly horses charging across the tray to the glowing sunshine.

Chapter 2

The Dynamics of the Psyche

In this section we will explore some of the significant interactions of the psychic structures we have defined above with particular emphasis on how they function to heal and transform.

Individuation and Differentiation

Freud (1933;1913/1966) originally described the ego as being driven by *eros* and *thanatos*. Eros is the drive toward pleasure and propagation. It is expansive. Thanatos is the death instinct. It is the force that wants to retire, to come to rest. It contracts. Jung (1971/1977) re-conceptualized the motivations of the ego, theorizing that the ego is driven by the actualization of the Self. According to Jung's observation, the individual's potential life objective is to realize as much of the archetype of the Self as possible. This is accomplished by assimilating as much of the shadow as possible, thereby diminishing the layer of the personal unconscious that separates us from the collective unconscious. This process is what he called *individuation*.

Individuation involves another psychic process which Jung (1971/1977) called *differentiation*. Early in his work Jung observed that the four functions, *thinking, feeling, sensation* and *intuition*, must separate from one another in the process of growth and development. From his experience, Jung concluded that the ability to distinguish thinking, feeling, sensation and intuition allows a person to clearly identify a goal or course of action. Jung saw that when two or more of the functions were confused, the individual was unable to move in a meaningful direction, because he or she could not distinguish what is either relevant or irrelevant to the goal. In his later work Jung emphasized the differentiation between conscious and unconscious material as more central to the process of individuation. Individuation is the process of forming a relationship between the ego and the collective unconscious. Because the unconscious compensates *and* compliments consciousness, a clear understanding of their differences greatly facilitates individuation. Although he placed less emphasis on the differentiation of the four functions in his later work, Jung continued to see the development of the fourth, or inferior function, as important to the overall individuation process.

As we might suspect, individuation and differentiation are characterized by the growing ability to form meaningful, appropriate relationships with other people and with the collective culture. This is significant in sandplay, and it is frequently seen as the growing presence of meaningfully related figures and elements in the sand tray series.

Jung's concept of individuation was a profoundly significant contribution to Western psychological theory, for it implies an inherent *meaning and purpose* to individual development. Individuation embraces a form of meaning that honors the uniqueness of each person and, at the same time acknowledges the common source of all being. Jung's theory essentially integrates a spiritual purpose for human passage into Western developmental theory.

Individuation must be distinguished from the process of integration, which concerns the ego's becoming conscious of cast off, or shadow elements of the psyche. The process of individuation, while it entails a growth in consciousness, always concerns the ego's alignment with the Self as the center of the personality. A substantial degree of integration of the shadow might be said to be a healthy prerequisite to individuation, as a stronger ego is better equipped to withstand the arduous undergoings of individuation and the re-ordering of the ego to the Self. However, the integration of elements into consciousness alone is not individuation. Individuation always involves the re-ordering of the conscious position to accord with the Self.

The process of individuation entails the individual's appreciation of his or her uniqueness and wholeness in a world that may or may not see things in the same way. At the same time, individuation necessarily entails the humble recognition of the individual's human ordinariness. The danger in not acknowledging one's shadowy qualities and limitations leads to serious inflation, while the failure to truly value one's uniqueness and wholeness results in deflation.

Jung originally thought that individuation was unique to the second half of life, but later theorists have extended the concept to early development. The sandplay process with young latency age children appears to provide ample evidence that individuation can indeed occur early in life. The sandplay of 9 year-old **Aaron**, well illustrates the early phases of individuation in a child. A review of **Aaron's** work reveals the wholeness of centering in the Self, the discovery of his own gentle form of masculinity, and a healthy acknowledgment of his need to control his temper. The characteristics of the process of individuation are all present and visible in the sandplay work of this boy.

Sandplay therapy facilitates individuation by integrating cast off shadow elements, by centering the psyche in the core archetype of the Self and by creating an environment into which the Self is invited and addressed with intention.

Compensation

Compensation is the dynamic that concerns the ego's relationship to the collective psyche. It is a life long process that works to achieve balance in the psyche by compensating for the over-emphasis on consciousness. Through the process of compensation the collective unconscious acts on its own to react to the conscious position of the ego, providing an on-going commentary on how well the ego is doing. Compensation can also occur through communications received from the collective conscious world.

Let us recall the ego's drive to Self-actualize and its reluctance to surrender to the fact that it is the servant and not the king of the land. While sometimes the ego is properly aligned to the wholeness of the Self, there are always occasions where it is not. When the conscious position is out of sync with the needs of the Self, a counter tension forms in the unconscious. The process of compensation provides the ego with the quality or psychic product that is opposite the one with which it is misidentified. This initiates the ego's fluctuation between two conflicting identifications that are alternately held in conscious awareness. This process is known as *enantiadromia*, from Heraclitus' notion that anything followed to its extreme will turn into its opposite. Jung commented,

> I use the term enantiadromia for the emergence of the unconscious opposite in the course of time. This characteristic phenomenon practically always occurs when an extreme, one-sided tendency dominates conscious life; in time an equally powerful counterposition is built up, which first inhibits the conscious performance and subsequently breaks through the conscious control (1971/1977, p. 426).

Enantiadromia is not under conscious control, but it occurs of its own accord. During the alternation between the opposing identifications of the ego, one pole is conscious while the other remains unconscious. In its own time, without rhyme or reason, the shift occurs and the poles exchange places. This oscillation between poles continues until such time the process comes to a standstill through the ego's ability to hold both in conscious awareness at the same time and the psychic energy descends into the unconscious to activate material that has the potential to resolve the conflict. This leads to symbol formation, which we discuss below.

Adaptation

Adaptation is the dynamic that concerns the *ego's relationship to outer circumstances.* Life events and daily affairs continually present the individual conscious awareness with challenges and choices of response. How each person responds or adapts to these challenges is of great concern to the process of individuation. It is certainly possible, and not at all uncommon, for people to react unconsciously or by rote to environmental demands. In the process of individuation however, the individual's concern becomes to adapt to these outer circumstances in concert with the direction of the Self.

The process of individuation is that of utilizing life's challenges to move deeper into the truth of the Self. Honoring the directives of the Self makes the process of adaptation a sacred process, as the adaptive choices one makes are in concert with deeply centered inner directives. When we consider the Self as both the goal toward which each individual heads and the source from which all being emanates, adaptation in concert with Self has profound individual, as well as global implications. As the source of all of being is in the Self, Jung's theory, not unlike Eastern spiritual traditions and the more recent theories of quantum physics and mechanics, might be said to indicate an essential inter-connectedness among all of being (Goswami, Reed and Goswami, 1993; Walker, 2000). It thus appears that, as the individual honors the directives of the Self in his or her daily life, so all of being is re-ordered by the concomitant respect accorded the collective Self. The rectitude we attain as individuals has a very real, material impact on all being.

Symbol Formation

Symbol formation begins when the ego's alternating identification with the polar opposites is stilled. As we discussed in our review of the process of compensation, this occurs when the ego is able to simultaneously hold both poles of the opposites in conscious awareness. A great tension develops, as the ego can no longer identify with one pole over the other. The psychic energy builds but has nowhere to go, so it is forced down into the unconscious. This is what psychologist, Pierre Janet (1903) called the *abaissement du niveau mental*, the lessening of mental clarity.

The descent of the psychic energy is fueled by the power of the oppositional dilemma. Running through the Self as the organizing center, it finds the archetype that corresponds to the crisis. The images that are attached to the activated archetype are drawn from the individual's unique personal experiences, as well as from the individual's absorption of cultural experiences. These images form the *symbol*. The symbol emerges out of these archetypal images as the response from the unconscious to the adaptive crises of the ego. The symbol bridges the ego's original misaligned position and the resultant compensatory product from the unconscious, providing a new perspective for addressing the particular crisis.

Symbols enter the ego's awareness in many forms. They can appear in dreams or in fantasies. Symbols may appear as sudden inspirations or intuitions. Physical or somatic symptoms may also function as bodily carriers of symbolic information. Unexplained changes in mood may be indications of symbol formation. And, of course, symbols appear in sandplay therapy.

The Transcendent Function

The *transcendent function* refers to the deepest order of human transformation. It is the ability to climb across, or transcend, the gap between the opposing positions of consciousness and the unconscious in adaptive and psychic crises. Considered one of the most significant concepts in Jung's theory, the transcendent function is a distinguishing characteristic of sandplay therapy, particularly in relationship to symbolic process. We will briefly define this concept here, then we will explore it more in depth in the following section on how symbols work to heal and transform.

The transcendent function is the dynamic through which new psychic energy emerges out of the symbol. As we discussed in the previous section, the unconscious produces compensatory products in response to the ego's misalignment to the Self. This gives rise to the vacillation of the polar opposites in the process of enantiadromia. The *transcendent function* is at work when fate or circumstance forces us to hold both of the two misconstrued opposing views or psychic contents in consciousness. This results in the impossible situation of the ego's mutual and simultaneous certainty of a conviction and its antithesis. When this occurs the fluctuating identifications between the poles halts, the psychic energy builds and dives into the unconscious to activate the symbol, which emerges to resolve the oppositional conflict.

The transcendent function is a repeated process that requires the participation of consciousness, however it is a function of the unconscious psyche over which we have no control.

LILLY Seven year-old **Lilly's sandplay** is a good example of compensatory dynamics. **Lilly** was dealing with the issues surrounding her absent, drug-addicted mother. In **Tray 5 Lilly** cages the saber-toothed tiger in the far left corner of the tray, as an angel appears on the near right. In the angel, the compensatory heavenly counterpart balances the old and dangerous mother image, which is now safely caged. By **Tray 10 Lily's** psyche finds its own safety and nurturing in the same container as she tenderly places two tiger cubs and two pelicans in the protection of the cage. Through the symbolic process she is able to find new, archetypal mothering in the sand-play work.

MAIZIE Eight year-old Maizie's process concerned issues regarding her absent birth mother and a controlling step mom. Maizie's Trays 9 and 10 are a beautiful example of confrontation of the ego's limitations. In the sand trays she deals with the issue of her own identity as feminine. After somberly and ceremoniously anointing everything in the sand tray with water, she proceeds to drown the Barbie doll identity. In this sequence of trays, Maizie released and transformed the caused personality, or persona, expected of her by her parents.

Chapter 3

Symbolic Process: How Symbols Work to Heal and Transform

Definition of a Symbol

The term *symbol* is commonly used to mean something that represents something else. This is not what is meant when we speak of the symbol as an element of depth psychology or of sandplay therapy. The symbol must be thought of, not in a static way, but rather as an *active function* of the psyche. Jung used the term *sign* to mean something that stands for something else.

In our discussion of the process of compensation and symbol formation, we explored how symbols arise when the conscious position of the ego falters in a crisis that it is unequipped to handle. We recall that the ego's misalignment with the Self results in the production of a compensatory product by the unconscious. The ego's misidentification then alternates between the misaligned identity and its compensatory product in the fluctuating condition known as enantiadromia. This alternation of false identities is arrested when the ego is able to hold both of the polar opposites in conscious awareness simultaneously. Being unable to identify fully with both or one over the other, the ego is stymied and comes to a temporary standstill. This initiates the transcendent function. The mounting pressure of the ego's crisis creates a great deal of psychic energy. This energy plunges into the unconscious to activate the archetype relevant to the resolution of the ego's dilemma. Drawing upon the many images and experiences the individual has attached to that particular archetypal core, the psychic energy courses from the archetype, through the Self and re-emerges into consciousness as a symbol.

The symbol holds a counter-balancing position to both the ego's conscious position and its compensatory polar opposite. The symbol is paradoxical, holding both sides of the psychic opposition, as well as something new that bridges the existing conflict. The symbol does not align with either pole of the opposition; rather, it offers the opportunity for an entirely new way of addressing the precipitating crisis. In a conscious, or visible, form symbols hold unconscious material, which if made conscious and reflected upon, supports and furthers the individuation process.

A symbol is partially conscious and partially unconscious. The conscious part is, obviously, that aspect of it that we see or of which we are aware. If for example, the symbol of the cat is activated for an individual, the conscious aspect of the symbol is the furry, be-whiskered, bright-eyed animal. The deeper, archetypal underpinnings of what the symbol of the cat holds or carries for this person, however, remain unconscious until integrated into conscious awareness.

What functions as a symbol for one person may simply function as a sign for another. In the case of our cat, its image is compelling and endlessly intriguing to the person for whom it is working as a symbol. For someone else, it may simply represent another household pet, or wild animal.

It is not possible to create a symbol. To do so would be a conscious effort that overlooks the unconscious aspect of the symbol. The symbol always points to something beyond itself. The portion of the symbol that is conscious indicates something yet unseen and unknown.

In *Psychological Types*, Jung (1971/1977) described the symbol as presupposing the best description of something relatively unknown, but known to exist, or postulated to exist. It points to something that is unconscious and cannot be more directly represented. The symbol seeks to become something. It bears a hidden meaning and is not derived from anything. The symbol is alive and is moving. Jung observed that,

> The symbol is alive only so long as it is pregnant with meaning (p.474).

Once the symbol becomes fully conscious, it ceases to function as a symbol.

The Transcendent Function of the Symbol

The symbol works as a bridge between the ego's limited position and the compensatory product offered by the unconscious in response to the ego's limits. Neither the ego's limited perspective nor the compensatory product holds the answers needed to solve the ego's crisis. Instead, they create a condition of two opposite poles, neither of which provides an adequate solution. The symbol is the energy that connects these two polar opposites, yet its center, unconscious and deep within the psyche, is the archetypal constituent the ego does need to find resolution.

It is important to make a distinction between the production of a symbol that arises in the transcendent function and the unconscious compensatory psychic products that occur when the ego is out of alignment with the Self. During enantiadromia, when psychic energy bounces back and forth between the opposing poles, the ego adopts one side over the other. When this occurs, one side of the identification moves into a conscious position and its polar opposite reverts to the unconscious resulting in the ego's loss of energy. Thus, the compensatory product emanates from the unconscious as a result of ego energies that are *out of balance.*

In contrast, during the course of the transcendent function the symbol arises when both sides of the polar opposites are *simultaneously experienced with equal tension in consciousness.* The symbol provides a resolution to this otherwise insoluble dilemma, expanding and developing the personality by integrating more of the Self into conscious awareness. Symbol formation occurs through an *increase of psychic energy,* powerful enough to activate previously unknown contents in the unconscious that will work in the service of growth and development. The symbol carries the dynamic tension that arises between the ego's position *and* the compensatory product created by the ego's limitations. The symbol thus arises from an archetypal core, which is being stimulated to expand the ego's position. The qualities held by the archetype are those the ego needs to grow and change and to address the current crisis. They are the qualities the conscious position currently lacks, does not see, or fails to identify with.

The symbol's bridging function is critically important. A powerful tension builds up between the two poles of a psychic conflict. The ego, still attempting to identify with a particular position, oscillates back and forth between the two poles. Neither pole satisfies the ego any longer. But the dynamic tension between them compounds as the ego's crisis continues to demand resolution. If the symbolic process progresses toward transformation, the ego reaches a point where it *realizes*, or *sees,* that it cannot identify with both poles of the conflict at the same time, so it comes to a standstill. The ego's position is suspended between the two sides of the conflict. Jung told us that psychic energy cannot stand still. Thus, the tremendous pressure created by the two sides of the irresolvable conflict forces the energy downward into the unconscious to the archetypal core of the symbol. The new product required by the ego to address the crisis situation is thus energized and brought to conscious awareness.

The experience of the transcendent function may feel like a death, because it entails an irrevocable alteration of the ego. It may be felt with despair and hopelessness as the ego's conscious hold is surrendered to an, as yet unknown, new alternative. Undergoing the transcendent function requires the willingness to release the ego's hold when called for, trusting that the outcome will be a fuller life.

Let us create an example to illustrate the symbolic process. If a young man grows up with an abusive, rejecting father, the boy may identify himself as worthless. Because this worthless nature is far out of alignment with the central archetype of the Self, the unconscious compensates by sending an opposite, offsetting identity of grandiosity. In this example the ego has identified with the persona in order to survive. The resulting compensatory identity is as equally off balance as the original misperception. Nonetheless, the young man lives his life in a futile struggle between the false identities, batted back and forth between the two polar identifications, vainly attempting to find his wholeness. One day the ego is able to reflect both positions at the same time, acknowledging that it is both worthless and grandiose. The contradiction is not viable, but this is all the ego has ever known. Although the ego sees no other possibility, it can no longer identify with either pole. The conscious recognition of both sides of the polar swing suspends the movement of energy between the two false identities. The psychic energy dives down into the unconscious to the core archetypal father. We will presume that when he was a little boy, our young man was fascinated with television wildlife documentaries, particularly with lions. During the course of his development, the male lion image became affixed to the father archetype in this boy's psyche. Now, with the activation of this issue in his continued development, the powerful psychic energy from the negative father image attaches itself to the inner image of the mighty, fierce and quiet lion. In this way, the lion is activated as a symbol in our young man's psyche. The lion is now a highly charged psychic image that spans the breadth of the violence and savagery of the rejecting father, the compensatory over-valuation, and a new, empowered image of himself as a man. The symbol of the lion bridges the wounded image of his masculine self and holds a new identity, which is more truly aligned with the Self. In this example, the lion is activated symbolically for the young man. It is imbued with a vital charge that captivates the fatherly aspect of his psyche and facilitates the development of the lion-like qualities. The symbol remains alive, or active, until the qualities it carries are integrated into conscious awareness. When this process is complete the young man will see himself as more worthy and empowered.

Observing Attitude

Jung noticed that it was primarily the attitude of the observer that determines whether or not something functions as a symbol. Speaking of the conscious and unconscious components of the symbol, Jung noted,

> It is the symbolic attitude of the observing consciousness that endows them both with the character of a symbol (1971/1977, p.477).

Returning to the example of our cat, it is the symbolic attitude of the observer that determines whether or not the image of the cat functions in a symbolic way. I like to think of symbolic attitude as a form of reverent contemplation, during which consciousness is positioned to suspend the hold on rationality sufficiently to become receptive to information from something deeper. This might be likened to the liminal awareness of play, somewhere between conscious awareness and unconsciousness that is referred to in developmental and learning theories. We explore this topic in more depth in our considerations of development and the free and protected space. D.W. Winnicott described this state of awareness in relationship to the tensions of balancing inner and outer reality.

> It is assumed ...that the task of reality-acceptance is

> never completed, that no human being is free from the strain of relating inner and outer reality, and that relief from this strain is provided by an intermediate area of experience which is not challenged (arts, religion, etc.). ...This intermediate area is in direct continuity with the play area of the small child who is 'lost' in play (1958/1992, p. 240-1).

With this same attitude of quietude we enter the mysteries of the unknown aspects of ourselves through the symbol. Like the child deep in play, the reverent orientation of symbolic attitude positions the psyche to experience the directives of the Self.

Because of its archetypal core, Jung observed that the symbol touches a similar aspect of every psyche. If several people, or a social group, regards a particular image with the symbolic attitude, the symbol will work to activate similar psychic qualities in each of its observers. The archetypal constituents of a symbol activate the corresponding archetypal component of the individual or group psyche. There are cases, of course, where an individual has unique attributions attached to a particular image, which carry a stronger energy for that person than do the collective meanings of the symbol.

Jung also asserted that the symbol,

> ...compels ... unconscious participation and has a life-giving and life-enhancing effect (1971/1977, p.476).

This is highly interesting. What Jung recognized in this concise observation is that once the visible, or noticeable part of the symbol appears to conscious awareness and is regarded with symbolic attitude, the symbol goes to work on the observing psyche. When the observer's attitude is properly attuned, the energies bridged by the symbol begin to activate and move the psyche of the observer to effect change and growth.

With this understanding of how symbols function, we can begin to see how compelling the healing and transformative aspects of sandplay therapy actually are. The power of the production of the three-dimensional sandplay is incomprehensible. The symbolic content of a series of sand trays in a full sandplay process is so vast as to be unfathomable. The fact that a sandplay is made in concrete form and carries with it the relational content possible only to a three-dimensional medium, gives rise to a uniquely powerful symbolic construction.

The range of figures available to the sandplay client allows the possibility of a symbolic production unique to that individual's growth and transformational needs. Additionally, the three-dimensional nature of this form of symbolic construction exerts a powerful and palpable influence on the client's psyche. The sandplay as a symbolic construction is an act of body, mind and spirit. That the sand is formed and moved, and that the figures are selected and placed in their unique relationships by the sandplayer's own hands, moves the psyche in profound ways.

Chapter 4

The Role of The Therapist In the Symbolic Process

In our previous discussion we explored how the attitude of the observer of a symbol functions to activate its transformational potential. We also considered how the symbol works, in turn, to move and re-configure the psyche of that observer. In sandplay therapy there are two people simultaneously engaged in the symbolic process: the sandplay client and the therapist. This unique therapeutic arrangement of *active, concurrent participation* in the client's symbolic process gives rise to some highly interesting dynamics and accounts for the profound therapeutic potential of sandplay.

The therapist is the most important tool in the sandplay room. Acquiring the sand trays and amassing the sandplay collection are the simpler tasks of doing sandplay therapy. Having these tools is certainly important, but it is the unseen work of the therapist that is the key factor in the overall quality of the sandplay process. Given what we know about symbolic process and observing attitude, it is the *quality of the therapist's presence* that functions as one of the key factors in the overall quality of sandplay work.

The quality of the attending consciousness of the therapist has a material effect on the healing and transformative process of sandplay therapy. The therapist must position him or herself in such a way as to enter into a conscious agreement to hold and understand the client's symbolic work. At the same time, the therapist must be willing to undergo the demands made upon the therapist's own unconscious by the client's sandplay. The therapist thereby joins with the client to create a co-operative, overlapping field of psychic energy to hold the client's symbolic undertaking. Through the impact that the observing attitude has upon the symbolic process, the therapist and client conjointly enter the symbolic field. Their joint effort serves to strengthen the action of the symbol and to increase its potential to effect psychic transformation. The therapist's presence has the capacity to greatly influence the client's symbolic transformation.

In our discussion of the transcendent function, we explored the hazardous conditions undergone in the psyche when the ego's position is no longer tenable and new contents are brought up from the unconscious. When the client reaches this stage of the process in sandplay, he or she must literally surrender the hold on reality. Exactly how terrifying and treacherous this is defies the limits of words. Because observing attitude affects the symbolic process, the therapist's presence works to stabilize the psychic field during this undergoing. Although it is invisible, the stability of the observing ego of the therapist quite literally holds and contains the client's psychic process during this precarious time. By being sufficiently outside of the particular psychic constructs of the client and by bringing more conscious awareness to the process, the therapist's observing attitude has the potential to provide the containment needed by the sandplay client to undergo this violent psychic disunion. We might say that the psyche of the therapist has the potential to function as the sturdy cauldron in which the alchemical transformation takes place.

It is evident how, if properly positioned, the therapist's presence provides strength and stability to the client's symbolic undergoings. By the same token, it becomes apparent how a misplaced or inadequate presence on the part of the therapist can do substantial disservice to, if not gravely endanger, the client during the tumult of the symbolic process. The responsibilities and obligations undertaken by the therapist who chooses to work in sandplay therapy cannot be over emphasized. For the therapist, sandplay demands total presence and complete attention, not only to the symbolic work, but to the therapist's own inner work and life journey. Engagement in the symbolic process at this level demands continual examination of the therapist's own orientation to the Self along with a ceaseless re-ordering to deeper purpose. Anything short of this commitment to inner truth will stand in the way.

To undertake the work of sandplay is to enter a life engagement. The client's work and sand trays are unique and by definition, there is no limit to the meaning of symbols. The sandplay therapist does not *do* something that is left at the office. Rather, he or she enters into active relationship with the symbolic life. This relationship is for life, if not beyond, for essentially such an engagement with the Self is eternal and not about time at all.

Once witnessed, the client's symbolic work in the sand tray is borne by the therapist as a living presence until it becomes conscious to the client. Recalling Jung's distinction between a sign and a symbol, it is only when the work undergone in the sand tray becomes conscious to the client that its symbolic activation ceases and comes to a rest. Until this moment, the therapist is entrusted with the sacred obligation of carrying and containing the tensions of that symbolic mystery together with the client.

The conscious integration of the work undergone in the sand tray may take the client several years. In addition, I strongly suspect that the therapist may continue to carry sandplay far beyond the time its content is consciously integrated into the clients' lives. The therapist bears sandplay creations as embryonic psychic development, which evolves and matures until it is consciously born in the client's psyche. During its active period, the sandplay therapist is profoundly affected by the symbolic material that gestates. Even after this psychic content is birthed and on its way in the clients' lives, the therapist's psyche remembers its children.

The symbolic content of sandplay is vast and limitless. Sandplay therapy does not demand that we know or understand everything that transpires in a process. What it does require is that we remain open to being informed by it and about it. While studying in Switzerland in 1988, I asked Dora Kalff if it was necessary to understand everything going on in a sand tray. I can still hear her words when I recall her remarkable response,

> It is not necessary that we understand everything. But what we must do is *be engaged in the process of coming to understand.*

Doing as Dora Kalff advised, *engaging in the process of coming to understand*, makes several demands of the sandplay therapist.

Doing one's own sandplay work is essential. In order to engage in the medium of sandplay with a client, the therapist *must* have experienced the full movement of his or her own psyche by the same means. Knowing what we do about symbolic process and the profound significance of being a witness to that work, it is clear that the experience of one's own sandplay process is a critical part of the therapist's psychic participation in the process. To attempt to engage in sandplay with a client without having undergone one's own sandplay work is a grievous act of unpreparedness.

The sandplay therapist must study and work with the symbols arising in the clients' work. The symbolic material presented to the sandplay therapist through the clients' work becomes a part of the therapist's own life inquiry. The therapist's engagement with the sandplay work depends in great part upon his or her active association with its symbolic content. With conscious intent, the sandplay therapist must enter into relationship with the client's symbols. The therapist must read about, mull over, play with, dream about, discuss, and in all other ways imaginable, consider and come to understand these mysterious therapeutic allies that present themselves as symbolic configurations in sandplay.

The sandplay therapist must consult with other sandplay therapists. It is essential to review sandplay case material either in a secure group setting or on an individual basis with a trusted sandplay therapist. The symbolic content and process of sandplay therapy is far too great for a single therapist to contain. The input and support of others is very important.

The group or individual consultant functions as an extension of the holding environment. By viewing the case material, the consultant joins the sandplay therapist's role as witness and engages in the client's symbolic process. It is essential there be consistency in the group membership and that trusting relationships be formed between the colleagues sharing in this format. This functions to stabilize and strengthen the therapeutic holding environment. To have the membership in a consultation group constantly changing would not provide the steady holding climate that is required to pursue symbolic process. Also, it would be disrespectful to the client's work to dilute and diffuse its containment with such flimsy conditions.

The benefits and joys of ongoing consultation in sandplay cannot be overstated. Regular consultation both deepens our understanding of our client's work and strengthens our psychic holding of their processes. It is not at all uncommon to see dramatic shifts or deepening in a client's sandplay soon after the therapist has brought the case to consultation. This is a powerful testament to the material effect of the quality of witnessing on the client's sandplay process. The deepened understanding gained by the therapist through consultation and the added containment of the holding power of the consultants both work to move the client's psyche. Additionally, it can be profoundly comforting to have a trusted circle of consultants with whom we can share the uncertainties of sandplay. Sandplay can be frightening. It is important to confer with colleagues to help clarify what is transpiring and to rectify our own positioning as therapists, wherever necessary.

The sandplay therapist must engage in continual study and work with his or her own symbols, arising from dreams, fantasy, synchronous events, and life experience. Using the words of Jungian analyst Edward F. Edinger, the sandplay therapist must be committed to *living the symbolic life* (1972, p.117ff). The symbolic dimension of being must be listened to and heeded in all of its manifestations. And the demands made on the sandplay therapist through the symbolic mystery must be honored as a sacred duty.

The sandplay therapist must engage in continual self-examination of all dimensions of his or her life. Fundamentally it is the quality of the therapist's being that is the tool brought to the sandplay process. Ultimately the sandplay therapist must cultivate the capacity to draw deeply from within in order to co-facilitate the symbolic process with the client. The therapist must effect a cooperative alignment of his or her conscious and unconscious to support and to be moved by the client's symbolic undergoings.

To be properly ordered to the work of sandplay, what we hope to achieve is an abiding attitude of reverence, an open presence to the sacred, and a willingness to be informed by the symbolic process. For ultimately, sandplay is a conscious engagement with the divine presence in the client, in oneself, and with the mystery that informs all of being.

~ Conclusion ~

PART ONE
Theoretical Concepts—
How Sandplay Therapy Works

This concludes our exploration of the theoretical concepts that provide a guideline for the structural components and dynamic movements of the psyche, as well as for the functions of symbols and the therapist in sandplay therapy.

Now we turn to the subject of *process concepts*, in order to deepen our understanding of the many faces of healing and transformation in sand-play.

PART TWO

Process Concepts: Healing and Transformation In Sandplay Therapy

PART TWO

Process Concepts: Healing and Transformation In Sandplay Therapy

Introduction

In the previous chapters we have examined the theoretical concepts of the workings of the psyche, paying particular attention to the role and dynamics of symbols in psychic transformation. These concepts form the foundation we need to ground our further exploration of the *processes* of healing and change that occur in sandplay. In this section we will explore the growth and development of the psyche in sandplay. We will examine the themes through which this healing and change manifests in the sand tray, as well as means of coming to understand this process in sandplay therapy.

Overall, sandplay process consists of a descent into the unconscious to the Self, followed by a re-emergence into consciousness and a re-ordering of the ego to the Self. It is a re-alignment of consciousness to the primordial wholeness from which we come and to which we return. As we discussed earlier in our exploration of the Self, such a conscious alignment of the ego to the Self invests life with meaning and gives purpose to its challenges and circumstances. In sandplay, the process of the re-alignment of consciousness to the Self may occur in several ways. Although it is possible to discern general patterns of process, it is important to remember that each sandplay case is essentially unique and must be allowed to inform the viewer.

The developmental considerations that apply to sandplay bridge several disciplines. While our primary concern is that of intrapsychic growth and healing, other dimensions of development factor into the sandplay process. Matters such as age, gender, and individual history all influence the course of development in sandplay. In the chapters that follow, we will address the subject of development through the lenses of three primary points of view: psychological, mythological, and neurobiological.

Our *psychological* examination of development in sandplay will draw primarily upon the work of Erich Neumann (1953/1973, 1971, 1972 & 1973) to whom Dora Kalff (1980/2003) turned for an explanation of the intrapsychic processes she witnessed taking place in the symbols of the sand tray. In Neumann's work, Kalff found a theoretical structure that keenly articulates development from the depths of the psyche. Although Neumann's work can be challenging to understand, coming into deeper relationship to the workings of sandplay demands that we have an adequate road map of the inner machinations of the psyche's change process. After completing this examination of the more interior aspects of growth and change, we will study some features of developmental differences as they outwardly appear in the sand tray. This will include consideration of issues of client age and gender in sandplay.

In a departure from these more rational considerations of development, we will look to *mythology*, the psyche's own language, for an image-rich understanding of the inner workings of change. While countless mythic sagas depict patterns of healing and transformation, I have selected the ancient Norse tale of Yggdrasil, the world tree, to facilitate our understanding of sandplay for its parallels with Neumann's and Kalff's theory. The roots at the base of Yggdrasil illustrate the steps involved in psychic development, and they serve as points of entry into the change process. Both considerations have bearing on our work in sandplay and deserve close examination.

Finally, we will take a very different approach to sandplay, bringing to our inquiry some contemporary findings in the field of *neurobiology*. Although I can personally make no claims to understanding the sciences beyond a layperson's interest, we will attempt a cursory examination of recent research that has dramatic parallels with Kalff's and Neumann's earlier observations. We will explore findings in the hard sciences that document critical aspects of interpersonal relationship in brain growth and development. In addition, we will examine scientific work that explores the central organizing features of the mind we refer to as the Self.

As we proceed through our discussions of development in sandplay, it remains critical to remember that our sole goal is to deepen our relationship to the sandplay process. Nothing we say is cast in stone, and everything we discuss is intended as a guide to facilitate that relationship.

Section I
Developmental Considerations in Sandplay Therapy

Chapter 1
Developmental Theory in Sandplay—Neumann and Kalff

Introduction

Dora Kalff (1980/2003) drew upon theories of early psychic development from Erich Neumann's 1973 work *The Child: Structure and Dynamics of the Nascent Personality*, to explain the process of healing and transformation as it occurs in sandplay. In this section, we will examine Neumann's psychological theory in order to cultivate a structure for understanding the sequence and characteristics of intrapsychic growth and change that Kalff witnessed.

Neumann's theories provide a tool for understanding the inner mechanisms of change involved in infant development, as well as in the adult's healing and growth processes. Neumann's postulations assume the Self as a central organizing principle. As a means of coming into relationship with these unseen elements of psychic change, Neumann's theories work well.

It is important to note that, as a European, Neumann described the process of inner growth in the Western psyche, which holds conscious awareness as its goal. However, the distinction between conscious awareness and the unconscious presumed as a measure of development in the West, is not prominent in the East. Hayao Kawai (1988) noted Japanese sandplay scholar, observed that the Asian psyche differs by striving to see the whole, thus maintaining vague boundaries between the unconscious and consciousness. The differences in psychic development between the West and the East are an intriguing area for exploration, but they are beyond the scope of this work. I mention them here, as therapists from non-Western cultures, as well as Western therapists working with Asian clients, need to be mindful of these essential differences as they manifest in sandplay.

Neumann was a personal student of C.G. Jung and an acquaintance of Dora Kalff. *The Child* is one of Neumann's (1973) later works and is considered a pinnacle of his distinguished career. In *The Child*, Neumann integrates theories of development by Freud, Klein, Levy-Bruhl, Piaget and others into an intrapsychic, Jungian conceptual framework. The result is a minute, detailed account of the earliest emergence of personality, which is under the direction of the central organizing principle of the Self. Whereas Jung's work is primarily concerned with the adult individual in the second half of life, Neumann's work details the earlier psychic foundations of the later emerging ego-Self relationship.

A wealth of research in child development has emerged since these earlier beginnings in the field. While contemporary research may pose many arguments regarding the particulars of Neumann's ideas regarding infant development, his observations continue to provide a valuable working guide to psychic growth and development from birth to the stabilization of the conscious ego and adaptation to outer, collective life. In fact, those readers who are familiar with object relations and self psychology theories may discover some similarities to Neumann's observations.

Neumann's work provides us with a powerful tool for recognizing the subtleties of the earliest phases of inner development undergone by the growing infant. Understanding this material is essential for our work in sandplay. Frequently, the clients' wounds require them to return to the beginnings of experience, to re-order and re-build the psychic foundations for sturdy personality development and healthy functioning. A firm grasp of early psychic development is also essential in order to understand the inner work characteristic of the healthy individual during the individuation process of the second half of life.

Kalff and Neumann recognized that every expansion of conscious awareness involves the psyche's re-tracing the course of development from the beginning. With each inner transformation, the ego dies and must be reborn in greater and greater conscious relationship to the Self. In order to be fully integrated into the personality, *each new awareness must progress through all phases of psychic evolution.* Thus, as we consider the process of psychic development, we are looking at three dimensions of change:

I. The initial development of the psyche in the child
II. The healing of intrapsychic wounding and arrest
III. The development of each new expansion of conscious awareness that occurs throughout the life span.

Dora Kalff's (1980/2003) work emphasized the critical significance of the foundational relationship between mother and baby. What Neumann referred to as the *primal relationship*, Kalff called the *mother-child unity*. Kalff observed that the healing and transformative work of sandplay takes place on these early levels of development. Through her profound intuition and deep awareness of symbols, Kalff was able to trace the intrapsychic movement of her patients through the most primal phases of development in the sand tray. Time and again, Kalff observed that the sandplay imagery evidenced early wounding in the mother-child relationship. By carefully following the movements of psyche in the sandplays of many people, Kalff discovered that their healing processes frequently re-traced the phases of early child development described by Erich Neumann.

The pattern that Kalff observed entailed evidence of a secure mother-child unity, followed by a relationship to the mother figure. This is followed by the centering of the psyche in the constellation of the archetype of the Self. Healthy ego development comes next, resulting in an abatement of symptoms and restored functioning.

Dora Kalff was not a theorist by nature. That task having been well-handled by Neumann, Kalff referred to the developmental phases she saw in sandplay by the *symbolic imagery* through which they manifested. The following table compares Neumann's theoretical terms with Kalff's symbolic observations.

Early Phases of Psychic Development

Neumann	Kalff
Primal Relationship with Mother	Mother-Child Unity
Separation of the World Parents	Relationship to the Mother
Centroversion	Constellation of the Self

Ego Development Follows

A comparison of Neumann's and Kalff's understanding of the first three phases of the psyche's developmental process.

Phases of Ego Development

Neumann	Kalff
Phallic-Chthonian Magic-Phallic	Animal-Vegetative
Magic-Warlike Solar-Warlike	Battle
Solar-Rational	Adaptation to the Collective

A comparison of Neumann's and Kalff's understanding of the early phases in the development of the ego.

Erich Neumann's Theory of Psychic Development

Now let's turn to Neumann's (1973) theories regarding child development from his work *The Child* and make connections to their application in sandplay. I have attempted to summarize and outline those elements of Neumann's concepts that are of particular significance to understanding sandplay.

Phases of Early Psychic Development

The First Phase of Psychic Development: The Primal Relationship

Neumann (1973) based his perceptions of psychic development on the concept of the Self as the directing center. The Self is *a priori* and unfolds during the course of life in relationship to the environment. The Self exists before development. It is the source of being and development, the guiding center of development, and ultimately, the goal of life itself.

Neumann (1973) described the earliest phase of development as the *primal relationship*. Dora Kalff would later refer to this as the *mother-child unity*. We will use the terms interchangeably. The post-birth mother-child unity is a *participation mystique*, in which the child has no sense of self and other. The child and the mother read each other's unconscious. It is a unified field where the child has no perception of a separate body or of individuality. These do not develop until around one year of age. It is this point that provokes debate in contemporary research. Daniel Stern (1985), among others, argued that even the youngest infant has its own experience of perception, albeit in a less-defined, more global form than will be available with later brain development. Not to dismiss the significance of inquiry into these specifics of early development, the critical feature for our work concerns the relationship between the infant and the primary caregiver, so we will not direct our attention to this debate.

This primary relationship is the foundation of all subsequent relationships. The initial sense of security found in the primal relationship forms the foundation for emotional relatedness in all contact with other people and things.

The Great Good Mother

The primal relationship of the mother-child unity is the foundational phase of development that exists before the development of ego awareness in the child. Due to the archetypal nature of the pre-ego psyche, during this early phase the infant perceives the mother as the great mother and mother goddess in human form. She is an archetypal constituent. In fact, Neumann (1973) observed that the mother remains an all-powerful figure to the child until the child is individualized and the ego develops. The archetypal great mother is indispensable to the child's development. While the child's ego remains suspended in the sheltering wholeness of the mother-Self, it is the great mother that provides the security and confidence that is essential to the sound development of the personality.

Neumann (1973) posited that the mother represents, or carries, the Self of the child. He observed that the neotenous traits evoke tender parental interactions with the child. Neotenous features of babies include the round head, tiny, foreshortened facial features and prominent cheeks and forehead (Gould, 1977; Montague, 1981). Limited body movements are also included with these characteristics. The mother's instinctual caring behaviors initiate complex psychic functions in the child. Although they are very early in the developmental process, Neumann described these as the beginning of psychic development between the ego and the unconscious.

Neumann (1973) theorized that in early childhood, the child's experience is as a body-self. He suggested that the child experiences the outer world through the skin, and the inner world through the alimentary canal. The recurrent contact with the mother gradually brings awareness of the body as a separate self. According to Neumann, the young child has less feeling in the trunk area. This is why small children will frequently draw people with heads, arms and legs, but without a body. Neumann notes that food is a symbol for this relationship; however, it is not an adequate substitute for it.

Neumann (1973) continued this line of reasoning, observing that in this early mother-child phase, the child experiences all spiritual and psychic elements as bodily and tangible. Outer reality has not yet split off from the inner reality of soul and spirit, and they are experienced as a unity. Thus, Neumann observed that the child apprehends the world mythologically. That is to say, the child 's experience is from *within* the mythic. He or she has not yet developed the ability to reflect upon the mythic experience with thoughts, words or distinct mental images. The child lives without the ego, much as the dreamer's ego is suspended while asleep.

The Significance of the Primal Relationship

The nature of the primary mother-child relationship determines the quality of all forms of relationship. This includes relationship to other people, things, and events, as well as to one's own intrapsychic experience. Thus, the relationship of the child to him- or herself is determined by the quality of the original mother-child relationship.

Self confidence depends almost entirely on the primal relationship to the mother. Of great interest however, is Neumann's (1973) observation that, because the child's early experience of the mother is archetypal, the infant is open to other positive, maternal archetypal influences. Neumann suggested that, in addition to the positive containment of the mother, or in spite of mother-child insufficiency, the child can be positively influenced by the archetypal maternal qualities of such things as trees and gardens. Neumann's observation is helpful in understanding how it is that some clients, with evidently poor early parenting, exhibit nonetheless fairly stable and solid personalities.

Neumann (1973) pointed out that it is the boundary-less, uroboric experience of early mother-child unity that becomes the prototype of the popular meaning of falling in love. In lieu of a solidly developed capacity to relate to another human being, Neumann suggested that the relationship behavior of many adults remains relegated to the dimension of the primary relationship absorption by the mother. Judging from the romanticized, alluring advertising material that is used in Western culture to sell products, it becomes painfully clear how few of us are capable of more mature forms of relating. Apparently, many people have unaddressed wounds of varying degrees stemming from early deprivations.

Neumann (1973) attributed the child's ability to perceive reality as an ordered whole, instead of as unrelated parts, to the Eros, the loving and life-giving energy of the primal relationship. Neumann defined Eros as an experience of order and meaning that is feeling-toned. This bond of love experienced in the mother-child relationship allows the child to invest his or her energy into life in a meaningful way. Neumann called this Eros-rich nature of the primary relationship the *matriarchal level of consciousness.*

Another aspect of a solid grounding in a secure mother-child relationship is the individual's capacity to tolerate deprivation or hurt. In the security of the healthy mother-child relationship, the mother acts as the Self for the child. In so doing, she acts in a compensatory manner to mediate the baby's inner and outer hurtful experiences. The mother assures the child that the negative qualities do not predominate his or her experience. In this way, the mother facilitates the child's growing ability to tolerate pain and difficulties. As development progresses and the mother and child begin to move apart, Neumann (1973) commented that the love *between* them increases. Neumann suggested that this further develops the child's capacity to tolerate tension.

A positive primal relationship later enables the developing ego to integrate crises that might arise in the transpersonal dimension, as well as in personal and individual development. That is to say that a positive mother-child relationship helps the child develop the emotional skills and character he or she will need to make profitable use of unconscious material that arises during the course of a lifetime. The solid grounding in the primal relationship positions the individual to be better able to understand and tolerate unconscious eruptions and to have the inner strength to allow such eruptions to move him or her toward greater levels of intrapsychic development. Without these emotional tools developed in early childhood, the individual is battered about by unconscious material. This may result in any degree of inappropriate acting out on unconscious impulses, or may be defended against by a rigid personality structure. In any case, the individual is cut off from both inner and outer world authenticity and relatedness. Neumann (1973) speculated that much of the disorder of Western culture results from this very inability to tolerate intrapsychic tension. Neumann wrote this many years ago, but it is not difficult to see how the violence and cruelty or the possession-driven qualities of contemporary life might be explained by his early observation.

Disturbance in the Mother-Child Unity

Loss of the mother during the critical time of the primary relationship constitutes the child's loss of contact with the world. This results in fundamental impairment in self preservation and the capacity to grow and develop. The loss of the mother during this early phase of development is essentially the destruction of the beginnings of ego development. During this phase of development, the child perceives rejection or condemnation by the mother archetypally. Because the child experiences the Self as body, acceptance or rejection of the body is also tied to acceptance or rejection by the mother.

Disturbance of the mother-child unity can occur as a result of difficulties experienced by the child. Physical illness or discomfort, such as with colic, may present fearsome obstacles to the child's sense of comfort and safety. Because the child does not yet have an experience of his body as separate from the mother's, he or she experiences these disturbances as the loss of the mother. Neumann (1973) reminded us that the crucial factors to consider in matters of psychic development are always the child's archetypal experiences, and not merely the objective data.

Aggression and Psychic Development

Within the primal relationship, the child becomes aggressive when his or her well-being is disturbed by hunger, pain or fear. This aggression serves as a means of self-defense, or as an alarm that communicates the difficulty to the mother. The child is able to integrate his or her aggressions when the personal mother responds appropriately and is able to channel and contain the powerful feelings. From within the archetypal experience, the child experiences this safe holding as the great mother.

Neumann (1973) observed that aggression appears naturally during the onset of any new phase of development. At the beginning of any new phase of psychic development, the sense of well-being is disturbed by the changes necessitated in the growth process. Whether in early child development or in later growth, the subjective experience elicited by change is the same sense of alarm, which is evoked by environmental deprivation in early life. In sandplay, it can be helpful to track themes of aggression in relationship to new phases of development. If aggressive themes seem to appear out of nowhere during the sandplay process, they may indicate the aggression Neumann described as accompanying new development.

Guilt and Psychic Development

Neumann (1973) made a distinction between pervasive forms of guilt and transitory guilt feelings that arise in the normal course of growth and transformation. Neumann observed that chronic feelings of guilt are symptomatic of a disturbed primary relationship. The mother is experienced as being lost, which results in the child's mythic experience of *him or herself* as the terrible mother. The child experiences the loss of the mother as being unloved, condemned, abnormal or revolting. Guilt becomes an all-pervasive feeling, because the child experiences these condemnations as a form of higher, archetypal judgment. On the archetypal level of the psyche this is subjectively experienced as condemnation by God.

With no healing or transformation in later life, the individual continues to perceive the denigration and condemnation as a given, a fact beyond question. Neumann's observations about the formation of primary guilt can be of great help to us in sandplay. By being able to equate pervasive guilt with profound, yet often elusive pre-verbal deprivations, the therapist is better able to contain the primal nature of the client's healing and transformation.

Feelings of guilt are also a natural component of the transformation process when the developing personality surrenders its hold on the material with which it formerly identified. Guilt feelings factor in as the sense of having abandoned what was formerly valued most highly in favor of conscious loyalties to new psychic material. So, every change in psychic development is accompanied by feelings of guilt and loss. In addition, there is a component of grief for what has been lost.

Narcissism and Early Wounding

Neumann (1973) observed that distress in early phases of development results in an ego-less form of apathy and decline in the baby. As the child's development progresses and some ego structure forms, the experiences of early distress result in subjective suffering and negativity.

In its extreme form, the highly disturbed mother-child relationship results in the subjective experience of being unloved. The absence of this essential basis for life sets in motion an insatiable longing to compensate for the lack of love. This loss is the province of narcissism, which Neumann described as the forsaken nature of a *negativized ego*. Neumann distinguished this from a weakened ego, which occurs as a wounding at a later stage of development when the ego has attained some degree of consolidation. The negativized ego shuts itself off from contact. The isolation works to increase the subjective experience of insecurity and forsakenness. In turn, this results in a vicious cycle of rigidity, aggression and negativity that alternates with feelings of inferiority and desolation.

As we recall from our discussions of Jungian personality theory, the ego's task is to represent the total personality in its confrontation with both the inner and outer worlds. The ego works to preserve consciousness and to be open to influences from the unconscious. The stable ego is capable of worldly continuity, as well as growth and transformation. The negativized ego, on the other hand, is rigid. It excludes unconscious contents, causing their energy to build. This results in periodic episodes of chaotic flooding and rage.

HAROLD **Harold's** sandplay case exemplifies this level of early wounding and narcissistic defense. Done when he was in his sixties, sandplay provided him the opportunity to address his very early losses. **Harold's** wounding occurred developmentally prior to his capacity to articulate or consciously understand. The non-verbal, symbolic qualities of sandplay allowed him to return to his grandiose, romanticized defenses, his losses, and his handicapping pain. **Harold's Tray 1** pictures a gravely wounded old man in diagonal opposition to an exaggerated sexy young woman.

Through the course of his sandplay process, **Harold** was able to acknowledge and grieve his loss and to form a healthy, intrapsychic connection to the feminine. **Harold's Trays 2 – 5** hold a profound and painful acknowledgement of loss and grief. In **Tray 5** an old, gray man assumes a central position on a park bench, directly facing the unrealistic, inflated statue of the feminine that he vainly sought his entire life. As he confronts the marble idol directly, a new source of nurture is presented on the table beside him. Now he can eat real food that will meaningfully sustain his spirit.

In terms of his psychic development, **Harold** was able to return to the beginning, to heal, and to begin his developmental journey again. Because of his chronological age, he would likely not be able to progress through all of the subsequent phases of development. However, his sandplay work re-ordered his foundational awareness of himself. Able to heal and transform his pervasive guilt and condemnation, for the first time **Harold** began to know that he was worthwhile as a human being and that he was loveable.

The Primal Relationship in Sandplay— The Mother-Child Unity

From within mythic apperception, the child experiences comfort as paradise. Conversely, the child archetypally experiences distress as being in hell. While it is never possible to ascribe any specific meaning to figures in sandplay in a formulaic manner, the general ambience of the beginning of a new piece of psychic development on the mother-child level is one of pure, quietude that fully holds and supports the newly emerging elements. In sandplay symbolism the mother-child unity may emerge as bucolic scenes with pairs of mothers and babies. These may be animal mothers and their young, or human mothers and babes.

ADRIENNE In her sandplay work, **Adrienne** symbolically addresses her mother's rejection rather directly in **Trays 11 and 20**. The sand tray becomes the gravesite for her painful losses. In **Tray 26**, the body of the sand becomes a womb for the birth of new potentials. **Tray 26** is a beautiful example of the mother-child unity, as the delightful babies crawl about on the surface of the earth mother, herself. Observe that the rounded womb of the earth body carries the figure of the pregnant woman.

IVY **Ivy's Tray 2**, which she called *Paradise*, is another beautiful example of the mother-child unity. In **Ivy's** work, these beginnings of psychic development manifest as animal pairs abiding in a serene garden. **Ivy's** transformed acceptance of her own feminine nature arises out of an earth womb, much as did **Adrienne's.**

AARON In **Aaron's** sandplay work, all three early phases of psychic development appear simultaneously in his **Tray 4**. Having symbolically clarified his wounding, his strengths and the direction of his inner work in **Trays 1, 2 and 3**, the initial three stages of his transformation appear together in **Tray 4**. The mother-child unity is held in the Native American mothers and their babies. The relationship to the mother appears in the community's circular assembly around the fire. The Self constellates in the archetypal configuration of the combined circle and the square of the landscape around the central fire.

Because the child is unable to distinguish between the ego and the unconscious in the earliest phases of development, the infant experiences everything through the body. Neumann (1973) conjectured that, to the very young child, all psychic and environmental factors are mythical and are experienced in alimentary symbolism.

Symbolism with feeding or nutritive themes is characteristic of the first stage of psychic development, the mother-child unity. When we see feeding and eating themes in sandplay, we may be alert to the primal level of the psyche that is being nourished. We may understand that the client has returned to the very beginnings of development, like those of a newborn babe. Irrespective of chronological age, the sandplay client enters a seamless field of nurture and support. Like the newly emerging psyche of the infant, the newly developing psychic quality is just beginning its emergence in sandplay. The client's new psychic product has not yet separated, or distinguished itself, from the ground of its birth. Yet, it has a palpable presence in the stillness of poignant expectancy.

Neumann (1973) speculated that for the child, the natural digestive processes of assimilation and elimination are mythic corollaries to the process of creation and transformation. From the vantage point of the child, creation and transformation are lived out daily. When the client is working at this level of the psyche in the sand, the same archetypal dynamics apply. The distress felt during the early phases of the transformation process in sandplay, when the ego's hold on reality begins to crumble, is the same as that which the infant feels when his or her entire world is threatened. In sandplay the intrapsychic distress induced by the changes and transformation that occur at any phase of development may give rise to hunger and devouring symbolism.

The core symbol for distress at this level of perception is hunger. Gnawing and devouring themes appear. In sandplay we may witness threatening forms of swallowing, such as threatening sharks and monsters. The many devouring arms of the octopus may hold this primitive level of threat, as well. To distinguish between a devouring form of swallowing and a theme of feeding and nurturing we must consider the figures used, as well as the affect of the work.

IVY **Ivy's Tray 4** carries the devouring aspect of the primal relationship in the figure of Jabba the Hutt, the licentious, ceaselessly hungry monster from the film, *Star Wars* (Lucas, 1977; Reynolds, 1998). As the earth swells with the potential for new birth and the two figures of Pegasus rise and roar, **Ivy's** psychic development requires the presence of the dark and devouring aspect of the archetype, which was able to activate her new growth in the safe container of the sandplay. **Ivy** completed this tray many years ago, but I still shudder when I examine it. The power it holds is phenomenal.

ADRIENNE **Adrienne's Tray 20** similarly carries the devouring monsters who stand in front of the ghostly apparition of the dead mother delivering a baby. In **Adrienne's** sandplay, the devouring aspect of the primal relationship is confronted in preparation for the new birth we see in **Tray 26**.

The Second Phase of Psychic Development: Separation of the World Parents

Toward the end of the first year of life, the child's psyche separates from that of the mother. Neumann (1973) referred to this phase of development as the *separation of the world parents.* Dora Kalff described it as the period during which the child is able to form a *relationship to the mother.*

During this phase of development, the child's awareness turns to the outer world, launching a desire for exploration and learning. No longer subsumed in the psyche of the mother, the child's psyche begins to polarize the world into opposites. Initially, these oppositions are very simple divisions of good and bad. They grow in complexity as the child matures.

Feminine and Masculine Energies in Early Development

In the language of Jungian psychology, the earliest experiences of the child are in the feminine. For this reason, Neumann (1973) and Kalff (1980/2003) referred to this dimension of the psyche as *matriarchal.* This is the quality of energy that is dimension-less, dark, unknown, and feeling-toned. It is the realm of the unconscious. The masculine qualities of definition, boundary, rationality, and conscious awareness evolve later with the development of the ego. Neumann theorized that in the early stages of development, the child experiences intrusions to well-being as masculine. These interruptions to the wholeness of the feminine are the beginnings of masculine energy. Disturbances may be either positive or negative experiences. Neumann postulated that the child is later able to distinguish between the positive and negative experiences, attributing positive experiences to the good mother and negative experiences to the terrible mother. Masculine energy subsequently coalesces and becomes more defined with later ego formation. Nonetheless, in the mother-child relationship, everything is experienced as coming from the mother.

The Terrible Mother

Neumann (1973) observed that the initial division of experience into polar opposites assumes the form of a split between the good mother and the terrible mother. Neumann explained that the child's continued dependence upon the mother at this tender age, and the toddler's subjective experience of his or her independence as loneliness, account for this initial split. In this process of growing into a healthy and natural sense of autonomy, the uncertainties of the new experiences create anxiety for the child. The toddler attributes these negative qualities to the mother, which the child subjectively experiences as the terrible mother.

As the child's development and exploration continue, the psyche progressively organizes into pairs of polar oppositions. The child learns patterns of pairs of things that give shape and order to his or her world. The differences between up and down, front and back, good and bad, in and out, and so on, begin to build an intrapsychic structural framework to help decipher the workings of the world.

Separation of the World Parents in Sandplay: Relationship to the Mother

In the sandplay process, this newly emerging psychic growth characteristic of this second phase of psychic development may emerge as pairs of figures. Figures may be placed in groups of twos, as if to call attention to the initial recognition of their being. For example, paths may be laid out in two alternating colors. The variations in symbolic appearance are endless, but the theme of this phase of psychic growth remains one of the new presence of something in relationship to others. The new product is emerging into being, and it is acknowledged. By being witnessed in relationship, its being-ness, its existence, is validated.

Wounding and deprivation at this phase of development may manifest as wicked, abandoning mothers and witches. It may appear as the antithesis of emergence and growth, showing death and loss. In any case, the appearance of the dark side of this phase of development in sandplay is an acknowledgement of its presence. Through recognition it becomes a part of the process of growth and development, albeit one that is accompanied by profound grief.

The Third Phase of Psychic Development: Centroversion

In the child's experience during the first phase of life, the mother holds the archetype of the Self. In the secure mother-child unity, the child experiences reality as a fully ordered, compensatory totality. From within this mythical position the child simultaneously experiences all of the inner and outer worlds as whole and complete. Neumann (1973) speculated that this subjective experience of completeness quickens an innate aptitude for order in the child's psyche that awakens as the Self in later development. As stated above, with continued healthy development, the child begins to experience the polar opposites inherent in manifest reality and develops a relationship to the primary caregiver.

At approximately age three in conditions of adequate love and security, the child's psyche undergoes a natural process of centering. The spark of wholeness ignited in the child's psyche by the experience of the wholeness of the mother, kindles the emergence of the Self in the child. Neumann (1973) called this process *centroversion*. Dora Kalff (1980/2003) referred to it as the *constellation of the* Self.

With this monumental developmental event, the child's psyche separates from that of the mother into an autonomous whole, guided and directed by the centering influence of the Self archetype. The child undergoes a profound inner experience of centering, subjectively recognizing his or her presence at the center of a tremendous pattern of life organization. Of course, at this age, the child has not yet developed the ego structure that allows him or her to reflect upon the experience. The subjective experience of the Self at this phase of development is completeness.

The experience of the Self in early childhood is a form of anthropocentricity in which the child sees him- or herself as the center of the world. To the child, the unconscious experience of the Self in early childhood is the experience of him or herself as a god. The early constellation of the Self defines a point of center, around which it is possible to organize all of human experience. Neumann (1973) commented that this is an indispensable foundation for all of human development and is unique to human beings. Although certain cat fanciers may disagree with Neumann, it is fairly safe to say that the capacity for conscious recognition of the Self as center, which becomes possible later in life, is the unique province of humans.

At the same time, the child experiences the enormity of the Self as overpowering. While the solidity of the mother-child relationship is what allows the child the safety required to surrender to the superior power, the completeness of the Self is an assault to the child's psyche. If the mother-child relationship is secure, the child is able to withstand the incursion. In this way, the healthy mother-child relationship permits a spiritual awakening in the child. This sets the ground for the child's later, more conscious development of the Self.

Centroversion in Sandplay: The Constellation of the Self

The constellation of the Self in the sandplay process culminates the pre-ego phases of psychic development. The newly emerging psychic quality, now having been adequately held, nurtured, and acknowledged as an emerging presence, is at this stage brought to the center of the psyche. For individuals for whom early deprivation and trauma impaired the constellation of the Self, the centering of the Self in sandplay restores order and meaning to life. With the centering in the Self, the client forsakes all doubts about belonging and purpose in life. With the initial constellation of the Self, the psyche is radically re-ordered to a center. While this does not mean that the individual is fully enlightened in the sense of a conscious, ever-after perception of him- or herself and all of reality as divine, it does awaken a profound awareness of centeredness, of core and of purpose, that may be archetypally experienced as the abiding presence of God. The cultivation of a more evolved awareness of Self is dependent upon the individual's continued attention to the ego's conscious relationship to the Self, which is possible further along in the development process. As we have discussed in our exploration of Jungian personality theory, this is the task of the individuation process.

At this point of the discussion, our concern is mainly the centering in the Self as it pertains to the initial process of child development and its role in subsequent growth and change of the psyche. As the third phase in the pre-conscious emergence of new psychic material, the Self serves as the center point for organizing and assimilating the new qualities. For the integrated personality, what is new must run through or touch the Self, before working its way into consciousness.

If we were to compare this process to the development and maturation of a community member in a feudal kingdom, we might liken this phase of the process to being presented to the king. Growing up in this kingdom, it is essential to acknowledge the source of our heritage, before taking our place in the world. It is also essential to be acknowledged by the king, as being a member of the realm. In addition to remembering our beginnings and receiving sanction to participate in life, it is critical to remember whom we continue to serve when we move out into the world.

My experience suggests that the Self may be touched many times and in many ways throughout the course of a sandplay process. My preference is to distinguish between the initial *constellation of the Self*, as a momentous occurrence of great magnitude, and the *manifestation of the Self* as subsequent returns to center. For my own work I make the distinction as a means of acknowledging the foundational level of wounding and repair undergone by the client when the Self is initially constellated. To argue the differences and distinctions, however, seems completely unimportant. The Self is the Self, no matter how we experience it.

The manifestation of the Self in sandplay cannot be subject to formula. Because of its archetypal nature as central, the Self frequently appears in a mandala formation. However, not all mandalas are Self manifestations and not all Self constellations are mandalas. Dora Kalff (1980/2003) observed that the Self manifestation in sandplay was primarily distinguished by its numinous energy.

To attempt to argue what is or is not a Self manifestation seems to me unnecessary and is, perhaps, disrespectful of a client's work. After all, everything that manifests in the sand tray is a reflection of the Self in some way. As the Self is the source of all being, even the most egregious wounding and disorder is held by the Self, as the client moves to heal and re-order the psyche. To hold sandplay work with this awareness seems far more respectful than attempting to account for Self trays. If a presentation in the sand tray is numinous, then it is numinous. If it is not numinous, it is still legitimate work and is still grounded in the Self as source.

Dora Kalff's training cases were filled with constellations of the Self. Whether we can attribute this phenomenon to who she was as a personality, who the clients were whom she treated, or to the particular cases she chose for teaching, is unknown. In any case, it is my experience and that of many of my sandplay colleagues, that while the Self is often touched in sandplay, the Self constellation is a not-too-frequent occurrence. Even so, substantial processes of healing and change do take place. Why this is so may become clear in our discussion of the Yggdrasil myth in the upcoming section.

Ego Development: Formation of the Conscious Functions of the Psyche

Following the separation from the mother and the centering of the Self, a process of ego development is set in motion. We recall from our discussions of Jungian theory that the ego is the organ of consciousness. Until this time of development, the child has lived in a relative state of unconscious participation with the parental psyche.

The ego begins to form when the child has successfully developed a sense of separateness from the mother, is capable of having a relationship with the mother, and has constellated the Self as the center of the individual personality. Under these conditions, the ego then moves through progressive phases of development until it reaches a level of independent conscious functioning.

As with the centering in the Self, Neumann (1973) observed that the true beginnings of the ego actually occur in the very early phases of development, before they become evident in the personality. Neumann observed that in the course of normal child development, an integral ego forms slowly over time. It begins to emerge while the child still lives in a situation of identity with the good mother. Gradually this becomes the ego pole of what Neumann referred to as the ego-Self axis. This development begins in the first phase of the primal relationship and achieves its central position in the second phase of the mother-child unity, at approximately one year of age, when the child's psyche begins to separate from the mother. For the purposes of study, however, Neumann identified ego development in stages that occur *after the centering of the personality in the Self.* Neumann observed that centroversion creates the possibility for not only the centering of the Self, but for the future development of the ego as the center of consciousness as well.

Dynamics of the Development of Consciousness

Whereas Neumann (1973) identified the process of ego development in terms of *psychic dynamics*, Kalff referred to the *symbolic images* that typically characterize these dynamics. Neumann defined five phases in the emergence of consciousness. Dora Kalff (1980/2003) consolidated these into three, based upon their symbolic appearance in the sand tray.

Neumann's Stage 1 Ego Development: The Phallic-Chthonic Phase

According to Neumann (1973), the beginning phase of ego development is passive and is directed by the archetype of the great mother. The matriarchal unconscious still predominates during this first level of ego development, as the masculine consciousness begins its emergence from the participation mystique. At this early phase of development, the child's subjective experience is both omnipotent and impotent. The child is unrestricted by the limits of a developed consciousness, but he or she is also helpless. Neumann described this as an omnipotence of feeling, be it positive or negative.

Neumann's Stage 2 Ego Development The Magic-Phallic Phase

Neumann (1973) theorized that during this phase of development, the young ego begins to be active on its own, but remains essentially determined by the mother archetype.

During this phase of development, the symbol of the circle appears in the child's psyche as a mandala. The circle holds the budding ego as it begins to set itself apart from the uroboric, undefined wholeness of the earliest phase of psychic development. The symbol of the circle carries the ego as it begins to coalesce and set itself apart from the world. Neumann (1973) said that the ego still senses its belonging to the totality of the Self in this early phase of development, thus lending a magical sense of empowerment to the budding conscious autonomy. During this phase of development, the ego experiences the omnipotence of power over the body and has the subjective experience of dominance over the world. Becoming conscious, yet still rooted in the Self, the child's subjective experience is of being at the center of the world. The child's experience is colored by emotionality rather than conscious awareness.

Because the growing child still experiences him- or herself as the center of the world, the orientation is still a mythological one. Categories of experience are grouped as mythic apperceptions of symbols and archetypes. From the orientation of the center emerge the mythic directions of heaven and earth on the vertical axis, and the perception of the passage of time on the horizontal plane. The child's psyche thus begins to structure its conscious reality through the mythic experience of the directions. The subsequent construction of a conscious relationship to life builds upon these rudimentary and mythically experienced coordinates.

Another mythic element that is central to this phase of the ego's emergence is the dependence of the individual on the world and the perception of the world's coincident dependence on the individual. Neumann (1973) observed that the acquisition of food is central to the individual. The budding conscious awareness of this need in the still-magical matrix of the Self gives rise to parallel perceptions that not only is the individual dependent upon the world, but that the world is dependent on the individual. This is observed in mythic themes such as the slaying and devouring of the youthful lover-son by the great mother, or in sacrificial blood rites to keep the sun in motion.

In many ways, it is difficult to discern Neumann's (1973) first two phases of ego development from the first and second phases of pre-conscious psychic activity. In addition, Neumann's observations regarding the appearance of the circle as a centering point for the emerging ego, are difficult to distinguish from the earlier appearance of the circle Kalff (1980/2003) spoke about in conjunction with the constellation of the Self. In bringing psychic content into conscious awareness, the early developmental processes are repeated. The difference is that during the phases of ego development the element of reflective awareness evolves to accompany the new content on its journey. This repetition of developmental phases that occurs during ego emergence is much the same as the process we witness in the life stage development of adolescence, wherein the adolescent psyche appears to re-experience early life events with the added task of integrating them into conscious awareness. In intrapsychic development, each emerging content is initially gestated in the unconscious, then is birthed into consciousness.

The significant thing to remember at this phase in the development of conscious awareness is the mythic, magical nature of the still-connected Self and ego. The consciousness is emerging, but it remains rooted in the mythic regions. It is magical and not reflective. In sandplay, it must be held and allowed to continue its movement into conscious awareness.

Kalff's Animal-Vegetative Phase of Ego Development

Dora Kalff (1980/2003) combined Neumann's (1973) first two phases, calling them *animal-vegetative* for the types of symbolism the psyche uses to organize these early phases of consciousness. Phases one and two appear symbolically as animals and vegetation, as the budding consciousness enters the primeval world for the first time. The material that originates in the uroboric sea of the unconscious emerges into material form in a primal way. Symbolically, the new content, on its way to becoming conscious, assumes a primordial form.

As it begins its journey into consciousness, the psyche revisits the evolution of the world. It is important to remember that this process occurs during early child development and with every new psychic development that becomes conscious. Consciousness at this level of development appears in sandplay as scenes of forests and jungles, animals, plants, and earth. It is rich with life and primal energy. The atmosphere of the animal-vegetative phase of ego emergence has a quiet, almost moist stillness about it.

LENAE Following the constellation of the Self in **Lenae's Tray 14** and its presentation to her intrapsychic family grouping in **Tray 15**, she returns to marine life in an animal-vegetative world of **Tray 19. Lenae's** growing conscious awareness of her own value and center, even amidst her highly divisive, fractured family unit, are carried into her new awareness by the heart and gold pieces she includes in her underwater paradise. Continuing in her progression into consciousness in her **Tray 20, Lenae's** family, while still horizontal, is now invested with the heart of her own centeredness in the Self.

IVY After touching the center of the Self in **Tray 10**, Ivy's psyche rapidly assimilates her budding awareness of healthy feminine and masculine energies by combining two phases of ego development together in **Trays 11 and 12**. Atop her serene hilltop landscape, **Ivy** proudly stands

> an infant mermaid holding a pearl. **Tray 11** simultaneously carries the subsequent phase of ego development. The distant totem pole and the prominent funereal chimney bear testament to the battle and confusion regarding her value as a woman, consigned to her through her family's fundamentalist religious heritage.

Neumann's Stage 3 Ego Development: The Magic-Warlike Phase

During this phase, Neumann (1973) observed that the ego begins to overcome its dependence on the matriarchy. This is the early stage of the separation of masculine energy from the feminine, during which the conscious ego is moving toward identification with the masculine energies.

Neumann (1973) observed that the need to master nature, or the outer world, is mythologically evidenced in symbols of the hunt, wherein the hunter overcomes wild tigers, lions, and so on, as aspects of the terrible mother. Symbolically viewed, the masculine force surmounts the devouring force of the feminine during this phase of its development. Neumann described this phase as an earlier form of consciousness, which is later replaced when the ego is freed from the dominance of the mother archetype.

Neumann (1973) said that the entire realm of archetypes appears to the ego as the great mother. Each phase that must be overcome is thus the symbolic dragon, which threatens regression to a lower or less conscious dimension. The growing ego, as a masculine energy, must do battle with the dragon to maintain itself and move on. Mythically this is the classic hero's journey. This is the mythic story of the initial development of the infant's capacities to be conscious. It is also the story of the career of every aspect of our conscious awareness as it emerges from the darkness of the unconscious into the light of awareness.

When wounding or arrest occurs at this phase of development, the conscious ego remains fixated on dominance by and over the feminine. Neumann (1973) described this as a failure in transition from the *matriarchate* to the *patriarchate*, or from a state of unconsciousness to one of fully evolved conscious development. Neumann observed that wounding during the magical phase of ego emergence results in a permanent fantasy relationship to the masculine, wherein what he terms *upper, or solar manhood* is confused with *lower, phallic manhood.* Neumann observed that this is clearly evident in men he called *Don Juans*, who engage in endless serial romantic conquests, while lacking the ability for real relationship out of fear of being overwhelmed.

While Neumann's (1973) example applies to male development, a corresponding dynamic is seen in the wounding of females, who are denied the ability to completely develop their conscious autonomy. Not unlike the Don Juan syndrome, this results in dependence on men and a compensatory bitterness. For now, bypassing debates as to whether or not restraints on development beyond this phase for females are culturally sanctioned, the dynamic remains the same. Arrest in the development of the individual at this stage results in a continual struggle for dominance, which is fueled by an underlying terror of being subsumed. Similarly, intrapsychic arrest of any emerging product at this phase manifests as an analogous inner struggle.

Neumann's Stage 4 Ego Development: The Solar-Warlike Phase

At this phase of development, Neumann (1973) described the ego as having completed its separation from the unconscious, feminine energy. Neumann explained that the ego is now able to move from identification with the mother archetype to that of the father. At this phase of its development, the ego is established as a separate, conscious entity.

Neumann (1973) observed that a fundamental conflict exists between the development of ego consciousness and the inertia of the psyche to adhere to a position once attained. This is because one of the first aims of ego awareness is power and mastery over the outer world. At the same time, the growing ego is still saddled with the responsibility to harness and contend with the unconscious dimensions of the inner world. Symbolically, Neumann observed that this appears as the clinging aspects of the mother archetype. He explained that this results from the tendency of the dominant archetype of each successive phase of development to attempt to hold the ego fast. The archetype of the next phase tends to show its good aspect, or light side, while the archetype of the phase being transcended shows its dark, or terrible, clinging side.

Kalff's Battle Phase of Ego Development

Dora Kalff (1980/2003) observed that symbolic imagery at this phase of conscious development assumes the characteristics of battles. In the sand tray, this is the phase of conscious emergence where warring sides face each other in direct opposition. At this point of psychic development, the ego has separated out from the maternal energies of the unconscious. Now functioning as a growing, autonomous psychic entity, the ego identifies itself with the masculine conscious energy. This establishes a condition of polar opposites, the feminine and the masculine, the dark and the light. The emerging psychic content was formerly identified with, or subsumed in, the dark and undefined realm of the unconscious feminine energies. As it emerges into the light and distinguishes itself in conscious definition, it must abandon its former home in the darkness. Energetically, what is moving into consciousness becomes masculine. By virtue of its emergence, a polarization is established between masculine and feminine, light and dark.

What was once without form in the sea of the unconscious emerges into pairs of opposing energies that interact in a seamless motion, which manifests as form. This is conscious awareness that has the capacity to reflect back on itself. Symbolically it appears as one pole of a pair in opposition to its opposite. In sandplay, consciousness that has arrived at this phase of its development will frequently appear as two warring teams confronting each other in shows of equal force. There will frequently be good teams opposing bad teams. This may also appear as images with light characteristics opposing those with dark features.

In her sandplay work, Dora Kalff (1988) observed some differences in the trays of girls and boys during the battle phase of ego development. Whereas the sandplays of boys contained battle images, the trays of girls frequently held images of horses. Kalff speculated that the gender differences evidenced the predominance of relational styles of conflict for males and those of nurturing or care giving for females.

The battle stage mirrors its predecessor in the pre-conscious phase of development, where pairs of figures manifest in relationship to each other. The defining difference between the earlier relational phase of pre-conscious development and the battle stage of ego development is the striking role of consciousness manifested in the display of polar contrasts. In the symbolic dimension, consciousness becomes apparent when it is fully able to recognize its antithetical opposite. When black sees white, black *recognizes* that it is completely different. When the good guys encounter the bad guys, they *acknowledge* the difference. The operative element in this phase of development is in the conscious awareness of the recognition.

IVY As **Ivy** begins to consciously integrate her newly discovered feminine nature and body image, an energetic herd of horses is released in her **Tray 9**. The new psychic qualities that emerge into **Ivy's** consciousness take place in the tranquil domestic setting of Native American village life. As her awareness moves toward solidification in consciousness, it is carried by the animal instincts and is brought home.

AARON **Aaron's Trays 6 and 7** reflect a similar movement toward conscious awareness. **Tray 6** holds the squaring off of soldiers into warring teams of opposites, while **Aaron** declares, "I'm going to make a war going on." **Aaron's** newly developing consciousness clearly confronts itself in the symbolic dynamic of opposition, characteristic of masculine development in males. Just as in **Ivy's** Indian village, **Aaron** brings the newly conscious product to the tranquil home place of his own room in **Tray 7**.

Polar Opposition in the Transcendent Function

In our discussion of Jungian personality theory we also observed the symbolic encounter of polar opposites during the transcendent function. We must be careful that we do not confuse this with the appearance of opposites that occurs in the emergence of consciousness. In a sense, the polar opposition that occurs during the transcendent function is the reverse of the forward moving developmental process. The polar opposition of the transcendent function takes place when the already-developed position of the ego is no longer tenable. The psyche recognizes the utterly unviable position of conscious awareness and forces a return to the unconscious for further growth and development. The polar opposition occurs when the symbol of the ego's position separates into its archetypally opposing elements, bringing the psyche to a grinding halt and forcing energy downward to access new resources. The newly tapped psychic quality must then progress upward through the developmental stages into consciousness. My experience is that the transcendent function sometimes appears as an evident polar opposition in sandplay, but not all of the time. My sense is that the polar opposition of the transcendent function is present in the symbolic matrix, precipitating the downward rush of psychic energy, but that it is not always apparent.

Whether or not we will be able to discern all of these phases of transformation and development in sandplay is open to question. It is also improbable that the sandplay therapist will necessarily see them in the sequence of their theoretical explanation. We must remember that the theory is abstracted from experience in order to provide a means for understanding. The mystery and beauty of sandplay is the richness of the symbolic process in which the psyche unfolds and reveals itself in endless ways. In some of our case examples we have noticed that the developmental steps and stages sometimes appear out of order, repeat themselves, or occur simultaneously. In **Aaron's Tray 4**, for example, the mother-child unity, the relationship to the mother and the constellation of the Self all appear at the same time. Each case is unique. We must remember to let it speak to us.

Neumann's Stage 5 Ego Development: The Solar-Rational Phase

This fifth and final phase of development is the conscious, developed ego that has a will to survive and maintain itself in the world, while being simultaneously constituted to grow toward the Self. At this final phase of development, the ego exercises relative freedom of will and functions independently of the unconscious.

Neumann (1973) reflected that in each phase of development, the Self incarnates in an archetype that guides the process but does not become identical with it. Neumann referred to the Self as the supreme, directing quality of each developmental phase. Neumann recounted that through the process of development, the Self first appears as the mother archetype, then as the father archetype, then as a group Self, then as an individual Self. We might think of this as first being merged in the darkness of the matriarchal unconscious and gradually moving into the light of masculine consciousness. Having arrived at conscious awareness, the growing individual, or the emerging psychic quality, is able to take a role in the greater body of being. With continued development the individual uniqueness of the person or psychic quality is embraced in the midst of the collective.

Neumann (1973) wisely reminded us that the transformation of the Self through its various phases of development compels the developing ego to annihilate what has hitherto been the supreme value. For conscious awareness, this results in anxiety, guilt and suffering. All of human development, both inner and outer, is dependent on a creative openness that allows a person to be creative and heroic, and at the same time suffering.

The Ego-Self Axis

Neumann (1973) visualized a line connecting the autonomous ego and the wholeness of the Self, which he referred to as the *ego-Self axis*. Neumann imagined this as an axis of personality that connects the Self as the center point of the total psyche, and the ego as the center of a smaller circle of consciousness. Through the phases of psychic development we have examined above, we have seen how the ego separates out of the Self as a derivative. The ego-Self axis achieves its independence and sets itself apart from the unitary reality of the Self. The two circles, however, belong together with the Self at the root of the ego. During the second half of life the ego and the Self move back together again. The objective of growth in wholeness in later life is to develop and maintain a *conscious* connection between the two.

The ego-Self axis is the center of a complex of parallel and opposing processes. It takes place between the directing totality of the center of the Self on the one hand, and the consciousness of the ego, on the other. The ego-Self axis comes into being during the first half of life when the psyche separates into the conscious and unconscious components. A healthy ego-Self axis, or relationship between the ego and Self, is important in the daily experiences of movement in and out of unconscious material such as in dreams and images.

Neumann (1973) observed that insecurities experienced during the mother-child relationship result in an insecure ego-Self alliance. In these cases, the ego may be overly defended against communications from the Self. This results in the individual's refusal to heed or resistance to the messages being sent from the inner truth of the Self. A weak ego-Self axis may also result in a negative Self image and its consequent exaggerated conscious defense mechanisms. A weak ego-Self alliance that over-emphasizes the unconscious direction may result in psychosis.

Of note, Neumann observed that the issue of power is always concerned with the ego and its derivatives. Neumann reminded us that power is never related to the authentic personality structure. Preferably, in a healthy relationship to the Self, the ego always remains open to the experience of the unitary reality of the Self. This concern is not about power over or powerlessness, rather empowerment that proceeds from the ego's alignment with the central archetype of the Self. In the individuation process, the ego gives itself up to the Self, however the ego does not cease to be. Rather, it *becomes* the total personality and is no longer its derivative.

Kalff's Adaptation to the Collective

In sandplay, the imagery that appears during this phase of ego development is what Dora Kalff (1980/2003) called the *adaptation to the collective* or to the *marketplace*. This is the final phase of ego development, in which the newly conscious quality of psyche assumes its place in ordinary, outer life. This is the phase of ego development where the ego presumes a sense of completion. Conscious awareness feels it has arrived. It knows who it is and what is what, so breathes a sigh of relief and enters a temporary repose.

Scenes of ordinary life appear to announce the assimilation of the new conscious product into everyday awareness. The new psychic product becomes the consciously perceived *reality* of who, what and where we are. In the sand tray this may be reflected as villages or towns with people going about business as usual. The struggles are over and the archetypal constituents of psyche have gone underground. Figures and symbols used during this completion phase of a piece of work are generally contemporary and otherwise undistinguished.

In early childhood, the first arrival at this phase of ego development, establishes the child as an individual with thoughts, feelings and a will of his or her own and a sense of belonging to the outer world. In subsequent growth of consciousness, this is the culmination of a component of inner work where the conscious awareness integrates progressively greater awareness of the Self as its guiding center and source. What was formerly unknown and unconscious has now entered the accumulating body of what is known. The ego comes to a temporary rest, until it is called to further development by the pressures of the Self.

IVY Ivy's final sandplay, **Tray 13**, is a beautiful example of a return to the marketplace. It pictures a village, unconsciously drawn from her Native American heritage. The adobe buildings form an inviting town square. It is quiet and peaceful, awaiting the arrival of the villagers.

AARON Aaron's **Tray 15** pictures a return to ordinary life on the right side of the river. On the left, he leaves behind the relics of the struggles he suffered to arrive at his new level of consciousness.

HAROLD **Harold's final tray** symbolically returns to ordinary life, celebrating his discovery of a source of inner loving and a new beginning. A jubilant cheerleader welcomes a parade of elephants, as a weary old man prepares to rest. Elephants are powerful path clearers and are devoted mothers. The artifacts of his life-long quest for idealized femininity stand nearby. The powerful wonder woman figure reflects a conscious and humorous reflection on the vanity of his wasted pursuits and the Venus is honored as a statue nestled in a grove of trees.

~ Conclusion ~

Chapter 1
Developmental Theory in Sandplay
Neumann and Kalff

Drawing upon the psychological theories of Erich Neumann and of Dora Kalff in the foregoing discussion, we have traced the complete progression of the overall growth of the psyche and the course of healthy development undergone by all elements of psychic expansion and transformation. Our objective has been to deepen and refine our comprehension of the underpinnings of the therapeutic processes operating in sandplay.

Dora Kalff (1980/2003) recognized that, when properly contained, sandplay removes all environmental obstacles to healthy, orderly, sound psychic development. The free and protected space described by Kalff re-creates the archetypal conditions of the original mother-child unity. The significance of this simple statement cannot be over emphasized. The sandplay method makes it possible to intentionally engage the full range of psychic healing and development. The free and protected nature of sandplay allows the client to return to the primal psychic conditions where all growth and development begins. As a secure container, the sandplay method creates conditions that facilitate the safe maturation of reordered psychic contents through all phases of the psyche's course of development.

In the free and protected space, the client is able to enter an unconscious engagement on the archetypal level. When this happens, a synthesis occurs. Neumann (1973) pointed out that every entry into an archetypal field results in an *abaissment du niveau mental*, a term from the French meaning a lowering in the level of mind. In the archetypal dimension, consciousness is lessened and there is an intensification of phenomena. The boundaries between subject and object become blurred. During this experience, a unitary reality replaces the ordinary reality of conscious awareness. It is a form of *participation mystique*. In sandplay the two psyches of client and therapist merge in the preverbal, symbolic context of the sandplay, re-creating the conditions of the mother-child unity. The activities and movements of the symbolic images in the sand tray allow the client to recapture and retrace the path of psychic growth from its inception in the mother-child unity through the developmental phases we have just explored.

In sandplay, the client's psyche may return to very early periods of development. It is critical that we regard the clients' experiences from what Neumann referred to as the child's mythological apperception. We are better prepared to hold the archetypal dimensions accessed in the sandplay process when we are aware of the shifts in awareness that accompany them. Our ability to contain the work is greatly strengthened when we are able to hold it from the within the mythic experience of each phase of psyche's evolution.

Not every sandplay process will follow the entire course of development we have explored. Nor will the phases of psychic development necessarily manifest in distinct, sequential form. In fact, much sandplay work appears to address only bits and pieces of the full developmental process. While work of this abbreviated nature may not cover the full spectrum of psychic development or constitute a completed case, I am of the opinion that it remains a legitimate, worthwhile process. The abiding concern as therapists is to contain the work as wholly as possible and to recognize the ways in which the psyche is at work.

Chapter 2

Sandplay Therapy and Other Significant Developmental Theory

Similarities to Neumann's and Kalff's observations of early infant development can be found in the writings of a variety of classic developmental theorists. Having explored Neumann and Kalff in some depth, we will now take a brief look at other significant developmental theories and their relationship to sandplay.

J.H. Pestalozzi

Educator J.H. Pestalozzi (1895) was seminal in the development of child psychology in the late nineteenth century. Pestalozzi proposed that the design of early childhood education should facilitate development of the child's inner capacities for observation and perception. Given that the common thought at the time regarded children as empty vessels who were to be filled with facts through rote memorization, some of Pestalozzi's theories were startling.

To his credit, Pestalozzi recognized that children learn in environments that allow safe and free exploration. These theories led to the proliferation of kindergartens and expanded interest in young children's development and their learning processes. The free and protected space of sandplay reflects Pestalozzi's early work. Dora Kalff (1980/2003) credits Pestalozzi with the simple but penetrating observation,

> "...that it is through genuine love by the mother that the child finds his way to inner unity and thus gains access to the divine" (p. 7).

J.F. Herbart

J.F. Herbart (1901) also conducted early studies in child development, recognizing that children pass through a series of developmental stages, each with its characteristic challenges and outcomes. Although this is taken for granted today, Herbart's and Pestalozzi's observations regarding child development were revolutionary at the time. Their work set the precedent for continued research and understanding of mental development in children and the environmental conditions in which it is fostered. In addition, their work underlies later explorations into the parallel processes of psychic development characteristic of adult growth.

Jean Piaget

In the early part of the twentieth century, Jean Piaget (1928/1976, 1929/1975) made inquiries into the nature and progress of children's cognitive processes. His work emphasized the essential role of *experience* in growth and qualitative change. Piaget's observations have particular bearing on sandplay.

Piaget (1928/1976, 1929/1975) observed that development consists of progressive constructs of reality that arise from the child's active interaction with the environment. Piaget reasoned that qualitatively different changes in cognitive structure come about through encounters with the environment in a process he referred to as *equilibration.* Equilibration is the self-regulatory system whereby the child maintains an adequate balance between his or her existing mental capacities and outer world experiences.

Piaget theorized that the child uses two primary strategies to achieve mental equilibrium as he or she grows (Flavell, 1963). One is known as *assimilation,* wherein the child employs his or her existing cognitive strategies to understand outer experience. In some instances, the child's existing capabilities are adequately able to comprehend experience and to solve dilemmas that they encounter. In other cases, where the child's mental tools are not sufficient to the tasks faced in the environment, the child mentally alters the external stimuli to assimilate it to his or her existing cognitive structures. When the tension from conflicts between existing mental capacities and outer experience become too great, the child undergoes changes to the cognitive structures, which allow him or her to make sense of incoming data. Piaget called this process *accommodation*. The newly developed cognitive abilities resolve the tension and restore equilibrium between inner and outer experience. Over the course of development, through the interplay of accommodation and assimilation, the child gradually passes through four successive levels of cognition.

Piaget (1970) recognized that *relationship and action* are necessary for cognitive development and that the child plays an active role in his or her development. Piaget commented,

> …to know objects, the subject must act upon them, and therefore transform them. He must displace, connect, combine, take apart and re-assemble them (p. 704).

Piaget's observations regarding the relationship between action taken upon outer objects and the motive powers to transform the psyche are evident in the sandplay method. In sandplay, the client acts upon elements in the outer world, the sand and the figures, thereby moving and transforming his or her inner world. In sandplay, this manipulation of outer world objects occurs in the dimension of play, wherein the existing constraints on reality are suspended, making possible new and expanded perceptions.

Contemporary researcher L.E. Jones (1982) looked directly into Piaget's stages of cognitive development in sand trays. Jones investigated the developmental structure in sandplay by combining measures of development on Bowyer Pickford's (1970) scale of normative development in sand trays (the *Sandtray Assessment of Development*) with Piaget's definition of the stages of cognitive development. Jones postulated that the study demonstrates a cognitive developmental methodology for the analysis of sandplay. Jones's work makes the valuable contribution of cognitive assessment to the understanding of sandplay.

Sigmund Freud

Sigmund Freud (1933) emphasized the importance of childhood experience in shaping the adult personality. This emphasis exercised a strong influence on the field of child psychology. Freud, Klein, and Erikson all emphasized the importance of early infant experience.

Freud made groundbreaking inquiry into the mental drives and forces beneath the surface of human awareness. Among his many observations, Freud postulated that human mental activity is characterized by the two opposing drives of *eros*, the drive toward life, love, connection, and so on, and *thanatos*, the drive away from life, love, connection and toward death.

Freud's work opened the field of psychology to a wealth of penetrating insights into how the mind and brain work to configure human mental health and pathology. Freud's contributions to the field of depth psychology were foundational to its later evolutions into the symbolic workings of the unconscious by his student, Carl G. Jung. Even these early theories already bear the underpinnings of the later explorations into the energetic polarization of symbolic process.

Anna Freud

Anna Freud, daughter of Sigmund Freud, was a pioneer in the field of child treatment. As early as 1923 Anna Freud began psychoanalysis with children. Throughout her distinguished career, Anna Freud investigated, wrote and taught about the application of psychoanalytic theory to the treatment of children. Anna Freud encountered theoretical differences with another early child psychoanalyst, Melanie Klein, regarding the timing of the phases and stages of child development. Freud and Klein subsequently pursued their different approaches to child treatment.

Melanie Klein

Melanie Klein (1932) was one of the first clinicians to use play as a means of treating children psychoanalytically. Klein theorized that normal development in early childhood occurs through the interaction of conflicting instincts of self-destruction and self-preservation. Klein observed that these fundamental instincts gave rise to defensive techniques of projection, introjection and splitting as means of dealing with conflict and anxiety.

Klein noted that development is based upon the early childhood occurrence of a division between the good and the bad object. When this differentiation is sufficient to create a distinction, but not so powerful as to overwhelm, the child forms the fundamental basis for mental stability. Klein's observation parallels the polarization of energetic opposites recognized by Neumann and Kalff in early development, as well as in all psychic change processes.

Erik Erikson

Developmental theorist, Erik Erikson (1950/1963, 1959/1980) observed a series of crises that must be resolved in order to progress through eight distinct stages of development. Like Freud and Klein, Erikson theorized that two fundamental opposing drives result in an ongoing struggle between forward moving and reactionary inner forces. Erikson observed that it is this struggle and its resolution that results in progressive development.

According to Erikson, change and development takes place through a progressively complex series of conflicting developmental challenges or *tasks*. Erikson (1950/1963) referred to this process as *epigenetic*, a step-by-step development of psychosocial tasks that are inherent potentials in the human organism. The development of subsequent phases is dependent on the successful fulfillment of the preceding tasks. However, Erikson emphasized that the successful negotiation of one developmental task does not forever eliminate the negative aspects of the polar qualities surmounted in the challenge. Erikson cautioned,

> The personality is engaged with the hazards of existence continuously, even as the body's metabolism copes with decay. As we come to diagnose a state of relative strength and the symptoms of an impaired one, we face only more clearly the paradoxes and tragic potentials of human life (1950/1963, pp. 273-4, note).

Erikson also noted that play is a significant feature of early development, as it allows the child to organize his or her experience.

D.W. Winnicott

D.W. Winnicott (1958/1992) referred to the early bond between mother and child as a *primary maternal preoccupation*, during which the mother is exclusively devoted to the new baby. Winnicott observed that this is a temporary, normal and critical aspect of development. In his words,

> The mother who develops this state that I have called 'primary maternal preoccupation' provides a setting for the infant's constitution to begin to make itself evident, for the developmental tendencies to start to unfold, and for the infant to experience spontaneous movement and become the owner of the sensations that are appropriate to this early phase of life (p. 303).

Winnicott (1958/1992) also emphasized the importance of the mother-child bond in subsequent development. He applied his observations of early child development to the field of psychoanalysis. Particularly, he examined the need for adequate ego formation as a prerequisite for the formation of a transference neurosis in traditional psychoanalytic therapy. He observed that the ego comes into being when there has been *good enough infant care* (p. 295). He observed that subsequent features of ego development are based upon this initial condition and that, in cases where there has not been adequate care, the true self is unable to develop during the infant's emergence from the primary identification with the mother. The true self remains hidden and what Winnicott referred to as a *false self* develops to interact with and react to the environment. The true self remains dormant for preservation, while the false self develops patterns of behavior to cope with outer reality. While the false self may appear from the outside to have continuity and integrity, Winnicott observed that it is unable to experience life as real.

Winnicott (1958/1992) realized that the traditional methods of analysis are unsuitable for such individuals, but he observed that their healing can come about through what he called the *setting*. Essentially, the setting is the way the therapist is present in the relationship to the patient. Winnicott said:

> The behaviour of the analyst, represented by what I have called the setting, by being good enough in the matter of adaptation to need, is gradually perceived by the patient as something that raises a hope that the true self may at last be able to take the risks involved in its starting to experience living.

> Eventually the false self hands over to the analyst. This is a time of great dependence, and true risk, and the patient is naturally in a deeply regressed state.
>
> ...One characteristic of the transference at this stage is the way in which we must allow the patient's past to be the present. ...Whereas in the transference neurosis the past comes into the consulting-room, in this work it is more true to say that the present goes back into the past, and is the past. Thus the analyst finds himself confronted with the patient's primary process in the setting in which it had its original validity.
>
> Good enough adaptation by the analyst produces a result which is exactly that which is sought, namely, a shift in the patient of the main site of operation from a false to a true self (pp. 297-8).

In sandplay, the symbols carry the client's historical experience, as the client and the therapist conjointly hold the symbolic field. The symbolic nature of the sandplay method provides an ideal *setting* in which the client's inner and outer historical experience can be safely held in a non-rational, pre-verbal manner. In my experience, the dependent transference Winnicott refers to is obviated by the mutually shared symbolic context of sandplay. In this way, the symbols move the client's psyche, resulting in far less need to work through the transference directly with the therapist.

John Bowlby

In 1969, researcher John Bowlby penetrated to the core of early mother-child relationship in his renowned work, *Attachment.* Bowlby advanced his theory of attachment behavior and broke new ground by stating that early child development was not drive dependent, but rather it was the result of the activation of behavioral systems in the infant by his or her interaction with the mother. Bowlby observed that the behavioral systems involved in this process make proximity to the mother the objective. They are highly organized and act in such a way that the child is *sustained by this proximity.* Bowlby laid the theoretical foundation for what would later be explored neurobiologically. His work underscored the essential nature of the mother-child relationship and its bearing on all future development.

Kalff's (1980/2003) observations about the activation of the matriarchal level of the psyche in sandplay provide a concrete testament to Bowlby's account of the role of mother and child interactions in the early phases of development. Kalff recognized that the sandplay allowed direct access to the same critically necessary behavioral activation systems of early development through the free and protected space. Kalff recognized that even older clients in later life were able to revisit and reorder developmental wounding and deficits of this very early period, thus providing a means for rectifying psychic disruptions that would otherwise affect the rest of their lives.

Margaret S. Mahler

In her efforts to understand the developmental arrests and the regressive, symbiotic behaviors she observed in psychotic children, researcher Margaret S. Mahler (Mahler, Pine & Bergman, 1975) realized she first needed to understand healthy patterns of individuation in early childhood. This launched her well-known studies of the interactions of normal mother-infant pairs, which have contributed richly to the field of child development.

Mahler and her co-researchers observed that the mother and child undergo a *symbiotic phase* during the infant's early life from birth to 18 months (Mahler, et al, 1975). During this time, the mother serves as the ego for the child, by setting boundaries and mediating frustrations. The mother acts as a buffer between the infant's inner and outer stimuli, helping to organize them for the child. During the symbiotic phase, the mother does the tasks that the child will later be able to do for him or herself.

Between approximately 18 to 36 months, Mahler concluded that the child undergoes a *separation-individuation phase*, during which the infant begins to experience his or her separateness from the mother in increasingly complex ways (Mahler, et al, 1975). Mahler theorized that what is first perceived by the infant as purely kinesthetic stimuli through the body is gradually recognized as objective, and ultimately separate from the mother. Mahler observed that separation-individuation commences when the child begins to walk.

At about age three, separation-individuation is followed by an intrapsychic separation, which results in the child's self perception as separate from the mother (Mahler, et al, 1975). Mahler emphasized the critical importance of the child's first successful completion of the separation-individuation process, observing that it results in a psychological birth, which is decisive in the success of subsequent development.

While Jungian theory attributes archetypal significance to the inner process of psychic centering that occurs with the separation at age three, the parallels with Mahler's early stages of symbiosis and separation-individuation are evident. During this time, the child's psyche undergoes the centering process of the constellation of the Self.

~ Conclusion ~

Chapter 2
Sandplay Therapy and Other Significant Developmental Theory

Our review of these theories of early development, while brief, illustrates many similarities with the observations postulated by Neumann and Kalff. The theorists we have reviewed were concerned with various aspects of the development of the child's inner capabilities and outer skills and their impact on later life functioning.

It is important to recognize that Neumann and Kalff focused primarily on intrapsychic growth and change. Their work emphasized the return to and repetition of, the stages of early development undergone by each new piece of psychic growth throughout the life span. Our understanding of the processes of healing and transformation in sandplay is strengthened and deepened by input across the boundaries of these respected theoretical perspectives.

Chapter 3

Patterns of Chronological Development In Sandplay

Having examined the intrapsychic components of development, we now move to the issue of developmental differences in the sandplay work of children of various ages.

The sand tray productions of children assume rather predictable characteristics, based upon the chronological age of the sandplay client. For the early research in this area we look to the work of Scottish psychologist and academician, Laura Ruth Bowyer (Pickford) (1970), whose studies in sand tray phenomena remain valuable guidelines regarding developmental norms for age and gender.

Laura Ruth Bowyer's Developmental Norms

With Margaret Lowenfeld's encouragement, Bowyer (1970) made an avid study of the World Technique. She wrote a comprehensive survey of the history and uses of the World Technique and made significant contributions to work in the field.

Among Bowyer's many studies of the World Technique is an investigation of the elements of sand tray content and process that change over the course of normal development (Bowyer, 1970). Bowyer's norms accurately summarize the age differences I have experienced in sandplay and are a helpful tool for acquiring familiarity with what is considered a *normal* production for a child of a particular age. As with so many aspects of sandplay, however, nothing is absolute. There are always exceptions to normal or typical productions in the tray. Keeping this in mind, in order to properly hold the sandplay work, it remains important to be aware of the differences in structure and content between the work of younger and older children. Knowing what typical sand tray productions look like with advancing age can help us recognize developmental disturbances and arrests in older children and adults. For ease of reference, I have summarized and listed Bowyer's norms.

Bowyer's Developmental Norms Summarized by Age Group

Ages 2-4

- Use of only portions of the tray
- Figures poked or tossed into sand
- Chaotic and disordered worlds
- Use of animal figures rather than people
- Great similarity of worlds from child to child
- Spilling of figures over sides of the sand tray
- Pouring sand or burying
- Pounding on sand

Ages 5-7

- Islands of order
- Increased use of space
- Predominant use of animal figures
- Dramatic and active play
- Themes of food and eating
- Beginning of fenced and rigid worlds
- Pouring sand over people and figures
- Beginning of fighting stage (age 7)

Ages 8-10

- Fighting stage continues
- Fenced and rigid worlds peak at age 10
- Greater emphasis on reality
- Development of themes
- More constructive use of sand

Ages 11+

- Whole world works together as a scene
- Organization of patterns and interdependence of parts
- Landscapes with human settlements common
- Conceptual and symbolic representations of towns or villages
- Jungle animals reappear, more realistically (Age 11)

Laura Ruth Bowyer's summary of changes in World Technique content and process over the course of children's chronological development.

Bowyer's study of children's sand trays remains a significant contribution to the literature and is supported by contemporary research (Pennington, 1996). Although the bulk of her work tended toward a diagnostic application of the sand tray, Bowyer's developmental norms do provide substantive guidelines for the sandplay therapist.

MARTINA **Martina's** work is a wonderful example of developmental changes in sandplay constructions through childhood. **Martina** began her sandplay as a girl of five, and ended her process at age 12. As a young woman of 15, **Martina** returned to therapy for a brief period and did one sandplay. As we progress chronologically through **Martina's** sandplay work, we see increased organization and relationships. **Martina's** work in **Tray 1** is characteristic of a five-year-old child. It is sparse and minimally integrated. Her final tray culminates in an integrated personality structure and indicates a deeply spiritual nature.

The Interactive Play of Children in Sandplay

Between the ages of three and five, children frequently engage in what I call *interactive play*. This is active play with the figures, acting out the themes and scenes, rather than the representative placement of figures in the tray. In interactive play, the child holds the cat, moving it toward the empty food dish, crying out, "Meow! Meow! I'm hungry!" In later more evolved representative play, the child places the cat by the empty bowl *because* it is hungry. These changes in play result from the child's progressive cognitive development. Because interactive play is a common component of sandplay work with younger children, it is important that we examine the phenomenon more closely.

In the early 1940's, developmental psychologist, Heinz Werner (1940/1973) began exploring what he called a *physiognomic* period of childhood, wherein the child's experience is one of a high level of fusion between person and thing, subject, and object. Werner observed that children between the ages of three and six years experience the world around them largely through motor and affective channels. In this phase of development there are far fewer boundaries that distinguish and separate subject from object. Werner speculated that young children in the physiognomic mode of cognition perceive things as animate. To the young child, things have an inner life, feelings, intentions and desires. Werner characterized physiognomic cognition as an immediate, deeply felt bodily-affective participatory experience of the object. It is important to note that physiognomic perception precedes personification of objects, as personification entails an awareness of the attributions to the object.

The physiognomic perception of the young child results in a total surrender to play. A young child enters into and is not separate from the objects and dynamics of the play. The young child feels deeply immersed in his or her play and experiences life intensely in the body. In early childhood, between approximately 18 and 45 months, the child's play consists of a physiognomic transference of his or her inner experience to the object of play. This literal transference of experience onto the toys is gradually replaced with make-believe, *personified play*, as the child develops. Overall, Werner (1940/1973) concluded that physiognomic perception decisively decreases between ages three and four, at which point the child moves from the physiognomic experience of play objects to more personified play. In personified, make-believe play, the child becomes increasingly aware that he or she is pretending.

Personified play retains a high degree of the child's identification with the objects of play, as he or she continues to grow in awareness that the object, for example, is not really sick, because it is laying on its side. These are gradual changes and there is not as clear a demarcation between the two types of play, as we might ordinarily think. While the older child is aware that the sharp, pointed lightening bolt in the sandplay collection is not wholly the terror he or she experienced during the storm last night, that lightening does carry the same fear and power in the play. The personification, characteristic of young children's play is not a representation of what the person or figure might say, or do, but *is the activity itself.*

Werner's (1940/1973) studies showed a predominance of personified play in children from about age 18 months through early childhood, gradually changing character and tapering off by approximately age six. Werner's work included a chart by Charlotte Buhler, showing the progression of personified play of one child from age 18 months to six years. Werner indicated a gradual diminishing in personification to physical objects over time, increase in personified play with plants and animals to age six, and a rise and fall of personifications to natural events, peaking at about age three and a half.

Referring to children's drawings, Werner observed,

> The graphic representations of children are not merely optical phenomena, but are precipitates, so to speak, of a whole attitude which reaches expression in the physiognomy of the drawn object (1940/1973, p. 74).

In this mode of perception, any movement is an expression of feeling, or a gesture of intention or action. In the sandplay process, the movements of the figures in interactive play are replete with the child's affect, emotion, and experience.

Werner's observation of young children indicated that the coupling of the child's physiognomic experience with objects and his or her need of something from the object gave rise to the child's more evolved capacity for personification. Werner said,

> That is, things become persons as soon as something is desired of them (1940/1973, p. 78).

Translating this perception to sandplay, it is not difficult to assume that the emotional and psychic needs of the young child give rise to the child's choice of figures and his or her resultant animation in interactive play in the tray. The inner forces to heal and develop stimulate the child's choice of figures, based on the child's *need for healing*. The child's perceptive investment in the figures allows him or her to work actively through the wounding to fulfill the need.

Apart from the thundering canon fire and gunshots in the battle scenes of some older latency boys, animated, interactive play with figures usually subsides by age six.

Gender Differences in Sandplay

Another aspect of development in sandplay concerns the progress in capacity for relationship to self and to others. In this section we will look at this subject, focusing primarily on the sandplay client's developing relationship to the outer world and the role that gender plays in this development.

Kalff (1988) described the second phase of ego development as a battle. In the course of unimpaired chronological development, this occurs at about ages seven to nine years. Kalff noted differences in the trays of girls and boys, observing that boys mark this phase of development as battles and aggressive encounters, whereas girls tend to evidence themes of nurturing. Kalff taught that she saw many scenes of caring for horses in the sandplays of girls during this phase.

Kalff's observations regarding gender differences in sandplay during this phase of development are mirrored in the work of two contemporary researchers, V.J. Burke (1996) and D.P. Cohn (2000). Burke studied the sand trays of children ages seven through 11 to discern thematic differences between the work of boys and of girls. Burke found significant gender differences in relationship themes in the work of the children. Aggressive interaction themes were common in the sand trays of the boys, whereas dyadic, or family relationship themes were predominant in the work of the girls.

Cohn (2000) investigated the themes and behaviors of children during the battle stage of sandplay. Cohn's research found that males commonly verbalized themes of aggression and conflict during this phase of their work. In addition, they showed pro-social behavior and problem solving tendencies. The females made fewer theme verbalizations, and the content of their trays included curiosity, discovery, and fantasy. Themes of passive observation and victimization were also frequent in the sand trays of the girls.

Kalff's (1988) observations in sandplay correlate with Neumann's (1973) theory that girls identify with their mothers in the primary relationship and that their relationships are, therefore, characterized by identification. Boys have a different experience. Because of their gender differences from their mothers, relatedness becomes essentially confrontational.

When we consider the development process from the standpoint of the capacity for relationship, Kalff's observations of gender difference in sandplay might be understood as the intrapsychic component of the character of relationship differences in males and females. In healthy development, this phase occurs during the pre-adolescent period, just before the emergence of sexual functioning and the genetic and social forces that bear upon males and females.

The dissimilarity in symbolic presentations in the work of males and females represents the difference in the nature of the male and female relationship to inner and outer world. What we see in the sandplay is that males and females are in relationship to outer and inner reality in very different ways. Whereas females appear to meet their worlds with alliances and nurturing, males compete, vying for territory and supremacy.

While more contemporary theories of gender differences have a wealth of information to contribute to this subject, the differences in relational symbolism that occur in sandplay during this phase of the ego's evolution are notable and bear further scrutiny. For now, the significant consideration in the practice of sandplay is the symbolic content that emerges as the ego progresses in its development.

~ Conclusion ~

Chapter 3
Patterns of Chronological Development in Sandplay

This concludes our exploration of the developmental process of healing and change in sandplay therapy through the lens of psychological theory. Now we turn to the paradigm of mythology for a very different view of the same psychic terrain.

Chapter 4

Mythological Considerations of Development in Sandplay—Yggdrasil, The World Tree

Introduction

On the basis of our grounding in psychological theory, we will now explore the change and transformation process more directly through the psyche's own language of mythology. We will look to the mythic account of Yggdrasil to shed light on some of the subtleties of the change process in sandplay work.

The tale of the World Tree, Yggdrasil, comes to us from the *Prose Edda*, an account of ancient Icelandic mythology first recorded from the oral tradition by Snorri Sturluson (1954/1984) in the twelfth century. Presented as a poetic series of questions and answers between a king, Gylfi, and three wise beings, the *Prose Edda* is a seminal text in the mythology of early Northern European peoples.

Read as the archetypal language of the unconscious, this rich and magical tale of giants and gods unfolds as a key that holds the potential to unlock the mysteries of the inner world. Within the limbs and roots of Yggdrasil lie the means to psychic growth and change (Metzner, 1994). This beautiful creation myth tells of the first man and woman, made from two trees, an ash and an elm. The great god Odin and his wife, Frigg lived in the land known as Asgard, along with the gods known as the Aesir. Odin is called the "All Father," the father of all gods and people. Frigg, known as the earth, is Odin's daughter and wife.

Of particular interest in the tale is the ash tree known as Yggdrasil, the sanctuary of the gods. A World Tree, Yggdrasil stands at the center of the world. Its branches encompass the whole of the world and arch up over heaven. A wise eagle sits at its top. Between its eyes sits a hawk.

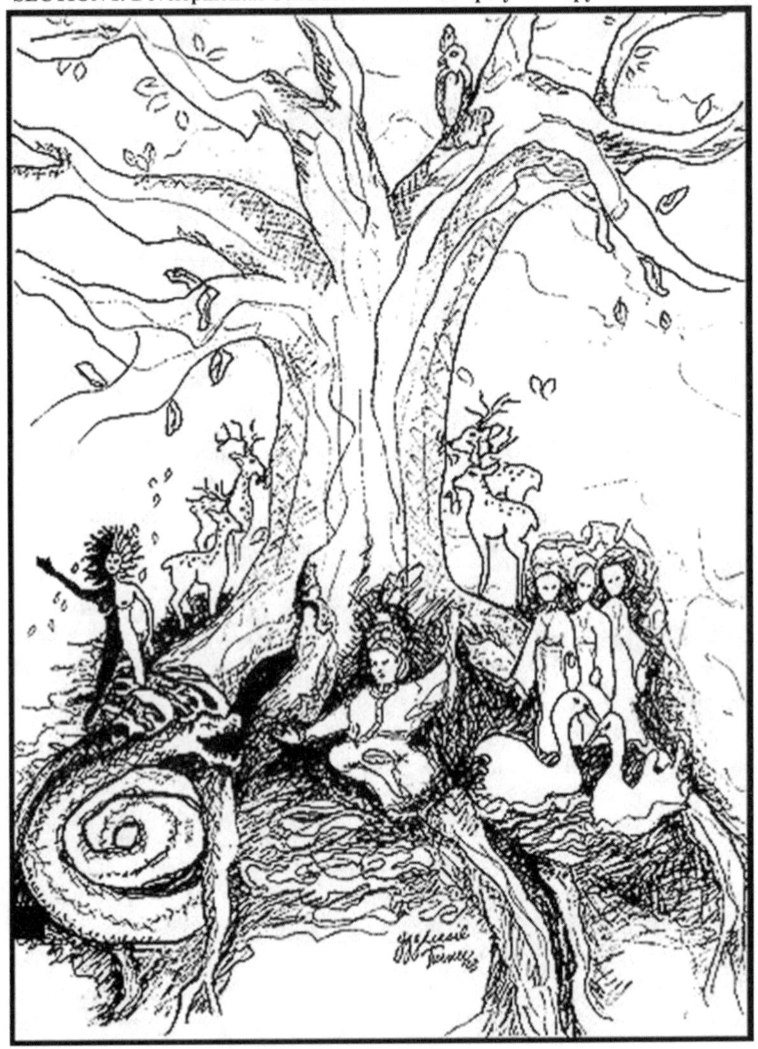

The Three Roots of Yggdrasil
Pen and ink drawing - B. Turner, 2003

Yggdrasil concurrently carries the entire cycle of life and death. It suffers great pain. The deer bite off its bark, the serpent Nidhogg eats at its root and the trunk rots on its sides. Its mortal passage is not without a price, for, as there is growth, there is also suffering and loss. A squirrel runs up and down the trunk, carrying bitter messages between the eagle at the top and the serpent Nidhogg at its root. The eagle, the bird of heaven, and the serpent, creature of the earth, do battle as the masculine and feminine principles. The image of the World Tree holds the entirety of mortal passage through time and circumstance. At the same time, it carries the potential for eternal wholeness inherent in the individual's passage through life. Yggdrasil is concerned with the intersection of time and eternity. It has to do with how we as individuals use the circumstances of our daily lives to realize more and more of the Self. The myth reminds us that the manifestation of the Self into form bears with it a continual struggle.

As manifest being, the polar energies of the masculine and the feminine contend with each other in varying combinations of balance and imbalance. Their struggle threatens to destroy the tree, but the entire process is fed by something deeper and so is sustained. Yggdrasil is thus symbolic of the constant regeneration of the universe. It is always growing and always being destroyed. It is born of, continually informed by and ultimately returns to the primordial wholeness of the Self. Jung (1956/1976) said that as it is the tree of life, so it is the tree of death. The Yggdrasil story reminds us that material passage necessarily entails suffering. Mortal passage is an undergoing, but it is fed and sustained by the immortal principle of the Self, which transcends time and form.

Yggdrasil means "Ygg's horse." Ygg or Yggr is Odin. Yggr is "the terrible one," the god of battle, struggle, human sacrifice and undergoing. Yggdrasil is the "horse of the Terrible One," the vehicle for travel between the realms of reality, through the dimensions of consciousness and the unconscious. Yggdrasil is the vehicle upon which one can travel to the depths of the unconscious and return to conscious awareness.

Jung (1967/1983) commented that as the mandala is an image of the Self viewed in cross section, so its profile is the tree. That is to say that Yggdrasil is the Self in the process of growth and development. Rooted in the earth and growing toward heaven, the World Tree carries the union of the opposites. Its mythic presence indicates the possibility for the union of opposites for humankind. Archetypally speaking we come to be from the World Tree. Through it, we find our way back to the conscious embodiment of the wholeness of the Self.

Yggdrasil thus provides a mythic template of manifest being and its development. As a metaphoric map of the relationship of the ego to the Self, it guides us to the paths for consciously integrating more and more of the Self. The three wells at the base of Yggdrasil define the three primary phases of change and development we explored in our psychological considerations of development. In addition, the three wells that feed Yggdrasil also define three prominent patterns or ways of entering and engaging with the individuation process.

The Three Roots of Yggdrasil and Their Wells

Yggdrasil stands on three major roots that are fed by three distinct wells (Davidson, 1964 & Hveberg, 1962). The first root is in Aesir, the realm of the gods and humans. Here the well of Urdr, the well of fate, is presided over by three Norns, Urd, Verdandi and Skuld. The second root is Niflheim, in the realm of the dead. This is the underworld or the abode of darkness. Hel, the female trickster who is half black and half flesh-colored rules over Niflheim. Nidhogg, the serpent abides here. The well at this root is known as "Hvergelmir." The third root is in the land of the frost ogres, Ginnungagap, the land of the open void. Located here is the well of Mimir, ruled by the giant, Mime, which contains wisdom and understanding.

From these three footings and the wells that nourish them, the Yggdrasil myth instructs us about the three primary phases of transformation available to human psychic experience. These correspond directly to the stages of psychic development in Neumann's (1973) and Kalff's (1980/2003) psychological theories. In addition, the roots and their wells portray the primary modes of change we encounter in sandplay.

Neumann's (1973) theory provides a description of the complete process of psychic development from the inception of a new psychic quality, through every phase of growth, to its culmination in the fullness of consciousness. The three wells at the base of Yggdrasil embrace the three pre-conscious phases of psychic development and may be encountered in sequence for a full and complete instance of pre-conscious psychic work. The three wells at the foot of Yggdrasil may be likened to the phases of early development described by Neumann and Kalff as indicated in the following figure.

EARLY PHASES OF PSYCHIC DEVELOPMENT		
NEUMANN	KALFF	YGGDRASIL MYTH
Primal Relationship With Mother	Mother-Child Unity	Nidhogg's Well
Separation of the World Parents	Relationship to the Mother	Norns' Well
Centroversion	Constellation of the Self	Mimir's Well

Comparison of the early stages of psychic development as understood by Neumann and Kalff with the three wells of the Yggdrasil myth

It has been my experience in the practice of sandplay therapy that the course of healing and change does not always follow the phase-specific sequence of development described by Neumann (1973) and Kalff (1980/2003). Frequently, the process appears to move in and through the various phases, forward and backward, any number of times. I have also witnessed sandplay work that clearly does not progress through all phases of development. Nonetheless, these clients continue to heal, change and live fuller lives. As we explore the Yggdrasil tale, we will highlight the similarities with Neumann's (1973) and Kalff's (1980/2003) theories. Our primary concern, however, will be to examine the modes of healing or change available at each of the three wells.

While the fullness of the psyche's change process does exist in Yggdrasil's three roots, its wells invite us to drink from any one, or a combination of them, and appears to do so in no specific order. This ancient mythic allegory suggests that the unconscious or underground phases of psychic transformation assume three primary modalities, any of which constitutes a point of entry into a legitimate and profound change process. It suggests that the process of deep-order change may be engaged through any one of the three modes, and it may progress through the phases of inner change from these various points of beginning. The tale also suggests that, with some qualification, it is not always necessary to progress through all three pre-conscious phases of change.

The Well of the Underworld: The Sandplay Process of Transcendence

The first form of sandplay process is the pattern we recognize as the transcendent function. This is psyche's darkest beginning place. It is the place where psyche is merged in the matriarchal unconscious. For Neumann (1973) this was known as the primal relationship. For Kalff (1980/2003) it was called the mother-child unity. This form of transformation is described as taking place at the root of Yggdrasil known as Niflheim, or The Abode of Darkness. This is the underworld, or the realm of the dead. The well that feeds this root of the World Tree is known as Hvergelmir. Hel, a trickster and giantess, who is half black and half flesh-colored is ruler of this domain of change. The Yggdrasil story tells us that a huge serpent called Nidhogg, "The Striker That Destroys," gnaws at the root and is at war with the eagle that sits at the top of the tree. This serpent, as a dark feminine principle, opposes the conscious position of the masculine, which sits up in the light. Further, Nidhogg, as the unconscious position not content to rest, continually chews at the root to get its attention. The unconscious presses upon the conscious position of the ego in order to stimulate growth and development.

The story tells us that Niflheim was created long before the earth. The area of the psyche that the Yggdrasil tale describes here is the deepest unconscious (Metzner, 1994). It precedes conscious awareness and informs consciousness. One function of this area of the psyche and this manner of change is to compensate for the conscious position. Niflheim holds the collective wisdom. Through the serpent, Nidhogg, it gnaws at consciousness to align with and integrate more and more of the Self. We do not willingly choose to drink from the well of Hvergelmir. We are sucked down into its dark depths by the necessity of change when the ego's position is no longer tenable.

The manner of change at the well of Hvergelmir is that of *transcendence*. By definition, transcendence has to do with passing over or going beyond. It is from the root word *trans*, which means *across*, or *to go across*. To transcend is thus to go beyond the limits of something. In Jungian psychotherapy we speak of transcendence as going beyond the limits of the ego by the integration of a new product from the unconscious. As we observed in our discussion of symbolic process, the ego is reluctant to release its position. This manner of change is thus characterized by radical disruption. It is abrupt and often deeply frightening. Although the transcendent function occurs deep in the unconscious, consciousness must participate in the transformation. The ego or conscious position, becomes aware of its own failings and impending disintegration.

The goddess Hel commands this dimension of change. She finds her counterparts in other cultures in images such as Kali and Rangda from Hindu mythology. While Hel's fleshy half is of this world, she is equally and irrevocably constituted of the darkness from the deepest unconscious. Hel must consume what is living, that is, what is conscious in order to sustain her existence and maintain the circle of life. By consuming conscious awareness and hurling it into the bowels of the unconscious, Hel feeds her fleshy side. She expands consciousness by digesting the limited conscious position and feeding it with the previously unknown riches from the unconscious.

Under Hel's direction, the serpent Nidhogg grabs and sucks us down to the well. If we are able to survive, we undergo radical transformation. The violence of Nidhogg is the mythic description of the fierce disunion that occurs in the symbolic process when the ego comes to a standstill and the psychic energies are forced into the unconscious to the archetypal core of the symbol. This form of change generally sneaks up on us and is not entered willingly. Its undergoing is both hazardous and violent. This manner of change carries us over, or beyond the limits of our ego. It catapults us across to the other side of our known reality, abruptly opening our conscious awareness to more of the Self. It is an irrevocable alteration of our awareness of who we are and what we are about.

The Well of the Underworld in Sandplay

When the sandplay client draws from the well of Niflheim, he or she is engaged in the transcendent function. This process of change is profound and is characterized by chaos. It is concerned with the radical reordering of the individual's ego and conscious awareness of who he or she is. It is change that dramatically deconstructs the limits of one's perceptions, expanding awareness of what is or is not possible, all in accord with the central archetype of the Self.

This form of sandplay process is evidenced by a descent to the depths of the unconscious. The descent may occur in stages with intermittent ascents back to more comfortable levels of consciousness. It may be characterized by great darkness and tremendous energy as the poles of the symbol culminate their struggle in a highly charged opposition. The inadequacy of the ego is consciously observed during this process. With the paralysis of the ego and its ultimate death, new products, richly informed by the archetype that characterizes the issues at hand, emerge into conscious awareness. The ego is thus re-vitalized, expanded and more aligned to the Self.

With sudden change we must be mindful that the client may be inclined to act out. Time and careful therapeutic containment is required for the client to consciously integrate these radical changes in a meaningful and productive manner. It is important to remember that chaos and creation exist in a compensatory relationship, much like the unconscious and consciousness. The tension of opposites is a precondition of psychological growth. Chaos is necessary and unavoidable. Chaos prefigures order and consciousness. In this sense it is sacred. It has everything in it. The dark aspects of the psyche are the source of richness and growth to wholeness. In the process of individuation it is of great importance for the ego to develop the capacity for an adequate relationship to the unknown, that is, to chaos. Psychological disturbance often results from the ego's inadequate relationship to the darker aspects of the psyche.

As mentioned above, change at this root of the World Tree is often sudden, hazardous and terrifying. When a client enters chaos at the root of Hvergelmir, the therapist's capacity for therapeutic containment is put to the test. The therapist must be able to psychically hold the tumultuous unknowns that arise in the client's process. He or she must remain steady, much like a sturdy vessel in a dark sea storm.

The radical disruption of the psyche at this level of change requires integration through the progressive levels of psychic development. What has deconstructed must be held and shepherded toward its integration into the psyche as a new product. Sandplay process that is entered at Nidhogg's well is deep-order work that must be carried through the succeeding sequence of developmental steps.

CARY Cary's sandplay work was entered through Nidhogg's well. Her process was characterized by a pattern of sudden descents to deep darkness, punctuated by intermittent ascents to less overwhelming psychic realms. For example, in Tray 7 Cary's work assumes an urgent, almost frantic quality as she rapidly constructs a radiate pattern of triangular islands. Although Cary describes her tray as "*…diamonds all the way around,*" it carries a sad darkness. Cary wept deeply as she constructed the tray, commenting that she felt nothing, but she was very cold.

Cary's sandplay process frequently carried both her and me to the limits of our holding capacities. Darkness and terror filled the room with each descent. During these sandplays, Cary's hands would tremble uncontrollably when she touched the sand. Often, as in this example, she would be catapulted into profound sobbing with no conscious awareness of its source. Cary's transformation at the root of Niflheim was tumultuous, yet deeply transformative.

The Well of Destiny
The Sandplay Process of Healing and Remembering

This root of Yggdrasil is in the sky among the Aesir, the realm of the gods and humans (Davidson, 1964, Hveberg, 1962, & Sturluson, 1954/1984). The well that feeds the root of the Aesir is called *Urd* or *Urdarbrunn*, which means *the spring of destiny*. This is the phase of development where manifestation begins and where what is moving into being begins to appear. For Neumann (1973) this was the separation of the world parents. For Kalff (1980/2003) it was the relationship to the mother.

Two swans swim in this well, which is ruled over by the three Norns. The Norns are three young maidens who determine the fates of the people and gods. Symbolically, swans have been thought to be hermaphroditic representations of the union of opposites, given their masculine, phallic neck and round, feminine bodies (Eliade, 1964/1974). As the balanced union of masculine and feminine energies, swans are symbolic of the mystic center. Considered a great bird, some traditions hold that the swan is the only bird an eagle will consider doing battle with. Some myths also hold that the Norns disguise themselves as swans to carry out their tasks. It is interesting that it is *two* swans that swim in the well of destiny. Two, as the number of manifestation or of duality, swim together in the well where the fates and destinies of people are made. The two swans carry the possibility of the union of the opposites within the field of mortal manifestation. As a pair of the greatest birds, they remind us of the possibility of balance as a goal of manifestation, as well as the wholeness of the center and source of manifest being.

The Norns are concerned with three aspects of mortal, embodied passage. They are frequently likened to the Greek Fates, as Past, Present and Future, or as Birth, Life and Death. However, this tends to confine their significance too strictly to the dimension of time. What is of concern to us as sandplay therapists is the dimension of meaning in the course of passage through time. As we saw with Nidhogg's constant bickering with the eagle perched on top of Yggdrasil, the work at the level of the psyche governed by the Norns is done in the context of relationship. The two swans swim together in the well, and the three Norns work in concert to inform us of our fates.

The Norns also work to put our fates into form. The area of the psyche that the three Norns address is that which concerns temporal passage and embodied manifestation. It has to do with conscious attention to worldly affairs. The water in this spring concerns our origins and our ancestors. It deals with ancient memory, deep in the collective unconscious and with making these memories a conscious part of the individuation process.

The function of this well is that of remembering. It pertains to paying debts and with healing wounds. This also has to do with our roots as human beings, concerning where we have come from. This is our temporal path; that is, our genetic, familial and cultural heritage. The Yggdrasil story tells of the gods riding from earth to heaven over the bridge known as *Bifrost* to hold their court of justice. What the myth holds for us at this root is the function of the psyche that connects mortal passage and events to the wholeness of the Self. It is the compensatory function, that dynamic which keeps account of the ego's alignment to the Self.

The three Norns comfort Yggdrasil with a salve of white clay from the spring to keep its branches alive. Thus, "...it stands ever green over Urd's Spring" (Sturluson, 1954/1984, p. 46). This is necessary, because four deer continually gnaw at its bark and leaves. The myth thus tells us that the type of nourishment provided by this well is that of comfort and of soothing. This nurturing sustains and allows material, worldly passage to continue. It salves the undergoings of duality and provides just enough comfort that we can tolerate the tensions of the struggle between the masculine and feminine forces.

The Norn called Urd presides over the dimension of destiny. This has to do with the uniqueness of who we are in light of the greater Self. Urd's domain is that which each of us brings with us as our unique potential. This potential is defined, not in terms of worldly greatness, but in terms of the unique embodiment of the Self. This might be likened to the Hindu concept of *dharma*, literally, "...that which holds together, or supports" (Reyna, 1993, p. 55). Our dharma is the material manifestation of who we are in truth. It concerns the real nature of phenomena as the highest universal truth in its particular embodied form.

Urd is concerned with the dimension of healing that deals with remembering. This includes *re-membering* in the sense of honoring one's dharma, as well as remembering in the conventional sense of recalling forgotten aspects of one's own history and past.

Urd asks the question,

Who am I in truth
in this unique embodied form?

Urd works to insure that each human being is equipped with the possibility of unique gifts and talents that, when recognized and manifest, serve as an embodied presence of wholeness. In other words, there is meaning and a way that meaning may be revealed in each person's life, through the discovery, acceptance and honoring of their own inner truth. Like the swans, the individual who heeds Urd's guidance comes to know his or her own mystic center, the Self, in the course of life.

Verdandi is the Norn of being and becoming. Her domain is that of acting in accord with one's own unique destiny. Verdandi oversees that aspect of mortal passage that demands a response. She is concerned with the transformative potential of being and with the conscious awareness that temporal passage is ordered to the Self. This might be likened to the Hindu concept of *karma*. Commonly misunderstood to simply mean, "a fate caused by my own actions," karma is truly concerned with the realm of action itself. This is action that is in accord with the individual's dharma and that is in proper response to the demands of the particular circumstance. It is when one is acting outside of his or her dharma, the Self, and is improperly attached to the outcomes of the actions, that future tasks and repercussions are created. These are properly known as *samskaras*, which we will give more consideration momentarily. Verdandi's concern is to use life's challenges to realize more of the Self. This is the dynamic of adaptation, which we considered earlier in our discussion of the dynamic components of the psyche. Verdandi's focus is healing through right action. Verdandi's concern is to establish and maintain inner and outer order through honoring of the Self in all circumstances. Honoring our greater being in the process of becoming through time and space orders our passage to the integration of the Self.

Verdandi asks the question,

Given who I am in Truth, what is my proper
response to this particular situation right now?

The third Norn is Skuld. She is concerned with the dimension of necessity, or debt and guilt. These are the debts we owe in this life from our own actions, from our ancestors, and perhaps from our past lives. These are the *samskaras* to which we referred earlier, the accrued debts that must be paid. These are the lessons we must learn. Skuld oversees that part of our passage that must take responsibility for past transgressions in the context of using them as our own lessons for re-ordering to the Self. Skuld is concerned with the aspects of healing that deal with grief, forgiveness, and assuming responsibility.

Skuld asks the question,

What remains unfinished?

The Well of Destiny in Sandplay

When a client draws from Urd's well in sandplay, he or she is dealing with change that is ordered to remembering and healing. This is change that is concerned with the client's actual passage through time. By definition, healing concerns the making whole or fit in the embodied condition. It has to do with becoming free from disease or ailment and with restoring health and soundness. Drawing from the well that feeds this root of being in sandplay brings *healing* by restoring conscious awareness to the past, thereby making possible any necessary grief and forgiveness. It allows us to remember what has been forgotten, to grieve, and to reorder these temporal undergoings to the Self. This healing restores to conscious awareness those parts of our past which, having been repressed or denied awareness, burden us as unresolved complexes.

It is clear that *healing* in this form is different from the form of deep order *transformation* that we see working in the transcendent function. Yet, it is an essential feature of the individuation process and one that we see very commonly in sandplay. Sandplay scholars frequently identify two forms of change in sandplay. Weinrib (1983/2004) referred to *processes of healing* and of *the expansion of consciousness*. Ammann (1991) distinguished between *healing* and *transformation* in sandplay. Amann observed that healing is undergone to restore wellness to damaged aspects of psychic development that impair further progress. She noted that healing results in a healthy ego. Transformation is characterized as beginning with a stable ego as a foundation for the further deepening and broadening of the conscious relationship to the Self in the individuation process. Bradway and McCoard (1997) referred to processes of *healing* and of *growth*, however they emphasized that the two may occur together.

We should be clear that the processes of remembering and healing might occur in conjunction with a classic transcendent process of transformation. This, in fact, frequently occurs in sandplay. The important point is that when a sandplay series consists of a remembering and healing process pattern alone, it is still a legitimate form of psychotherapeutic work and a credible sandplay process.

The remembering and healing process assumes many forms in sandplay. It may appear as the remembrance of wounds resulting from historical abuse or losses. I recall my first experience with sandplay as a clinical trainee in San Francisco. My weekly client meetings were scheduled in various locations in the clinic, based on room availability. On one occasion I ended up in the sandplay room. My client, a female law student in her thirties, asked if she could make a sand tray. Although I was unfamiliar with sandplay, I said that would be fine. Being completely ignorant of procedures, I took no photographs. In the following session, the client reported that the sand tray had really stayed with her and had touched something deep and old. She began to remember sexual inappropriateness from her father that occurred when she was a young child. Fortunately, we were both able to contain and work with these revelations and memories that arose from her sandplay. This ultimately resulted in substantial relief, healing, and empowerment on the part of the client. For the therapist, it resulted in a career in sandplay therapy!

The remembering and healing process may address physical illness and other bodily distress. Remembering and healing may take the form of recalling and honoring a religious heritage or one's ancestral or cultural lineage. The process may also be concerned with taking responsibility and grieving past wrongs, as can be seen in the case of **Elizabeth**.

ELIZABETH Elizabeth's Tray 6 is a beautiful example of the grief that frequently accompanies healing in sandplay. In this tray, the suggestion of a river separates the activity of the near right corner from the world of daily life, indicated by a remote village in the far left.

A casket containing seven tiny piglets sits in a sacred grove of flowers by a fountain, which is the source of the river.

At the time she did this tray, Elizabeth was a professional woman in her late forties. Although she loved children, she did not have any of her own. In reviewing her case material, she realized that in this tray she was grieving the loss of the children she would never birth.

A moving process of healing and forgiveness were inherent in this work. Upon completion of the tray, **Elizabeth** gestured toward the fountain saying, *"...from this sorrow, life flows."* Much later, during our review of her work, Elizabeth became fully conscious of the significance of the loss and the healing in her life.

CARY **Cary's Tray 6** provides an example of intense grief and healing. In the past, **Cary's** profession had required her to euthanize hundreds of animals. In this sandplay she constructs a series of twelve small burial mounds, interspersed with sacred figures, including angels and jewels. **Cary** scored a boundary around the edge of the entire tray, as if to hold it extra securely. Her final figure is the broken heart, which she tenderly placed in the near, left corner. Unknown to her consciously at the time, **Cary's** psyche takes account of the many deaths, which occurred by her hand, entrusting their souls to the care of the divine. Simultaneous with the initiation of this healing process is her deep experience of grief.

The well of healing and remembering may be accessed in a wide variety of ways. An example of healing and change from my practice that falls outside classic sandplay patterns is that of a young boy traumatized by an automobile accident.

CHARLIE **Eight-year-old Charlie** was referred to me by his physician for symptoms of anxiety and Post Traumatic Stress. **Charlie's Tray 1** features a car crash

> prominently placed on a central mound. The subsequent trays in his rather short series consist of various modes of lining up opposing forces. This takes the form of two soccer teams facing each other on the field, ready to start the game in **Tray 2**. In **Tray 3**, dinosaurs circle around a central point, marked by a small tree. In **Tray 4** a white soccer team vigorously plays against a red team. In **Tray 5** a variety of wild cats circles around a playful central cub, who safely wriggles on his back. **Tray 6** consists of **Charlie's** firm stamp of his hand prints in the sand. In his final **Tray 7, Charlie** put a variety of boxers and karate fighters in a central boxing ring. Asking if it was all right for him to do whatever he wanted with it, **Charlie** threw sand into the ring and poked at the players within it
>
> **Charlie** was finished. He loved his sandplay and found great healing and strength through it. Yet his process contained no manifestation of the Self or transcendent function. He was released from treatment after ten sessions with restored ability to sleep comfortably through the night and freedom to ride in the car without anxiety. Charlie was symptom free.

As we have seen in the examples above, it is evident that sandplay work can be entered into through the Norns' well. It appears that genuine healing can occur there without the necessity of either diving into Nidhogg's abyss, or of progressing forward through the succeeding sequence of developmental steps. To remember through the symbols and to establish a connection between this movement of the psyche and the Self, in the sandplay container constitutes real healing and legitimate psychic reparation. While a full constellation, or manifestation of the Self may not appear in such work, it is very important that the new material be somehow connected to or brought to the center. What has been healed must be related to the central wholeness. The psychic center needs to be acknowledged as the touchstone, or home base, to which all integrated elements are related. This may appear in any number of ways that indicate a radiate point of beginning, a source point or a point in the middle. In the example of **Charlie's** work, above, the psyche acknowledged the organizing principle of the Self in the central car crash in **Tray 1**, the growth of the central tree in **Tray 3** and the central safety and playful qualities of the cub in **Tray 5**.

Although work restricted to the well of healing and remembering clearly lacks the fullness of psychic development undergone from start to finish, experience indicates that healing and remembering by themselves are sometimes all the work a client needs to do. In any case, it is clear that healing and remembering work characterizes what many clients accomplish in their sandplay. It lacks many of the features of a classic sandplay process, but it is nonetheless healing and transformative. It is important that we acknowledge it as such for purposes of containing the work respectfully.

The Well of Wisdom
The Sandplay Process of Sacrifice

The third form of sandplay process is that of *sacrifice*. Unlike change at the root of Niflheim, which is entered unwillingly, this form of transformation is characterized by a willing, conscious engagement with the unconscious. In the Yggdrasil myth this mode of transformation is described as taking place at the third root of the World Tree, located in Jotunheim, the land of giants and frost ogres. Jotunheim is described as existing in the *open void*, an area called *Ginnungagap* in the old Norse tales (Hveberg, 1962). The well that feeds this root of Yggdrasil is called *Mimesbrunn*. It is ruled by Mimir, who drinks daily from its depths and is said to know more than anyone in the world. This is the third phase in pre-conscious development, which Neumann (1973) called *centroversion*, and Kalff (1980/2003) called the *constellation of the Self*.

The type of nourishment available at Mimesbrunn is hidden wisdom and understanding. Psychologically speaking, drinking from Mimir's well allows the individual to see beyond the surface appearance of things. The area of the psyche that is described by this root of the World Tree is the open void. This is the Self seen as the source of all. This is the area of being that precedes material manifestation. What it describes is the liminal space beyond the hold of consciousness. In its initial experience in child development, this is the centering of the psyche in the totality of the Self. In later development this has to do with the conscious awareness of the Self. The function of the mode of transformation at Mimir's well is concerned with a *conscious* engagement with the unconscious.

The image of the squirrel, who runs up and down the World Tree, represents the ability to travel between the planes of being. In its travels up and down Yggdrasil, the squirrel has a conscious engagement with both heaven and the underworld. Carrying messages between the eagle, the conscious masculine position at the top, and the serpent Nidhogg, in the depths of the unconscious feminine at its root, the squirrel symbolizes the human capacity to consciously enter into dialog with the unconscious position. The form of change described at the root of Jotunheim is a willing relationship with the unconscious.

Nordic-Germanic cosmology describes Yggdrasil as a three-fold world, with each of the three major planes consisting of three layers. It is thus nine-fold, with gods, giants, dwarves, elves, and humans all living in their separate realms. Like the squirrel who runs up and down the tree, only those who have attained special vision, the seers, are able to travel between the worlds.

Shamanic tradition provides us with a powerful model of this type of psychic transformation. Although lost and virtually unknown to modern Western society, the tradition of the shaman has a long and rich history that crosses wide cultural boundaries. Noted mythologist and religious historian, Mircea Eliade (1964/1974) chronicled a long history of shamanic tradition around the globe. As if drawing from the well of Mimesbrunn, the shaman typically releases his or her hold on conscious reality and travels between the worlds. This is undertaken at substantial cost to the shaman, who frequently risks great suffering and horror to make the journey. The purpose of these journeys is to garner deeper wisdom, as well as to obtain healing and diagnostic knowledge about individuals, or about society in general. In addition, the shaman frequently journeys to retrieve a lost soul, or to accompany a soul on its way to the land of the dead.

Of particular interest is that the cosmic tree figures prominently in the world of the shaman. Eliade (1964/1974) commented that the cosmic tree was planted with the creation of the first shaman. Wherever the world tree is located, it is considered to be at the center of the universe. The tree is thus the metaphoric means, the mythological template for making the shamanic journey to heaven, bringing heaven and earth together. Depending on the nature and location of the particular culture a shaman frequently possesses a representation of the World Tree. In some cultures this consists of a tall pole with steps notched in it for a shamanic ascent. Sometimes this is a small model of a tree in the shaman's quarters that he or she will *climb* in travels between worlds. In the water-oriented cultures of Malaysia, the shaman often has a small boat with a tiny World Tree at its prow, thought to carry him or her between the worlds.

The well of Mimir and its shamanic journey provide a mythological template for bringing heaven and earth together. In psychological language we would describe this as the development of consciousness of the wholeness of the Self in and through all of life. This manner of transformation entails a willingness to be informed by the unconscious. This is an abiding agreement to undergo change as necessary to remain in alignment with growth in the Self.

To drink from Mimir's well entails a sacrifice. The ego must willingly release its exclusive hold on reality as a means of initiation into wisdom. Shamanic transformation is characterized by a surrender of the conscious position in the context of gratitude for the wholeness of the Self, which sustains us. It is a radical act of listening, a mystical attunement to Self, others, and nature, which is only possible when the conscious position, that which is *known*, is put aside. The word *sacrifice* means the offering to the deity. It stems from the Latin words *facere*, to do or perform and *sacrificium*, priestly function (OED). Sacrifice is a surrender for the purpose of propitiation or homage. Sacrifice implies an altar on which that which is to be sacrificed is placed. To sacrifice is to surrender something valued for the sake of something having higher claim.

Although this manner of transformation is entered into willingly, it remains riddled with hazards. The individual elects this form of change because he or she is aware of the necessity of surrendering the limits of the ego in order to continue to grow in the Self. This form of change is undergone by a person who has sufficient experience with the individuation process to understand the need to release the ego's hold on known reality and to be able to consciously set the ego aside. Norse mythology gives us several accounts of transformation at the well of Mimir. In one tale, Odin, god who rules over all, asked for a single drink from the well. He did not get it until he sacrificed an eye. Odin is thus known as *The Father of the Slain* (Sturluson, 1954/1984). He had to sacrifice an eye, the purely conscious position, to obtain deeper wisdom. Odin sacrificed dual vision to obtain singular insight. Another account tells of the Vanir, the earth gods, feeling cheated in a war with the Aesir, the sky gods. They cut off Mimir's head and sent it to the Aesir. It appears that the earthly forces knew that their heavenly counterparts could use some more wisdom. Perhaps they were too much in their own heads, and needed to draw from something much darker and deeper. Tradition has it that Odin would consult Mimir's severed head for hidden knowledge.

In the poem, *Havamal,* Odin hangs himself on Yggdrasil nine days, pierced by a spear in voluntary sacrifice to gain hidden knowledge (Davidson, 1964). Poignantly he says,

> *I know I hung*
> *on the windswept Tree,*
> *through nine days and nights.*
> *I was stuck with a spear*
> *and given to Odin,*
> *myself given to myself…* (p.143-144)

What we see in this ancient verse is the account of Odin, the man, sacrificing himself to Odin, the god. The lower elements, the limits of the conscious ego, sacrifice themselves to the Self. Significantly, Odin is released from the tree when he discovers the *runes*, the Nordic tool for oracular divination. Subsequent to hanging from the tree, Odin has the means to access unseen truths and to acquire the wisdom and secret knowledge he sought. Odin's sacrifice on Yggdrasil is a ritual death on the world axis. It is a shamanic death and rebirth *voluntarily entered into.* Odin consciously engages with coming to know through sacrifice of the ego. His discovery of the runes is his new-found ability to see truth, the workings of the Self in and through corporal existence.

As in the Yggdrasil myth, accounts of hanged gods and the world tree figure prominently in tales of shamanic journeys across cultures. Odin's hanging himself on Yggdrasil might be likened to the sacrifice of Christ on a wooden cross. Like Yggdrasil, the cross is another wooden vehicle, that symbolizes the intersection of the planes of being. Its horizontal cross bar, representing the material plane, the circumstantial plane of being, intersects the vertical pole, or the divine possibility, which is the potential of the Self. It is at the crux that one is able to travel between the planes of being and bring the wisdom of the Self back to the material reality.

Jung (1956/1976) referred to the tree of life as the great mother, noting that sacrifice upon the tree is transformative. When sacrifice occurs on a tree, Jung said,

> *The dead are delivered back to the mother for rebirth* (p. 233).

Sacrifice upon the tree constitutes a renunciation of one's animal nature and is a successful redirection of psychic energy into the great mother. Jung observed that it is not a regressive gesture, but rather constitutes a spiritualization of this energy.

The Well of Wisdom in Sandplay

When the sandplay client draws from Mimir's well, he or she submits to being informed by the mystery of the unconscious. With conscious intent this client sets the ego aside to become more aligned to the Self. This is the work of the client who is quite familiar with his or her inner world and the workings of the psyche. This is the individual who already lives in conscious recognition of the Self as the guiding element of life. This is possibly someone who is already familiar with the domain of sandplay, who has deep respect for its capability as a vehicle for transformation. These will not be the greater number of sandplay clients, nor will these be children, whose cognitive development precludes such a conscious engagement in the abstract domain of the psyche.

In the sacrificial or shamanic engagement with the unconscious at the Well of Wisdom, the ego's hold on reality is voluntarily surrendered. To meet the unconscious in this way demands preparation and assumes a certain level of development and familiarity with the workings of the psyche and the inner regions of experience. The distinction we need to make here is between the conscious, intentional engagement with the unconscious and the *involuntary slip* into its grasp, characteristic of the mode of change at Nidhogg's well.

Because transformation at Mimir's well presumes some degree of psychic and spiritual development, it in no way means that this manner of transformation is in any way superior to the other means of change possible in sandplay. It is simply different. Opposite energies are encountered and integrated, and the ego suffers its requisite re-ordering to the Self. Jung (1967/1983) likened the symbolism in accounts of the shamanic journey to a projection of the process of individuation. Resembling alchemy, tales of shamanic journeys portray processes of inner development that are independent of will and consciousness, albeit they are willingly entered into. As in alchemy, Jung observed that the process frequently entails a union of opposites, such as a higher element with a lower, or a right with a left. Jung observed that any successful encounter with the unconscious entails such a union of opposites.

The primary difference between this manner of transformation and that undergone in the transcendent function is the position of the ego. In the operation of the transcendent function, the conscious position is forced into a standstill by the pressures exerted by the opposite poles of the symbol. The resignation of the conscious position comes about through forces outside of itself. The polar opposition of the symbolic material in question brings the ego to its knees and essentially obliterates its hold on consciousness. New material, generated by forces of the Self in the unconscious is released into consciousness, expanding the ego's hold on reality.

Just because transformation at the well of wisdom is entered into willingly, it is by no means free of hazards. Any encounter with the unconscious is rife with terrors. Any release of the ego, whether involuntary or by sacrifice, is horrifying to the ego. We need only picture Odin impaled on Yggdrasil with his own sword, or recall his cutting out his own eye, to get a clearer idea about the demands of this way of psychic development.

Sacrifice implies an altar on which the victim is placed. Sandplay so engaged with may serve as this altar of surrender. To consciously enter into sandplay with the intention of surrender for the sake of something higher is to make the shaman's journey between the worlds. It is to voluntarily engage in a process with the full awareness that great sacrifice will be required, that great terrors may be encountered and that one will be irrevocably changed. To engage in sandplay with awareness is to surrender to the greater Self. It is in a way, a means of paying homage to that which supports and sustains us, at the same time knowing that much will be demanded of us. It is anything but a passive offering.

An example of sacrificial work is that of a sandplay therapist colleague, who was having great trouble with a major academic paper that was required of her. Already having done extensive work in sandplay, she decided to return to do a few trays to address the unseen obstacles that had essentially halted her academic progress. She recognized that she had come to a standstill. The limits of her conscious position were prohibiting her from moving ahead with this significant accomplishment. A sacrifice was demanded of her, but she was unconscious of what it might be. It was with this awareness that she submitted to this sandplay work. Shortly after doing just one tray, she felt great clarity and was re-ordered to her work with great passion.

ELIZABETH Another example is **Elizabeth's** sandplay work. **Elizabeth** had already done extensive work in sandplay. In her late forties, she reached a level of exhaustion in her professional endeavors but was unable to see beyond the horizons of the career she had worked so hard to develop. Bridging a seven-year gap since her last tray, **Elizabeth** re-entered sandplay.

Doing one tray per year over the next three years, Elizabeth was able to recognize the limits of her conscious position and came to the conscious acknowledgement that her valued professional identity would have to be sacrificed in order for something new to arise. In **Tray 10, Elizabeth's** role as doctor lay dead in the center of the tray. Encased in a glittering star for a coffin, a trail of jewels marks the history of her valuable work that was now complete. The promise of something new lay in the jeweled path, leading away from this scene of completion. Although this was deeply painful to her, its glaring presence in the sandplay effected a dramatic transformation in **Elizabeth's** relationship to her inner and outer worlds.

~ Conclusion ~

Chapter 4
Mythological Considerations of Development in Sandplay— Yggdrasil, The World Tree

This concludes our exploration of the developmental process of healing and change in sandplay therapy through the language of mythology. Now we turn to the scientific paradigm for yet another view of the same psychic terrain.

Chapter 5

Neurobiological Considerations of Development in Sandplay

Introduction

Having examined intrapsychic development through the portals of psychology and myth, we now turn to the sciences, where contemporary researchers look to the intra-cellular world of neurochemical processes to penetrate the mysteries of how mind emerges from matter. I believe we will find many similarities between the three paradigms of psychological theory, mythology and neurobiology. Considered together, this interdisciplinary approach to development strengthens our understanding of the critical features of healing and transformation in sandplay and provides a balance of insight that nourishes the mind as well as the soul.

The Mother-Child Unity and Brain Structure Development in Sandplay

Contemporary neurobiological science lends insight into the necessity of *the relationship* in the physiological operations of human brain development. Allan N. Schore (1994, 2001a & 2001b) neuropsychiatric researcher at the University of California at Los Angeles School of Medicine, Department of Psychiatry and Biobehavioral Sciences, made remarkable observations regarding the relationship between the primary caregiver's regulation of the infant's affect and the genetic triggers for higher brain structure development. Schore synthesized and integrated an abundance of research from a variety of disciplines, noting that the relationship between the child and the mother has a material and permanent effect on the brain structures, which undergo critical phases of development during the early years of life.

Schore's investigations have direct bearing on our work in sandplay, particularly with regard to the significance and dynamics of the mother-child interactions and brain development during the first three years of life. Dora Kalff (1980/2003) taught that all healing and transformation occurs at the psychic level of the mother-child unity. In the only book of teachings Dora Kalff (1980/2003) left us, her primary area of focus was the indispensable role of the early phases of development in healing and transformation. Kalff clearly and simply stated that change takes place on the matriarchal level of the psyche. She emphasized that, in order to heal, the psyche *must* return to this early developmental level. Schore's study of the relational context of neurobiological development substantiates Kalff's observations and provides a deeper understanding of the mechanics of the holding relationship in the sandplay process.

Current research reveals that it is the adaptive regulatory functions of the mother in the context of the relationship that trigger genetic processes which, in turn, initiate cellular reorganization and development (Schore, 1994, 2001a & 2001b). Central to Schore's observations are that interactions in the relationship with the mother trigger neurohormones and neurotransmitters in the child that control the timing and initiation of progressively more complex brain structure development. Schore commented,

> ...by mediating and modulating environmental input, the primary caregiver supplies the "experience" required for the experience-dependent maturation of a structural system responsible for the regulation of the individual's socioemotional function. By providing well modulated socioaffective stimulation, the mother facilitates the growth of connections between cortical limbic and sub cortical limbic structures that neurobiologically mediate self-regulatory functions (1994, pp. 32-3).

Shore found that it is largely the *non-verbal communication of affect* between mother and child that governs these neurochemical and neurobiological mechanisms of development.

Daniel J. Siegel (1999) a colleague of Schore and professor of psychiatry at UCLA, asserted that both brain and mind are created in relationship, which he refers to as an *interpersonal neurobiology*. Siegel asserted,

> ...The mind develops at the interface of neurophysiological processes and interpersonal relationships. Relationship experiences have a dominant influence on the brain because the circuits responsible for social perception are the same as or tightly linked to those that integrate the important functions controlling the creation of meaning, the regulation of bodily states, the modulation of emotion, the organization of memory, and the capacity for interpersonal communication (1999, p.21).

Like Schore (2001a), Siegel's work affirmed that the *structure and function* of the brain are determined within the context of relationship. Siegel explored the product of the brain, commonly referred to as the mind, noting that *mind* comes about through the combination of relationship and neurobiology. Of particular interest in sandplay is Siegel's observation that mind arises from patterns of energy in the brain and *between brains in relationship.* Siegel observed,

> …even at a physical distance, one mind can directly influence the activity—and development—of another through the transfer of energy and information. This joining process occurs via both verbal and nonverbal behavioral responses, which function as signals sent from one mind to another. Both words and the prosodic, nonverbal components of speech contain information that creates representational processes within the mind of the receiver (1999, p. 277).

The notion that an unseen exchange of brain energy between client and therapist materially impacts the mind in the shared field of the sand tray assumes startling significance and may explain a critical element of containment. In sandplay, both client and therapist are in relationship with the client's largely unconscious symbolic process. The relationship between client and therapist in conjunction with their mutual experience of the symbols effects a relational field that contains both the therapist's subtle regulatory functions of client's affective states, as well as the interactive exchange of brain energies back and forth between client and therapist. All of this transpires within the symbolic field of the client's sandplay. It is difficult to begin to imagine the possible permutations of communications that are set in motion in the triad of client, therapist, and sandplay. Given their nature, the symbols move the psyches of both participants. This elicits an exchange of deep psychic communication in client and therapist, wherein brain energies are impacted, moved and further exchanged back and forth in all directions between the players, while, simultaneously, the therapist works to hold the entire process within a safe container. Siegel's research does much to affirm that what transpires unseen in a sandplay session must be truly remarkable.

Early Limbic Development—
Affect and Relationship in Sandplay

During the period from the third trimester in utero until 18 to 24 months of age, the infant undergoes rapid development of the right limbic brain, which is involved in social cognition, the regulation of bodily and affective states, as well as attachment and care giving behavior (Schore, 1994, 2001a & 2001b). This system remains dominant in the child's continued growth processes until approximately age three.

Limbic system growth is substantially influenced by interactions with primary caregivers (Schore, 1994, 2001a & 2001b). The infant and caregiver form what is called an *affective synchrony*, which effectively functions as a single biological entity to influence the infant's neurobiological development. This is evident in clinical studies that document parallel acceleration and deceleration in heart rates between infants and mothers during play. Interactive play and the mother's appropriate regulation of the baby's arousal levels facilitates brain structure development that eventually allows the child to self-regulate affect. Thus, through play and comforting interactions, limbic brain structure develops and attains to higher levels of organization.

The infant and the mother both change in the relationship. The mother's relationship changes in relationship to the child, as the child develops. In the developing infant, new affect accompanies growing and changing capabilities. The mother in turn, adapts and responds to the growing child's affect, while remaining in the containing or regulatory role.

The development from the merged condition of the mother-child unity that Kalff (1980/2003) identified symbolically in sandplay might be understood to occur in this adaptive, growing, relational context of limbic brain development. Bit by bit, the affective exchange between client and therapist, via the therapist's unconscious adjustments and energetic communications with the client's developing psyche, result in progressive development from a predominantly unaware merged condition in the archetypal mother, to the beginnings of a relationship with her. The therapist's psyche functions interactively with the client through the sandplay, to provide the feedback necessary for progressive growth, while the developmental changes are archetypally effected in the psyche of the client.

Early Affect Regulation and The Free and Protected Space of Sandplay

Dora Kalff (1980/2003) understood that all healing and transformation begins at the deepest level of the psyche. Kalff recognized that in order to access this pre-conscious, matriarchal state, the client must temporarily suspend conscious awareness and enter a play, or *ludic* state of awareness. While the miniature figures and the sand tray lend themselves to a loosening of the conscious hold on reality, Kalff also recognized that the client requires the assurance of safety and stability in order to be able to productively cross the threshold into the matriarchal level. Kalff thus defined the two unseen, but critical components of sandplay, *freedom and protection*, which exist, not by formula or training, but by the nature of the relationship between the therapist and the client.

Shore's (1994, 2001a & 2001b) insights into the significance of the mother-infant relationship in brain development lend a deepened understanding to the holding and containing relationship of sandplay. Sandplay facilitates a profound and powerful, yet largely non-verbal communication between the client and therapist. In a manner very like that between the growing infant and the mother, the sandplay client is held in the highly charged, seamless field of psychic communication with the therapist.

In what we refer to as *containment*, the therapist's psyche functions in a regulatory way through the subtle but formidable limit setting, known as the *free and protected space*. By subtly adapting to the changing needs of the client' s sandplay work, the therapist's holding and regulating capacity both stimulates and allows the psychic disorganization and reorganization required by the client to heal and to continue developing. It is perhaps not too far a reach to suggest that, in the psychic change process undergone in sandplay, the appropriate brain structures reorganize, in much the same way they do in the relationship between mother and child.

Hierarchical Brain Structure Development and Trauma in Sandplay

Schore (2001a & 2001b) asserted that child development can only be understood in terms of the progressive development of more complex brain structures. This advancing complexity accounts for the progression of behavior and capability normally referred to in child development. Neurobiological structures are continually organizing, disorganizing, and reorganizing in the developing infant brain. This parallels the process of the symbol and the transcendent function we are familiar with in sandplay work. Shore noted that as far back as 1931, John Hughlings Jackson theorized that the brain is organized horizontally in hierarchical levels. This early supposition conforms to contemporary observations that developing brain structures are, actually, more complex versions of their earlier, more primitive counterparts. Infant brain growth proceeds in a sequence of stages in which later cortical structures regulate the earlier sub-cortical structures. Increasing connections between lower structures allow processing at higher levels. The more developed structures function in an executive manner, yet all levels of the structure remain connected. This results in more highly developed means to manage and regulate affect

Neurologist Paul MacLean developed a model of what he called a *triune brain* (Cory & Gardner, 2002). Proposing that the brain developed evolutionarily to contend with successively complex tasks, MacLean suggested that the brain is actually composed of three brains. These include: the brain stem, which governs fundamental survival tasks; the limbic mid brain, the more developed emotional center; and the highest evolved cerebral cortex, the seat of more advanced cognitive functions.

When we figuratively stratify these sequentially complex layers of the brain in a hierarchal drawing, we have a structure that looks something like the following.

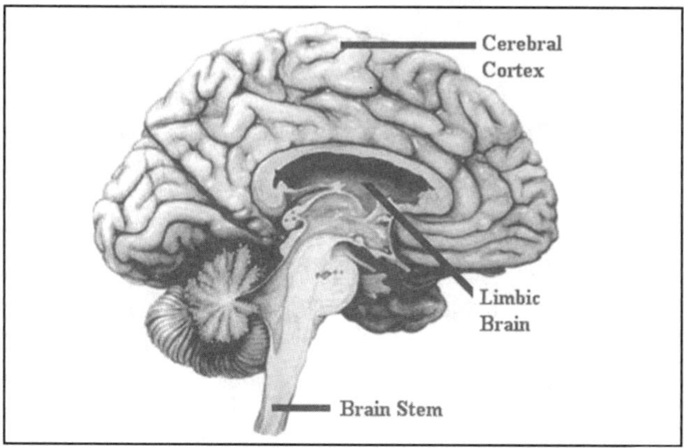

The three major areas of the brain.

Brain Level	Structural Components	Functions
Cerebral Cortex	Prefrontal Cortex Visual, Auditory, Sensory Cortices & Assn Areas Speech, Motor Cortices & Assn Areas	Complex Thought Intelligence Personality Sensory Impulse Interpretation Motor Functions
Limbic Brain	Amygdala Cingulate Gyrus Hippocampus Hypothalamus Thalamus Olfactory Cortex	Emotions Emotional Responses Hormonal Regulation Pain Pleasure Motivation Mood
Brain Stem	Midbrain Medulla Oblongata Pons	Autonomic Functions Breathing, Heart Rate Blood Pressure Digestion Alertness, Arousal

The components and functions of the three major areas of the brain

Reducing the highly complex structures of the brain to very simple elements for purposes of our discussion, we see that the brain grows from lesser to higher complexity. The structures necessary for survival are present at birth in the lower autonomic functions of the amygdala and brain stem areas. The more complex brain functions continue to evolve and diversify as development proceeds. Developing brain structures perform more complex functions than their underlying predecessors. Rather than simply replacing the underlying functions, the brain builds upon and incorporates the already-developed capacities into increasingly more complex abilities. As we progress to high orders of development, we re-visit the underlying layers of development that prefigured the advancements, augmenting the capacities of the lower structures with the newly developed mental tools.

I wonder if this hierarchal nature of brain development may, in part, explain the spiral archetype of growth and development. Perhaps we become aware of the spiral, as the newly developed higher-order capacities are able to reflect back on their structural predecessors. Another interesting neurological corollary to the archetypal figure of the spiral is that the nerve cell covering that speeds up signal transmission, known as *myelin,* grows in a spiral movement around the axon. It appears that spirals are physiologically built in to neurological processes of information transmission and connection.

Bruce D. Perry (2001, 2002), a brain development researcher focusing on the impact of trauma, observed that all incoming sensory information is matched against *templates*, or memories of prior experience at each level of the brain's organization. Matching new events against templates, or patterns of previous experience accounts for our ability to organize our existence in a progressively complex, but nonetheless coherent manner. By the same token, it is easy to understand how experiences of trauma create arrests in continued brain development, when incoming signals continue to be perceived as the original dangers. The traumatized individual remains in a state of fear and alert, which precludes the conditions of safety and relationship that foster higher order brain structure development.

The brain is dependent upon experience to develop and to organize its structure. Deprivation of experience may result in the death and elimination of neural axons and synapses. This is referred to as *pruning* and is a natural process of cell selection during early childhood when the brain has more neural connections than it will need. Genes program brain structure growth. Experience determines which genes are triggered and how they influence growth of the synaptic connections. Experiences of the family, the culture and so on, select out the neural pathways the child needs to survive and function in the particular environment, pruning out the unstimulated ones. In cases of environmental deprivation, where neural pathways growth is not activated by experience, important neural material is pruned away in response to the deprived experience.

The brain is the least differentiated organ of the human body at birth. Thus, early experience has a tremendous impact on its development. The earlier developing brain structures govern the ability to regulate fundamental survival affects, such as terror and rage. Although experience continues to affect how the brain functions throughout life, the core self-regulating structures form in early life. Trauma in early development may have a significant effect on these deeper brain structures, severely compromising the person's later ability to deal appropriately with stress (Perry, 2001, 2002).

During the first nine months of life, trauma or impairment to the developing mother-child relationship affects development of the amygdala and other limbic structures. This results in poor regulation of sub-cortical functions and poor autonomic regulation. One outcome of this condition is a reduced capacity to experience positive emotion, along with an impaired ability to regulate affect. Such wounding may manifest in later life as impaired emotional functioning and difficulty forming social connections. During the period from 9 to 18 months, trauma results in a poor integration of the differing layers of the cortico-limbic system. This results in a limited ability to manage and regulate levels of high stress. Shore (2001a & 2001b) contended that an organized, but insecure, attachment results from one of these experiences of trauma, and a disorganized attachment results from encounters with both types.

Schore (2001a & 2001b) observed that the areas of the brain responsible for integrating functions such as social relationships, meaning, awareness of self, and emotional regulation and response, continue to grow into adulthood. This area is the orbitofrontal cortex, which Schore described as a place of convergence where lower cortical functions meet with the higher cortical circuits. Schore contended that trauma results in excessive neural pruning in the cortical-sub cortical region, resulting in impaired capacity to self regulate.

In cases of severe trauma, deeper brain structures are wounded to such a degree that further growth is severely limited, if not impossible. In some instances however, safe interpersonal relationships formed in later life may foster healthy attachment experiences that trigger brain structure growth and organization, as they do in early childhood (Perry 2001, 2002).

Neuroanatomist Marian C. Diamond (1988) observed that brain growth and development is possible at any age with adequate challenges to the nerve cells. Diamond emphasized that the key factor in neural stimulation in later development is the *active engagement* with the environment.

This contemporary research leaves room for the prospect that, in cases where brain healing and growth are still possible, the sandplay client has the opportunity to re-visit and re-order neurobiological structural impairments and deficits that remain from infancy (Schore, 2001a, 2001b; Perry, 2001, 2002). It is not difficult to speculate that the free and protected space of the sandplay container creates the conditions wherein the client is able to re-constitute a healthy attachment in the archetypal mother-child unity. Through the active physical engagement with the sand and symbols, neurobiological structure growth may be triggered, mending wounded areas and allowing the natural progressive process of brain development to continue.

Patterns of Affect Regulation and the Development of the Self

Schore (1994, 2001a & 2001b) addressed the structural evolution of the psychic perception of oneself as an integrated whole, offering a scientific account for what Jung (1954/1981, 1959/1980, 1960/1981) called the *Self*. As we have discussed, the context of early development is the relationship between the child and the mother. Neumann (1973) and Kalff (1980/2003) asserted that the mother holds the Self of the young infant. Shore cited the earlier research of Diamond, Balvin & Diamond (1963), which observed that the mother functions as the child's auxiliary cortex. These researchers noted that the young baby is a sub-cortical creature, in danger of being shocked, or over-stimulated by powerful environmental stimuli. Lacking the structural features necessary to modulate the input, the mother does this task for the infant.

Schore (2001a, 2001b) noted that very recent research has determined that the mother's appropriate interactions set in motion the growth of connections between the sub-cortical limbic and cortical limbic structures. These connections function to bridge the deeply felt affective experience of the limbic region with the rational capacities to define and categorize them. These structures thus facilitate the infant's growing self-regulatory functions.

The developing child's sense of self arises from patterns of affect regulation that bring about a coherent sense of presence across fluctuations in affective states. Emerging out of the affective relationship to the primary caregiver, the development of the child's coherent sense of self is both a progressive and regressive procedure. It entails repeated patterns of brain organization, disorganization and reorganization within the context of the emotional connection and affect regulation between mother and child.

Of particular interest to the subject of growth and change in sandplay is the fact that the prefrontal cortex brain structures that are responsible for the creation of meaning, memory organization, and self-regulation of emotions are very closely linked to those that facilitate social perception. Translating this neurobiological finding into Jungian personality theory, we can infer that the coherent *centering of the Self occurs in the context of social perception.* Thus, the experience of the Self, as a coherent whole imbued with meaning and purpose, is inherently relational. The first experience of the Self occurs at about three years of age when the child's brain has developed sufficiently to permit the developing higher order brain structures to manifest the perception of the child as existing at the nucleus of an integrated meaning system, which is connected to all being.

Given the profound role played by emotions in brain organization and learning processes, it is likely that the relational, symbolic nature of sandplay operates in the non-rational, right hemispheric limbic system. This almost certainly would be the case at the earliest levels of psychic development, with more rational, conscious integration of newly developed material being made subsequently in the left hemisphere.

The Creation of Human Mind in Relationship and Sandplay

Siegel (1999) investigated the connection between neurobiology and interpersonal relationships, focusing on three central concepts. In Siegel's words,

> 1. The human mind emerges from patterns in the flow of energy and information within the brain and between brains.
>
> 2. The mind is created within the interaction of neuro-physiological processes and interpersonal experiences.
>
> 3. The structure and function of the developing brain are determined by how experiences, especially within the interpersonal relationships, shape the genetically pro-grammed maturation of the nervous system (p. 2).

It appears to me that the relational qualities of the free and protected space of sandplay facilitate the very exchange of mind Siegel (1999) described. In addition, the mutually experienced context of the symbolic work adds a powerful dimension to the faculties of change and transformation that are created within the relationship. Siegel observed that minds interact to influence one another and the signals sent from one mind to another have a direct effect on the flow of energy in the receiving mind. Siegel proposed that minds may overlap to form a mental *supersystem,* wherein each functions to strengthen, or deplete the other (p. 276). The overlapping field of psyche in sandplay is precisely such a mutually strengthening mental field, developed to support and fortify the newly emerging psychic material of the client.

Siegel (1999) reminded us that, in order to survive, even as adults, we need not only love and caring, "*...but to have another individual simultaneously experience a state of mind similar to our own*" (p. 22). Siegel observed that it is this congruity of mind in relationship that gives life its integrity of purpose and meaning.

The relationship of the therapist in the free and protected space of sandplay, where the client's symbolic creations are silently shared, is a profound experience of the meaning-making Siegel describes. The observing attitude of client and therapist join together in the symbolic field of sandplay to create a profound coherence of mind. The joint experience of the client's sandplay holds the possibility of bringing about the broadest and deepest condition of shared mind. It is not difficult to imagine how the vast meaning of the symbols and their simultaneous activation of the psyche at all levels might create conditions of shared mind that exceed our ability to grasp. Although the magnitude of the shared experience of the symbolic field of the client's sandplay is largely not conscious, it is of the greatest importance that it is ordered to the Self. Being anchored in the central archetype of the Self, the scope and simultaneity of the shared mind in sandplay thus serves the core vitality of life, integrity and purpose in profound measure.

Myth Making and Mystical Experience

The neurobiology of the Self is further elucidated by investigations into the mental functions of mystical experience and the operations of myth making. Medical researchers, Andrew Newberg and Eugene D'Aquili (2001), investigated the operations of brain physiology during episodes of mystical experience. Their research lends further scientific insight into the physical properties of what we refer to as the Self. Sadly, D'Aquili died before the completion of their book on the subject. Newberg however, continued the work. A physician and professor in the Departments of Nuclear Radiology and Religious Studies at the University of Pennsylvania, Newberg described the neurological mechanisms that account for religious and mystical experiences.

The Brain's Drive to Realize Wholeness

Newberg (2001) concluded that the mystical experience is based in neurology and is built into human experience. Furthermore, he found that there exists a natural human drive toward this unitary experience, which is biologically inherent in human brain function. What Newberg addressed neurobiologically is the psychological component Jung referred to as the *Self*.

Newberg (2001) examined the brain activity of several subjects during the experience of mystical states. The subjects of his brain scan studies included a variety of monks and nuns from differing spiritual traditions.

All were deeply religious or spiritual and described the subjective experience of the peak mystical states evidenced on Newberg's brain scans as either unitary states of awareness to all of being, or of complete absorption in the omnipresent divine presence. Newberg recognized that the research was showing neurological processes, which open the individual to the awareness of an absolute reality that underpins ordinary conscious awareness and that connects all of manifest reality. Newberg observed,

> Mystical reality holds, and the neurology does not contradict it, that beneath the mind's perception of thoughts, memories, emotions, and objects, beneath the subjective awareness we think of as the self, there is a deeper self, a state of pure awareness that sees beyond the limits of subject and object, and rests in a universe where all things are one (p. 155).

The deeper self that Newberg's brain scans reveal is in accord with the Self, described by Jung. In Newberg's studies, neurobiological science affirms psychological theory, as well as the mythic and poetic tenets of the perennial religious traditions.

Brain Activity in Mystical States and Symbolic Process

The cerebral cortex is characterized by right and left hemispheres. Each hemisphere is subdivided into four sections, known as *lobes*. Although the human brain is far more complex and integrated in its functions, the left and right hemispheres of the cerebral cortex are generally considered to specialize in modes of perception. The left hemisphere functions more rationally and analytically, and the right hemisphere is abstract and image-related (Newberg, 2001). The specific function of the lobes varies depending on their location in the right or left hemispheres. A broad overview of their purpose is as follows:

THE FOUR LOBES OF THE CEREBRAL CORTEX	
Lobe Name	**General Functions**
Temporal Lobe	Language, Conceptual Thinking
Occipital Lobe	Vision
Parietal Lobe (Location of Orientation Association Area)	Sensory Perception Visual-Spatial Tasks Body Orientation
Frontal Lobe	Attention, Reasoning, Judgment Personality Muscle Activity Initiation

In an effort to probe the neurobiological underpinnings of the religious experience, Newberg and his colleagues discovered that during transcendent or mystical states of consciousness, there is decreased activity in the posterior superior parietal lobe of the brain. To simplify the discussion, these researchers referred to this region as the *orientation association area*, or OAA. The primary function of this region of the brain is to define the limits of the individual in relationship to other people and things. In other words, the OAA delineates the *me and not me* of awareness. This is the region of the brain that locates us in time and space

Newberg (2001) defined a variety of higher cognitive processes, called *operators*, which it would appear, serve important functions in the experience of Self. The operators perform a variety of functions, which together work to transport the individual's conscious awareness beyond its current limitations by accessing the underlying neurology of the unitary experience. The eight operators are involved in the mental processes that identify and seek solutions to problems and conundrums, whose answers are beyond the individual's current understanding. When we translate Newberg's findings to Jungian psychology, we discover that the operators involved in mystical experience parallel the mechanics of what we typically refer to as the *symbolic process*.

The Eight Operators of Mystical Experience and Symbolic Process

Newberg (2001) maintained that, although there are many cognitive operators, or functions, working as the organizing principles that support human thinking, feeling, understanding, and so on, there are eight particular ones that factor into mystical experience.

> **The holistic operator** is the capacity to see the relationship between things and to perceive things as a whole.
>
> **The reductionist operator** is the capacity to see things in their component parts and elements.
>
> **The abstractive operator** assimilates separate pieces of information, drawing broader, general concepts from them.
>
> **The quantitative operator** is the ability to discern abstract patterns in time and space.
>
> **The causal operator** is the mental faculty that is able to understand experience in terms of causes and effects.
>
> **The binary operator** is the mental function that is able to reduce all components of experience to pairs of opposites.
>
> **The existential operator** is the mental capacity that allows the perception of things as real.
>
> **The emotional operator** assigns an emotional value to perceptions (pp.46-53).

Newberg (2001) observed that myth making is built into human neurobiology. He theorized that these neurological operators work together to create mythological accounts that address fundamental human questions and fears. Newberg postulated that the human mental capacity to perceive complex environmental threats fuels the need to understand them and to make sense of them. The anxiety created by perceived threats and unexplainable conditions, such as birth and death, drives the higher cognitive operators to find meaning and purpose. Newberg observed that this *cognitive imperative* to find meaning drives the mind to seek resolution.

The mind seeks a natural resolution to troubling existential mysteries through myth making. Mythic stories evolve from experience in order to provide relief from the existential anxiety and to describe the process of its resolution. The traditional mythic pattern begins with an existential problem that is unanswerable, such as the origin of life, what occurs at death, and so on. The mythic tale draws elements from cultural experience to contextualize the dilemma in terms of polar opposites. The tale then proceeds to resolve the dilemma through the intervention of gods, or forces beyond ordinary conscious awareness.

The mythic tale serves as a template that holds or contains our anxiety, while at the same time indicates the means of resolution. The mythic tale replicates the same process the brain undergoes in the processes of growth, development and learning. The universality of myths and symbols across cultures results from the basic brain structures and organizational qualities that make sense of existence. Perhaps the archetypes Jung described emerge from these same structural components of the brain.

Two of the cognitive operators, the causal and the binary, are particularly significant in the natural process of myth making. Newberg (2001) observed that what cannot be known or understood, elicits fear. This initiates the cognitive imperative to make sense of what is unknown in order to obviate the high state of tension. He noted that the causal operator seeks a reason for the particular unexplainable situation. Because no answers to the problem exist, the binary operator splits the components of the problem into polar opposites. This interrupts the high state of anxiety by equally distributing the energy between the two poles. The dynamic stasis of the polarized energy elicits left and right hemispheric activity that simultaneously, but independently attempts to resolve the dilemma to the unknown problem. While the left hemisphere grapples with the situation, seeking rational or intellectual resolution, the right hemisphere engages in a holistic, intuitive, emotional, image-rich attempt to come to grips with the problem. Newberg observed that both hemispheres engage in highly charged activity as they attempt to solve the problem. Resolution is reached when the elements of both hemispheres come together with the new elements that fit or match. The new understanding elicits a neurological resonance that results in a profound feeling of pleasure and peace. Newberg described the experience as, *…a rush of ecstasy and awe* (p. 72).

Newberg's (2001) description of the neuro-mechanics of myth making parallels the transcendent function, described by Jung (1960/1981), as well as what we frequently call the *symbolic process* in sandplay. The new product that emerges from the interruption of dialog between the two hemispheres is the transcendent product that emerges when the psyche is captivated by a symbol. Jung understood that to transcend meant to *go across*. It is fascinating that neurobiology describes a temporary separation of hemispheric communication, which is then *bridged* by birth of the new psychic component.

A beautiful example of bridging new connections is seen in the sand tray of **Lilly**, a young girl who had been abandoned by her mother.

LILLY Early in her process in **Tray 2**, **Lilly** gathers the psychic elements she will need to bridge the profound wounding she has suffered. At this phase of her work, the bridge is completely in the water. The new connections are beginning to form but will not surface until she has undergone further development. A shark swims nearby, underscoring the dangers of the crossing that remains ahead of her. Preparing for the journey across the bridge are the mother seal and baby, the snail family and a pair of sea horses. Two beautiful gold fish sit atop a prominent piece of brain coral. The brain had to be bridged in new ways in order to bring about the intrapsychic and archetypal union of family **Lilly** so urgently needed to be whole. In **Tray 10**, the bridging is fully accomplished, as the pelicans safely attend the cubs in the cage.

~ Conclusion ~

Chapter 5
Neurobiological Considerations of Development in Sandplay

Our overview of neurobiology has familiarized us with some of the aspects of brain structure development that account for variability in psychic capacity. Recent findings regarding shared brain activity in the context of relationship and its impact on healing and continued growth of the human mind, ground sandplay therapy in recent research in neurobiological science. We have seen how some of these functions may be the neurological foundations of symbolic process and the transcendent function. We have reviewed brain structure development that explains some of the changes and growth in psychological capacity that we observe in sandplay. We have explored the neurobiological aspects of the phenomenon of mind and its profound bearing on the relationship of therapist and client in sandplay.

Of greatest importance to us as sandplay therapists is the neurobiological reality of the necessity of human relationship in all phases of intrapsychic growth and change. Knowing how relationship facilitates neurological development crucially underscores the therapeutic potential created in the sandplay relationship. The freedom and safety created in the sandplay relationship recreates the psychic conditions of a mother-child attachment, thereby facilitating access to the earliest level of matriarchal consciousness. The shared symbolic field of sandplay creates the conditions for the mutual experience of the client's image-rich preconscious language. In the relationship, client and therapist directly experience the client's deep, inner psychic material. The concrete nature of the sandplay symbols permits the client to manipulate and reconfigure psychic structure in the immediacy of the relationship, facilitating affective resonance and the mental exchange of transactional feedback that supports the client's adaptive growth and transformation at profound levels.

Comparing Three Paradigms of Psychic Transformation		
Kalff	Yggdrasil	Neurobiology
Mother-Child Unity *Mother holds child's Self functions*	Well of Hel, Nidhogg/ Underworld *In darkest earth* *No separation* *Transformation through transcendence*	Sub-Cortical Amygdala and Early Limbic Growth *Care giver assumes higher cortical functions for child*
Relationship to Mother *Child relates to mother*	Well of Norns/Destiny *Polarities emerge* *Transformation through healing and Remembering*	Limbic Brain Growth/ Organization *Growing capacity to self regulate*
Constellation of the Self *Child's psyche centers in totality of being*	Well of Mimir/Wisdom *Connection to heaven bridged* *Transformation through wisdom and sacrifice*	Cortical-Limbic Connections *Coherent sense of presence across fluctuations in affective states*

~ Conclusion ~

Section I
Psychological Considerations of Development in Sandplay

Our understanding of what transpires in sandplay is deepened and strengthened by interdisciplinary study. The three templates for the psychic growth process we have examined—psychological, mythological and neurobiological—differ widely in methodology and language, yet each describes a remarkably similar course of development. Viewed together, the similarities are evident.

As Dora Kalff taught us, as the ancient poetry of Yggdrasil continues to inform us, and as contemporary neurobiology affirms, there is a tremendous possibility for healing and transformation in the relational field of sandplay.

I believe that Dora Kalff recognized the possibilities for both individual and cultural transformation in sandplay. To enter the relational healing space of sandplay with a client is an intimate, personal experience of transformation. While it might be said that sandplay with one patient at a time is such a small act, we must remember that the intimacy of relationship is essential to the transformation process. Transformation, in ourselves, our clients, their families, the community, the culture and the world, begins with this relationship. As Dora Kalff so clearly observed, transformation not only begins with this relationship, it cannot occur without it.

This concludes our examination of development, or how growth and change occurs in sandplay therapy. We will now focus on the thematic features of sandplay, in order to cultivate ways of deepening our relationship to and understanding of these processes.

Section II

Themes in Sandplay Therapy

Introduction

To track the processes of healing and transformation discussed in our last section, it is necessary for the therapist to develop ways of entering into a meaningful relationship with the sandplay. We recall Dora Kalff's observation that to provide adequate therapeutic containment of the client's process, the therapist must be actively *engaged in coming to understand* its unfolding mystery.

A helpful tool for developing a relationship with the sandplay process is to identify the thematic patterns that occur. Although it is impossible to apply any formula to the process of sandplay, tracking thematic patterns sheds a light on what the process might be about and where the client's work might be headed. For purposes of organization I have categorized thematic patterns under four general headings:

Content Themes
Spatial Themes
Affect Themes
Motion Themes

As we examine the themes, we must remain aware that these categories are not definitive. You may find many additions and changes that you prefer to make to better suit your own tastes and preferences. Important to remember is that we are attempting to find the means of engaging with the vast unknowns of a sandplay process. To contain it properly we must find methods of entering into dialog with its symbolic language. This relationship disposes us to being informed by it.

Although we frequently speak of symbols as if they were single, discreet items, we must remember that *the entire sandplay process* functions symbolically. By identifying thematic patterns we seek to tease apart elements of that symbolic process to arrive at some sense of its meaning. So, as we explore these thematic patterns, let us try to keep their possible symbolic significance in mind without attempting to impose fixed meanings on any sandplay case.

Chapter 1

Content Themes in Sandplay

Introduction

Examining themes of sandplay content provides another means of coming into relationship with the process, which can facilitate understanding and proper containment of the clients' work in the sand tray. When we consider the elements of content below, we must remember to think of them as pertaining to individual sand trays, as well as to themes that occur throughout a sandplay process.

Figures Used in the Sandplay Process

The figures that the client selects from the sandplay collection present an obvious focus of attention for the therapist's understanding of a sandplay process. The very fact that particular figures are chosen from the array of possibilities available in the sandplay collection is of great significance. With choices spanning the full range of life and fantasy, the selection of a figure, or of combinations of figures, is always a unique and remarkable event.

In the still atmosphere of sandplay, the psyche moves the client to see and select figures in physical form that embody the emergent edge of its transformative nature. With little or no conscious knowing, the client's psyche thus appears and moves. The material form of the full spectrum of possibility held by the collection of figures, as well as the motility of the sand, invites the psyche to a tangible, physical engagement that is concurrently witnessed and held by the client and the therapist. This conjoint conscious and unconscious holding of client and therapist creates and facilitates the conditions necessary for the psyche to move in its natural course toward an ego centered in wholeness and in service to the central archetype of the Self.

It is imperative that we hold this awareness when the client sees and selects figures for the sandplay. It is important to remember that even the choice of simple rocks or trees are the manifestation of psyche, who honors us with her appearance and entrusts us to properly hold her alterations and adjustments.

There are many ways we might go about examining the figures used in sandplay. The following suggests some preliminary considerations regarding the selection of figures. Our concern here is not the symbolic content of the figures, but rather the possible significance of the general types of figures selected by the client. We have separated them into figures from this world, figures from fantasy, and figures with archetypal content.

Figures From This World

Figures from Ordinary Life

Figures from ordinary life are figures and scenes typical of the client's world. As such they are likely indicative of material closer to conscious awareness. Among others this category includes figures from nature, such as animals and vegetation, objects common to the outer world, people, furnishings and buildings.

In all cases it is important to consider the client's personal relationship to the images selected, as well as their more characteristic symbolic implications. General classifications of objects may be related to specific aspects of psychic development. Animals and vegetation, for example, are likely to be concerned with matters of instinct. It is important to observe whether the figures are more of a wild, or domesticated nature. Movement between wild and domestic scenes over a series of sand trays may indicate the emergence and harnessing of a deeper, instinctual aspect of the personality. It may similarly have to do with apprehensions of being out of control and a need to restrain contact with the instincts. The choice of figures from the natural world must be considered in the unique context of each case.

Sandplays depicting scenes from ordinary life, such as houses, towns, and normal people going about every day duties, may typify what is called a *marketplace* tray. Marketplace sand trays are frequently done as the sandplay process nears completion. In this circumstance, the client's work in the sand has undergone a descent into the unconscious, contact with the central archetype of the Self and a reordering of psychic contents to the Self. The marketplace indicates a return to ordinary conscious awareness. Marketplace sandplays carry the client's readiness to leave the sandplay process and the ability to take the newly-integrated psychic work out into the world. Scenes from ordinary life may also make their appearance during the course of a process, as a significant piece of material is integrated.

> **AARON** A fine example of a marketplace scene occurring during a process is the creation of **Aaron's** bedroom in **Tray 7**. This sand tray, seventh in a series of 15, occurs at the conclusion of **Aaron's** resolution of conflict regarding his masculine nature. Following this temporary return to the surface of conscious awareness, **Aaron's** work descends into unknown reaches of himself, tapping his deeper spiritual nature.

In addition to indicating the conclusion of significant work at deeper levels in sandplay, the repeated appearance of ordinary, or marketplace content may serve as a defense against psychic descent. Each case must be considered within its own context.

Figures of people selected by the client for sandplay may suggest ordinary life and marketplace content, if they reflect the cultural characteristics of the client. When however, a client uses figures of people with a skin tone very different from his or her own, it is likely that the implications of this particular content are different from a typical marketplace scene. The choice of figures with a dramatically different skin tone may be better understood from a deeper symbolic perspective, rather than the more conscious marketplace scenes described above.

The gender and ages of the figures may also be significant aspects of the symbolic process. It is important to observe when the sandplay reflects a preponderance, or the absence of, a gender. When both male and female figures appear in the sandplay, we want to notice how they relate, whether they depict harmony or discord. When the age depicted by figures is significantly different than the client's chronological age, we want to take note of its possible significance in the client's psychic work.

Figures Remote in Time

Sandplay content reflective of times from history, of ancient, or primitive cultures may indicate the *age* of the particular issue in the individual psyche, the family lineage, or both. A typical example of this is a sand tray filled with battling knights in armor, or knights fighting contemporary soldiers. Sand trays with historical figures raise the question of not only what the content concerns, but how old the issue is. The age of the issue may be considered from an intrapsychic perspective in terms of the stage of the client's development when the wounding took place. In the case of the fighting knights, it might be that the wounding is old, or that it happened long ago. In the mixed battle of old and contemporary soldiers, it is important to consider the content held by the differences in the ages of the warriors. It may be that an old wound is doing particular battle with current development. It may be that a current struggle has reopened an old hurt. In the same way, sandplay content from incongruent periods in history may indicate confusion about the nature of the issues, or a disordered, uncertain stance in relationship to the issues. On the other hand, a mix of historic content may work as the celebratory integration of age-old issues. These are simply examples of the diverse considerations we might embrace.

When we see trays with dinosaurs and other ancient creatures, we must similarly consider the role of history in the client's wounding. It could be that the psyche is addressing a wound that occurred very early in the client's development. The prominent presence of dinosaurs may allude to a long family legacy of hurt and dysfunction. This may be particularly poignant when family groupings are regularly portrayed as dinosaurs.

Figures Remote in Distance

Figures from far-off places unknown to the client may appear with an almost mystical quality about them. Dora Kalff (1980/2003) indicated that when a client touches the spiritual plane, but has not yet developed a conscious relationship to it, the figures chosen will come from a form of spirituality that is far away from anything known to the client. They appear, as it were, from the other side of the world. We may witness serene constructions of oriental temples done by Westerners who are not at all aware of Eastern traditions on a conscious level.

It is not unusual for children from unsophisticated backgrounds to use buildings or religious figures from far away India, or China. When this occurs, we know that the client is reaching deep into a far, remote part of the psyche. The miracle of the psyche furnishes contents that hold the richness needed to nurture the client's continued growth and transformation. It is the beauty and magic of the psyche's capacity to manifest these symbols, so completely foreign to the client, yet invested with the energy to awaken the wholeness, that informs their mystical nature.

AARON Aaron's Tray 9 reflects his return from a serene and almost ethereal China. Led by a large blue dolphin, his boat begins its journey back home. Characteristic of **Aaron's** work, his next sand tray, **Tray 10,** has him back in the ordinary world of the classroom and school yard. This young boy's process in the sand takes him to the far reaches of spiritual possibility, then returns him home to integrate this newly acknowledged depth in the marketplace.

IVY Another example comes from the work of nine-year-old **Ivy**, who belonged to a strict and insular Western religious sect. In **Ivy's Tray 8** a Chinese Buddha appears along with masks from the Hindu epic tale of the *Ramayana.* Completely unknown to her consciously, **Ivy's** psyche drew images that held the very qualities she sought to embody in a holy and reverent way. Referring to the Buddha as *the fat guy*, she was completely unconscious that she had positioned this image of wholeness atop the characters of an ancient Indian tale concerned with the loss and recovery of the feminine. These were the deeper issues she confronted in her work. Within the context of her faith, her body and female sexuality were disparaged and repressed. Within the safety of the sand tray her psyche was able to access and embody the essential qualities she required to continue her growth and development.

Just as content from remote earthly locations holds deep and far away psychic content, so can inter-galactic figures and those representing space travel indicate connections with the nether regions of the psyche. When space ships or people from other planets land in the sand tray, it is fairly certain that something from far away in the client's inner world is making its appearance. When we witness the appearance of figures from far-off places, it is critical that we remain open to the possibility for the emergence of new psychic content. We must hold it with a quality of welcome anticipation. As with other aspects of sandplay, the opposite circumstance may also be true, as when space ships and rockets carry a more defensive or escapist quality.

> **AARON** In **Aaron's Tray 3**, two men in NASA space suits greet the round silver space ship that has just landed in the near right corner of the sand tray. In this example it is clear what was emerging in the psyche of this child in the form of the ship from outer space. This tray, with its concurrent scenes of death and of the subduing of monsters is followed by the manifestation of the Self, in **Aaron's Tray 4**.

Figures from Fantasy

Fantasy figures are frequently the normal friends and companions of the child's imagination. Cartoon figures from popular television programs or movies may hold the qualities of significant people in the child's life. They often assume the energies of the inner and outer villains, heroes and monsters that populate the experience of young children and help them negotiate their way through life.

The same fantasy figures in the sandplay work of an adult may indicate avoidance or lack of grounding. When fantasy figures appear prominently in the sandplay of adults, we must consider a tenuous grasp of reality, or a reluctance to assume more mature responsibilities. Because symbols span the distance between their negative and positive aspects, they may also carry the much-needed playful fancy that emerges to balance the overly responsible attitudes of a more rigidly-adapted adult.

Figures with Archetypal Content

Figures that bear archetypal content are those that embody a form or energy of what is otherworldly. Archetypal figures may appear as objects from nature, as animals or as human shapes common to this world, yet they emanate qualities that reach beyond the ordinary. Animal forms that appear as archetypal are frequently mythical creatures, such as the dragon, the satyr, and the phoenix. Archetypal figures depicted as human are gods and goddesses, monsters, and heroes, which assume their character in the deep psychic language of myth. Seminal shapes, such as eggs, crystal balls, stars, and jewels may also have archetypal content.

In sandplay, archetypal figures originate in remote regions of the psyche. They may evidence deeply dark, or profoundly light psychic qualities. Thus, when they are present in sandplay, they hold a numinous or mystical energy. Archetypal content is powerful, and its presence gives evidence that the very core of a particular psychic quality is being touched.

> **AARON** **Aaron's Tray 14** radiates a crystalline archetypal energy with its shimmering ice and snow. Although the figures used in the sandplay are from real life, all but the skiers are colored white or crystal. The archetypal content is held by the remote stillness of this creation that **Aaron** called *Winterland*. The unconscious juxtaposition of round and square shapes underscores the core energies tapped by **Aaron** in this sandplay.

Archetypal content may be used in sandplay as a defense against the messier, more authentic features of psychic exploration. When used in this way, the energy of the archetype is absent. The tray may have a very dark or shiny appearance, but retains a flat feeling about it. When this occurs, it is critical for the therapist to examine what he or she might be missing in the sandplay process in order to understand what the resistance may be about.

Symbolic Content of Figures

Addressing the subject of the figures' symbolic content is difficult, because the symbolic content of the figures is held within the context of nearly *everything we are exploring* in our examination of sandplay. A figure and its traditional symbolic significance must never be considered in isolation from the *total context of the sandplay process*. Nevertheless, we recognize that the figures do play a significant role in sandplay therapy. While the conventional symbolic connotation of a figure is indeed an important feature of sandplay, we do not want to fixate on meanings. By defining or identifying a figure's symbolic characteristics in too determined a way, we limit the possibility held by the symbol in general. Affixing a meaning to a figure also places serious limitations on the broader contextual symbolic process of which it is a part.

The commonly understood implications of figures arises from a variety of sources, spanning from the figure's instinctual, or habitual role in the natural world across the spectrum of possibility to the arcane reaches of the mythic and mystical. The meanings derived from nature are drawn from observation. Those of a deeper, intrapsychic nature arise from cross-cultural mythic themes that appear to be inherent in the common psychic experience of humankind, or what Jung (1954/1981) referred to as the *collective unconscious*. Symbolic significance is also drawn from literature, works of art, history, religion, geography, cultural habit, and so on. When we also consider that figures functioning as symbols bridge both light and dark aspects of the images, we begin to appreciate how merely affixing "meaning" to a figure is inadequate.

There are many symbol dictionaries, as well as encyclopedias of myth and folklore, that serve a vital function for quick reference. It is essential to be aware that these are *secondary source materials* only. They are compendia of selected, abbreviated, and edited references to original source material. For more substantial understanding, and for research purposes it is critical to go to the source materials. If for example, the symbol dictionary refers to a passage from literature, it is essential that we refer to the original work.

Some sources for deepened understanding of symbolism can be found in studies of the folklore, fables and mythology of various cultures. Art histories of ancient or remote lands can provide a wealth of information on symbolism particular to the culture. Religious scriptures can often lend insight into sandplay work that involves religious content. Nature chronicles of animal and plant life specific to various regions and climates are also richly informative.

The client's cultural heritage and socioeconomic history may greatly influence the significance of figures in the tray. Figures may have very different meanings to a poor immigrant child than to a middle class child whose experience is limited by exposure to just one culture.

What the client might say about the figure is also critical to understanding what symbolism is working in the sand tray. A figure we may know as female might be referred to as a male by the client. As an example, **Cary** used a figure of the lion-headed Egyptian goddess Sakhmet throughout her sandplay series. On every occasion she referred to this figure as *The Lion Man*. As far as **Cary's** work was concerned, he remained male. In this instance, the gender of the figure was not immediately evident. The matter would be entirely different if a client referred to an obviously female figure as *he*. In this case, the juxtaposition of the figure's appearance and the client's attribution adds emphasis to how the figure functions in the symbolic process.

Personal objects clients bring to the sand tray or crafts they make by hand emphasize their symbolic significance. Hand-made sandplay figures are invested with the client's psychic energy. Such figures are literally given form, or birthed, by the client's hands. We can infer that they play a profound role in the symbolic process. Objects that a client brings for use in the sand also carry a strong psychic charge. If this is something that the client has had for a while, such as a photograph, the symbol has been alive and operating in the client's psyche for some time. If the figure is one that he or she has just come across, it nonetheless holds a powerful synchronous function in the client's process in the sandplay.

As we recall from our discussion about symbols, we know that the symbolic process is not limited to single figures, but it is multi-layered. For instance, groups made up of figures that individually hold symbolic energy also function in a symbolic way as clusters. The groups then function together as larger clusters of symbolic content. Whole sand trays function in a symbolic way, and the entirety of a sandplay process works as a symbolic process.

While it is important to explore the significance of the symbolic content of the individual figures, it is also critical to build a relationship with the various layers of the symbolic content in sandplay. Exploring the commonalities and differences in the content of various figure groupings, of trays as a whole, as well as those between trays in a series, are all critical aspects of holding the sandplay process.

Sequence of Placement of the Figures

The sequence of figure placement is often a significant part of sandplay content. What is first or what is last in the sand tray often carries particular importance. In the same way, the first and last figures of a complete sandplay process can also have great weight. What is new in a sequence and what reappears can be significant.

It is important to consider sequences from tray to tray, and over the course of the entire series. For example, if a client always begins the sandplay construction by lining up two armies, an important feature of symbolic content might be to pay particular attention to any changes, however slight, in the tray construction. By doing this we may be better able to hold the subtle psychic changes that might be otherwise overlooked. As a consequence of these considerations, it is essential that we keep accurate notes of content and sequence of placement, so that we can reflect back on the sand trays in a meaningful way.

Change in the figure placement of figures is another feature of sandplay content that warrants careful attention. When a figure moves from a place of danger to a secure location during the construction of the sand tray, or from the periphery to the center, it is easy to understand how the changes in placement become critical features of sandplay content.

Figures may be placed in layers on top of one another, beside one another, and so on. The order of placement—which figure precedes or follows another figure—may be of great significance.

Martin Kalff (1993) advised the therapist to take note of figures that are not in their proper place. Boats and water life on land and cars and trucks in the water may indicate an uncertain capacity to discriminate or it may indicate a lack of clarity in relationship to the outer and inner worlds. As with all concerns in sandplay, the significance of things out of place must be taken into consideration within the context of the entire process.

LARRY **Larry** was a young four-year-old, who was brought in for treatment by his adoptive mother. Severely neglected, violated and traumatized in his family of origin, Larry's process begins in a sketchy manner in **Tray 1.** Adding water to the tray, **Larry** hastily mixes it in and shapes the suggestion of a mound in the near central region of the tray, backed by a sketchy lake-like area. He calls it a *Sandcastle*.

Larry's hero, Batman, makes a central appearance in **Tray 2**, which allows him to manifest scattered objects in **Tray 3**. As a final gesture in this sandplay, he placed a phonograph and a tiny vinyl record in front of a clock in the waterway. Certainly out of place in ordinary terms, we wonder now if **Larry** was beginning to hear the strains of a melody from within the depths of his psyche. In **Tray 5** **Larry** randomly placed figures of people, birds, and fish in a large lake. With enthusiastic interactive play, he competently announced that he was burying *...the goose, the kid, and the baby and the mama.* When finished, **Larry** said he was happy with his *sand-dan*, as he called the sandplay, unburied all of the figures and tidily lined them up at the end of the lake. Like the elements of **Larry's** early life and psychic development, the figures were out of place. In this process, he grew in his ability to confront, manage and reorder them.

AARON A very different example of things out of place is from **Aaron's Tray 14**. In this tray, done right before his 15th and final tray, **Aaron** intentionally puts things out of place. He calls it *Crazy Land.* Quite unlike the previous example, **Aaron** was finally able to see things in life from a new and humorous vantage point. He laughingly described cyclists riding in a river, a skier going uphill, and people inspecting a golf ball they suspect is really a bomb. He said this place, *...is not very safe. You can't get hurt, but you can't count on things.*

Five months after doing the tray, he spontaneously referred back to it during a session, likening it to his life. *Like my life, I can't always count on things to be the way I think they should.*

Whereas things out of place in **Larry's** sandplay initially reflect an uncertain relationship to the client's circumstances, **Aaron's** intentional irregular placements in Crazy Land demonstrate his firm centering in the Self and a flexible ego strength that is capable of dealing with the challenges of his outer world.

Another interesting feature of sandplay occurs when the client notices figures for the first time and asks if they are new to the collection. Recently, a twelve-year-old boy was thrilled to see several shelves of animals in my sandplay room. "Oh wow!" he commented, "You just got these!" Of course, those shelves had been there all along. The very important happening is that they are newly arrived for him. For the first time, in that moment of discovery in the sandplay room, this boy's psyche opened to many new possibilities for natural and instinctual expression.

I am careful about how I respond when clients comment on figures they are seeing for the first time. If they specifically ask if a particular figure is new, I will say, "No, but it's brand new for you." In the case of the boy above I said nothing and allowed him the full experience of the newness. This boy came from a severely deprived and abusive background, which left him with considerable limitations in the range of experiences common to normal development. His discovery in the sandplay room was a remarkable growth step. In silence we savored its newness together.

Perhaps a bit off the topic, or on a meta level of sandplay content is the use of the same figure or figures by several clients in the same day. I am not at all certain what this is about, but have heard several sandplay therapists acknowledge its happening in their practices. I even had two clients use the identical combination of three otherwise unrelated figures on the same day. I must admit this shook me up. Apart from making certain that we are not merchandising certain figures, or investing them with too much of our own energy, I cannot explain why this occurs. I do think it would make a fascinating piece of research.

Number and Color Content of Figures

Number

Symbolic content may be carried not only by the particular figures used in the sand tray but also by the number of items used. Frequently we will see sand trays where figures appear in pairs, or in threes, fours, and so on. To gain deeper understanding of the dynamics involved, it is important to investigate the symbolic content of the numbers themselves (Eastwood, 2002). A wealth of lore and literature has been written about the significance of numbers. To deal with number symbolism in any depth, it is essential to explore the subject further. As with any symbolic material, it is also important to consider both the light and dark aspects of the symbolic qualities. Eliade (1987/1995) highlighted some generalities, which are helpful to keep in mind in sandplay work.

The Number One **One** points to undivided wholeness, or unity that contains the possibility of manifestation. Depicted as a shape, it is a dot from which other figures begin or the empty circle, which contains all possibility.

The Number Two **Two** is the first division of **one**. It is the duality that constitutes the tension of all manifest being. As a shape it is a line, the flow of life.

The Number Three **Three** is the synthesis of **one** and **two**, and has to do with the plurality of being. It is the multitude of manifestation. It implies time, as it has a beginning, middle and end, a past, present and future. It is thus concerned with movement, or dynamism. As a shape it is the triangle.

The Number Four **Four** brings order out of chaos. It is both of this world and of the divine. The material world is ordered by its four cardinal points. Various spiritual traditions describe the heavenly plane as structured by four rivers or streams. Time is ordered by the passage of four seasons or by four great ages. As a shape, **four** is the square.

The Number Five **Five** is the number of the natural person, as the human form can be depicted as having five points: the head, two arms and two legs. Known as the *anthropos*, this archetypal representation of the human figure functions as an inner guide, and can be thought of as the wholeness of the Self in bodily form. **Fives** are found in the natural forms of leaves and flowers. In nature, **five** is associated with sexuality and reproduction. As a shape it is a star, or the pentagram, thought to have magical and rejuvenating power.

The Number Six As **two threes**, or **three twos**, **six** is the combined spiritual and material worlds. As two interlaced triangles or as the hexagon, **six** reflects that what is above is also below.

The Number Seven **Seven** is often considered a sacred number, as it consists of the plurality of **three** that is brought to order by **four**.

The Number Eight **Eight** is **four** doubled. **Eight** points to eternity, as quintessential order.

The Number Nine **Nine** is made up of **three threes**, and is concerned with perfection. As **three threes**, **nine** points to completion.

Number symbolism may appear in sandplay as groupings of figures clustered by number. An example of numbers used in this way would be a farm scene in which many of the animals appear in groups of three, four, and so on.

Number symbolism may manifest in the overall layout of the sand tray, such as in sandplays where four trees mark the four corners of the tray. Another example might be a road or bridging pattern that appears as a circle or a triangle. Number symbolism may also appear as characteristic shapes sculpted or drawn in the sand. The client may draw shapes in the sand, then place figures on top of them, or around them. The client may be immersed in number symbolism when he or she sculpts a shape, such as a cube, or a five-pointed star in the wet sand. Possible examples for the use of number symbolism in sandplay are endless. The important point is to be aware of this dimension of sandplay content as another means of deepening our relationship to the client's work.

ADRIENNE **Adrienne's Tray 26** provides an example where the number symbolism clearly supports the symbolic content of the figures used, as well as the sculpted shape of the sand. In this sandplay, **Adrienne** buries a pregnant woman beneath a rounded, central mound, on top of which she places four babies in a square shape, with the figure of baby Jesus in the center as the

> fifth element. The figurative content of the symbols indicates the burial of a mother figure, this one now pregnant with new potential, in a pregnant belly-shaped mound. New life adorns the top, with the babies and the divine potential of the central Christ child. Regarded from the vantage point of the number symbolism, burying the one (mother), it now becomes two (pregnancy). This birth bears embodied wholeness (four) and is completed with the fifth element (the divine potential).

Color

The presence or absence of color in sandplay can be a significant aspect of symbolic content. Some trays may be especially red, white, black, yellow, and so on. Some cases may appear utterly colorless. Thematic color patterns may suddenly emerge where there had been no color before. These thematic appearances and fluctuations of color in a sandplay case are another valuable way to deepen our relationship to the work underway.

Unlike the commonalities we found with number symbolism, the meanings associated with colors vary widely. In fact, red is the only color that has a consistent root word, *rudhro,* in all of Indo-European language (Eliade 1987/1995). Some cultures do not even have words for certain colors. At the same time, the Eskimo peoples have over fifteen words for the color white, depending upon the condition of the snow. Nearly all cultures distinguish the colors white and black, and when a third color is perceived, it is generally red. The meanings of color vary by both culture and history; thus, our psychological responses to color are thought to be conditioned. People who suffer schizophrenia frequently have abnormal perceptions of color. Developmentally, young children tend to prefer brighter colors, such as red and orange. Taking all of these factors into consideration, color still plays a significant role along with shape, space, and motion, in how we experience images in sandplay.

General color theory defines three primary colors: red, blue, and yellow. They are referred to as *primary,* because no other colors can be mixed to create them. Mixing two primary colors together creates the *secondary* colors: green, orange and violet. Adding or subtracting the amounts of primary colors in these combinations creates variants among these. Values of white or black can be added to the pure hues to lighten or darken the color. Colors in the yellow and red ranges are often referred to as *warm* and *energetic*, and those in the bluer ranges as *cool* and *soothing*.

In order to introduce the importance of color in sandplay, we will make a passing review of color symbolism in Western and Eastern traditions. As with our discussion of numbers, let's remember that a proper study of color symbolism is both vast and fascinating.

Early Paleolithic graves reveal an extensive use of the color red. Researchers believe that the red interiors of these small burial chambers symbolize the red of the mother's generative organs and a return of the dead to mother earth (Eliade 1987/1995). Jewish tradition uses the color white on Yom Kippur, the Day of Atonement, to represent humility and mortality. Kabalistic texts reveal a complex symbolism of color. Eliade (1954/1995) observed that since the Western religious traditions emerged from desert lands, the significance of the color green as foliage, oasis, and refuge is paramount. Islam refers to the color green as the cool, protective shade of tranquility.

Western liturgical tradition began to systematize the use of colors in the church in the Middle Ages, when Pope Innocent III (1198-1216) defined standards. White was reserved for festivals of the Virgin Mary, of Christ, and of unmartyred saints. Red was for martyrs and apostles and for feasts of the Cross and for Pentecost. Black, and later violet, was used for Lent and Advent and on occasions of death. Green was used for all other occasions. Black fell into disuse, as Church Fathers thought it the color of the devil. More recent reforms have ascribed red for use on Palm Sunday and Good Friday.

Pre-Columbian and Native American traditions described the earth as divided into four cardinal regions, each with a tree of a characteristic color. Each tree was shaped in the form of a cross and was topped by a bird. The Aztec and Maya peoples saw the tree of the eastern region as red, the western tree as blue, the southern tree as green, and the northern tree as yellow. Inconsistencies appear within various accounts of these traditions. For example, Eliade (1954/1995) observed that the Maya marked time and space by the movements of the sun across the horizon. They associated the color red with the east, black with the west, white with north and yellow with the south. The Apache nation ascribed colors to the four directions: white with north, blue with the south, black with the east, and yellow with the west. The Blackfoot peoples used the color red to symbolize the sun and black to symbolize the moon.

The Western tradition of alchemy assigned colors to the progressive stages of transformation of base metals into gold. The sequence begins with black, the stage of killing the original substance, to white, its purification, then to red, culminating in the production of the philosopher's stone.

In the Eastern traditions we find some overlap along with many different properties of color. In the Taoist tradition of China, yellow is the color of the center. The Yellow Emperor, the first emperor and ancestor of the royal family, was thought to live at the hub of the four directions in the center of the sky (Eliade 1954/1995). Chinese alchemy held physical immortality as its goal and associated the color red with the alchemical process. In the Chinese tradition, particular colors were also assigned to the five phases, or elements, that order the material world. Wood is green. Fire is red. Earth is described as yellow. Metal is white, and water is black. Corresponding directions and seasonal attributes also correlate to the five phases. We will discuss the directions further in our exploration of spatial themes in sandplay. In the Indian tradition, the dimension of color is considered an attribute of mind, or *manas*. The rising *kundalini* energy, which dissolves the ordinary self into the undivided consciousness of wholeness is described as bright red in color.

It is apparent that there are wide variations in color symbolism. When exploring color as a content theme in sandplay, it is wise to consider patterns of color through the series of trays, as well as dramatic changes in color usage. After making these initial observations in a sandplay case, other characteristics of content particular to the case may indicate the direction to follow for a more in-depth investigation of the symbolism held by the color.

Absence of Figures as Content

Not using figures in a sandplay may indicate a less-defined capacity to bring form to the inner and outer worlds. This may be developmentally normal for the very young child, as we see in early pouring and sifting play in the sand. The same absence of symbolic objects in an older client's sandplay may result from early developmental deprivation. It may indicate very low energy or depression.

On the other hand, a more highly developed, healthy client may also do a sandplay without using miniatures. The absence of figures in this situation may be an indication of the nascent formation of new qualities and capacities that have yet to emerge in more defined form. A tray without figures may also be a highly sophisticated psychic gesture, as is sometimes the case with a two-dimensional use of the sand tray.

REGINA A good example of the movement into greater figurative representation is seven-year-old **Regina's** work. **Regina** completed **Trays 1** and **2** in her first session. Following this highly figurative and evocative sandplay early in her work, **Regina** used the sand tray for cooking behavior. Having suffered significant developmental deprivation in her early life, this child's work necessitated a regressive form of play in the sand. Session after session, **Regina** cooked, and poured and stirred delicious foods for us to eat, as we see in **Tray 3**. When these early developmental tasks were sufficiently satisfied, **Regina's** play became more representative. Asking for my help with building, in **Tray 7** a castle emerges from the very body of the sand that had fed her in her earlier work.

ELIZABETH Another example of the scant use of figures in the tray is **Elizabeth's** work, where intrapsychic issues are accessed in their bare bones form. **Elizabeth's Trays 2** and **3**, for example, make poignant psychic statements, although their landscapes and figure content are minimal. In **Tray 2** a jester follows a path of pearls through a figure of the uroborous, leading to a central gold crown, attended by a guardian dog and her pup. Along the path is a dead mother and child. **Tray 3** shows another mother and child pair, this time they are primitive figures, apparently on a journey through a forest, suggested by a scattering of rocks and trees.

Elizabeth, a highly complex and colorful woman in her outer life, engages in the immediacy of the sandplay process devoid of any need for frills or trappings. While her work may appear sparse, it is not a result of psychic deprivation, but rather the urgency to address the inner issues with dispatch and clarity.

The Allegorical Content of Sandplay

Introduction

Having examined figures as thematic content in sandplay, we will now explore allegorical content. Our objective is to cultivate a working familiarity with a variety of voices, or languages, with which the psyche articulates its change process. In the material that follows we look at story, theme, and myth. We then examine some traditional paradigms of transformation, paying particular attention to alchemy, the natural elements, and the charkas.

Story and Theme as Content

The story or thematic content of sandplay can lend understanding to the overall process. Although allegorical content is not necessarily a part of all sandplay work, it is an important feature to bear in mind. As with the other dimensions of sandplay we have examined, it is important to think about the story or thematic content of an individual tray, as well as any movement or changes in symbolic narrative over the course of the entire sandplay process. For example, themes of journeys, of struggles, and battles, of discovery, of being lost or persecuted, or of leaving and return, may characterize a particular sand tray. The same themes may appear through the course of several trays with changes and evolving variations.

Sometimes the client verbally relates a story during the construction of the sand tray. Children, and particularly the younger ones, are frequently so immersed in the play that they open this very private sphere to the therapist through the verbal telling of the story as it unfolds. The honor of being invited into this magical space to concurrently share the child's experience is so precious as to be sacred. By giving words to the active creation of themselves emerging in the sand tray, the child extends his or her evolving being to include us. We must listen carefully, as their verbal accounts are a face of the symbolic process. Frequently these stories do not appear to hold together. There are often inconsistencies and contradictions that seem to make no sense. We must listen with a *symbolic ear*. These stories are like paintings made of images painted a stroke here, then there. They do not operate in temporal time and space; they emerge from the mythic dimension.

A client may relate a story after the sandplay is completed, describing what is going on in the tray. While it is very important to carefully note what the client says during or after a sand tray, we must be careful not to interfere with their process in any way by indicating that they *should* tell a story. We will discuss this in some detail in our consideration of Sandplay Procedures. For now our concern is primarily to follow the client's lead. If and when a client tells a story, we take careful note of it.

Adult clients do not tend to render involved stories like those that children craft, however there are always exceptions. More frequently, the adult client will make a comment about a figure or scene in the sand tray. These are equally important for the therapist to consider. With the adult client, these comments may arise from the same mythic level of consciousness as the children's stories, or they may be a more conscious reflection on something that is quite unconscious to them. In other words, the adult response may either be a part of the symbolic process, or be outside of it looking back with judgment or defensiveness. Careful listening and holding of the work on the part of the therapist will likely make this distinction clear.

As there are exceptions to nearly everything in sandplay, there are times when children will comment that their sandplay is the movie or television show they just saw. Just as with the adult's more conscious reflection, this is the child's outer awareness of what he or she has done in the tray. These sandplays still bear all of the symbolic significance of those the child shares more magically. After all, it is something operating deep within the child that has guided him or her to choose that particular story or movie for their sandplay.

What the adult client says during the session outside of the sandplay process may also factor into the allegorical content of the sandplay work. The sub text of the client's verbal therapy may lend understanding to a thematic content in the sandplay. The important thing for the therapist is to be quiet inside and listen carefully.

Mythic Themes as Content

Mythic themes are a common feature of sandplay. We recall from our discussion of symbolic process and dynamics of the psyche that myth is the language or story of the unconscious. Myth is the story line used to describe and explain the psyche's movements along the path to greater levels of integration, or *individuation*. Since sandplay is the three-dimensional depiction of the psyche's movement and change, mythic themes are frequently apparent in the sandplay content. It is essential to keep in mind however, that even if mythic themes are not readily evident in discrete scenes that are easily recognizable, the overall sandplay process *is mythic*, as it holds the psyche's movement toward wholeness.

Although there are many mythic themes, some common ones experienced in sandplay are of birth and death, quest, discovery, renewal, return, confrontation with darkness, integration, and centering. In some cases, identifiable myths, fairytales or folk tales are played out. This is frequently done with no conscious awareness on the part of the client. I am awed by the numerous cases in which Pegasus appears soon after the Medusa, or the Dark Mother, followed by a new phase of creative development, replicating the ancient Greek myth of Perseus (Hamilton, 1942). A perfect example of this occurs in the case of **Ivy**, the nine-year-old girl from a fundamental religious sect.

> **IVY** Struggling with her own budding sexuality in a repressive environment that placed severe limits on women's roles, in **Tray 4, Ivy** simultaneously confronts the devouring darkness as two figures of Pegasus rear up and roar. In the following **Tray 5**, the new energy of a herd of horses is released, as a central mound encrusted with golden instruments and jewels is topped with two golden crowns.

Ivy had no knowledge of the story of Medusa, the terrible Gorgon who had magical blood that could both create and destroy life. There was no conscious awareness of the mythic goddess, who was so fearsome that to look at her directly would turn a person to stone. Neither did **Ivy** have any conscious knowledge of the rise of Pegasus, the winged horse, from the blood of Medusa's severed head, or the creation of the fount of the Muses where Pegasus struck his hoof. Yet her psyche chose these images. As she confronted the fearsome qualities of the feminine during her transformation in the sandplay, **Ivy's** psyche opened to a new wealth of energetic possibility.

When the Story or Theme Appears Stuck

An important consideration of allegorical content occurs when the story or theme appears to relentlessly repeat itself and remain unchanged. Our first consideration is to examine the case even more closely to see if there are changes taking place, albeit small ones. When there is evidence of movement, although initially difficult to detect, we know that the process is moving along. Perhaps our studying it more closely will facilitate the work. Also we must ask ourselves what, if anything, this client might need from us that could help them move more quickly. Consulting on our work is essential when this occurs. Of course, it may simply be a situation in which the speed of the psychic movement is just as it needs to be.

When the theme remains the same with no perceptible change, we have to consider what it is that we as the therapists are failing to see in the process. A sandplay process may become stuck and go nowhere when the therapist is not able to hold a critical piece of it. This brings up some very interesting considerations. It is curious why one process may come to a grinding halt and others will proceed apace without the therapist consciously knowing what is taking place in either case. The difference concerns the unseen complexities of containment. In situations where the therapist has no conscious awareness of the client's work in the sand, but whose own psyche is sufficiently ordered to the Self, especially with regard to the particular archetypal constituents of the client's process, the therapist poses no impairment to the containment. However, when the client's symbolic work in the tray touches an area of the therapist's psyche that is wounded or otherwise compromised, an obstacle to containment is imposed upon the shared field of observing attitude. The client's symbolic work is thus thwarted and comes to a standstill. Albeit unconscious, the client does not feel safe or secure enough in the therapeutic container to have the freedom to move more deeply in the work. In this case, a block in the therapist's development has been touched and must be addressed before the client's work can proceed. The therapist may be able to address the blocked content through consultation and deep personal reflection. It may be necessary for the therapist to work the issues through in his or her own therapy, as well.

The nature of what is impeding the process is of great significance in the client's work, as well as in the therapist's work.

It is important to remember that the missing piece *is* a crucial content theme. The progress of the sandplay work depends upon this content, even though it remains unknown until such time as the therapist and client are able to move into relationship with this unconscious aspect of the client's work.

The magnitude of the missing piece can range from something the therapist is capable of seeing but has not yet acknowledged consciously, on one end of the spectrum, to deep wounds or shadowy material in the therapist's psyche, on the other. This factor underscores why the therapist's own inner healing and development is a critical consideration in preparation to work in sandplay.

If, in spite of sincere and thorough training, the sandplay therapist harbors psychic wounding that will impair a process, we can be assured that this inner material *will be activated by their clients' work.* While we hope to avoid this happening through rigorous training and preparation of sandplay therapists, it can occur. It will be recognized when brought into consultation. When our sandplay consultants say that it is our own issues that are getting in the way, we must respect that and take immediate reparative measures.

Traditional Paradigms of Transformation

In addition to mythological themes, other traditional paradigms of transformation may appear in a sandplay process. It is important to consider that the process of deep psychic transformation in a sandplay series may manifest with or without identifiable models of change. Our discussion here is to become aware of the possibility that traditional change paradigms may appear as thematic content in sandplay. Although there are many models of transformation from a variety of traditions, we will examine alchemy, the elements, and the chakras.

The Transformational Paradigm of Alchemy

The History of Alchemy

The practice of alchemy is a paradigm of inner transformation that has historical roots in the East as well as the West. Alchemy is frequently misconstrued as a primitive form of chemistry, or science, due to its reliance on laboratory apparatus and mysterious quasi-chemical formulations. The goal of all alchemists was to transform base material, or metals, into gold. The transmuted gold was thought to be the elixir of eternal life. Said in Jungian terms, alchemy consists of disciplines, practices, and procedures directing the inner voyage to the eternal Self.

Some scholars date the beginnings of alchemy to 500 BCE China, while others attribute its origins to early Hellenic Egypt (Multhauf, 1983; Eliade, 1978). The emergence of similar processes as allegories for deep-seated change at roughly the same time in cultures so widely different is very interesting. The goals of alchemists in all cultures was related to esoteric religious traditions. In China, alchemy was a central feature of Taoism. In India, alchemical practices were inherent in the Tantric traditions. In Hellenic Egypt, some of the Gnostics practiced alchemy. In Islamic cultures, alchemy was associated with the mystics. In the European Middle Ages and Renaissance periods, alchemy found its place within Christian mystery sects and Hermeticism, as well as among adherents of the Qabbalah. Early Hindu and Buddhist alchemies flourished between 700 - 1600 CE. Translations of Islamic texts brought the art to Western Europe around 1100 CE. The practice of alchemy in Europe ended with the scientific revolution of the 1800's.

Like alchemical gold in the West, the historical alchemists of China considered the red crystalline mineral, known as cinnabar or mercury sulfide, the desired elixir of immortality. Today, forms of inner alchemy are still practiced in China by Taoist priests. I recently had the honor of attending a Taoist temple in China where these practices still exist. It was riveting to listen as the priests chanted to the ancient strains of bamboo flutes, gongs, and sonorous drums, all the while standing on a large mandala, composed of the eight trigrams of the *I Ching*. Moving their arms and bodies in prescribed gestures and reverently burning inscribed papers, I felt the depth of their practice of what is called *nei tan*, or inner alchemy.

While performing the ritual within his body as a vessel, the priest inwardly holds the transformation of base material into what is called the *Chiao*, the *immortal fetus*. The *Chiao*, like the philosopher's stone in the West, is pure, divine, and eternal. The contemporary Taoist priest thus carries this in symbolic form for the community.

The term *alchemy* is derived from the Greek *chemeia*, which means *the art of transmutation*. The Islamic cultures developed the term *al-kimiya'*, either from the Greek, or the Southern Chinese word *kimiya*, which means *gold-making juice*. Eliade (1978) attributed the beginnings of alchemical symbolism to the work of the smith, who forged and thereby transformed metals. The symbolism of matter as suffering and the redemption to be found in the release from base matter emerged from watching the work of the smith. In Europe, the alchemists developed the view that all matter is alive and strives to perfect itself. They postulated that over time base matter will eventually arrive at a state of perfection. The perfection of base matter can be accomplished with the product of alchemy, which is known as the *philosopher's stone*.

The Philosophy of Alchemy

The underlying objective of alchemy was to overcome the limits of matter and time and thereby bring perfection to what was considered, by nature, a sullied material world. Whether the alchemist's practice assumed an outer or inner form, it was its practice that was significant, not its products.

In India, immortality was likened to gold. The ancient texts known as the *Brahmanas* proclaimed that the human body can attain the changeless nature of gold (Eliade, 1979). Indian alchemy, like the Taoist practice, assumed an inner focus. Buddhist alchemy, on the other hand, employed outward, chemical substances. The goal of Indian alchemists was *samadhi*, or return to the Absolute. The Taoist goal was union with the *Tao*, the Way. In Hellenic Egypt, alchemists sought to release the soul from its bondage in matter through the sacrificial practice of alchemy. Like the shamanic practices we examined earlier, these alchemists sought *gnosis*, the knowledge of God, by means of a mystical ladder that would release them from their earthly bondage and carry them to the divine above. The Hellenic Egyptian alchemists used a blend of inner and outer practices. Outwardly they endeavored to color substances gold, rather than make them into gold. In so doing, the alchemist professed a parallel transformation from body to spirit to soul.

The likening between the matter and spirit in humankind and these in metals was also drawn by Maria Prophetissa (Haeffner, 1994). Known as

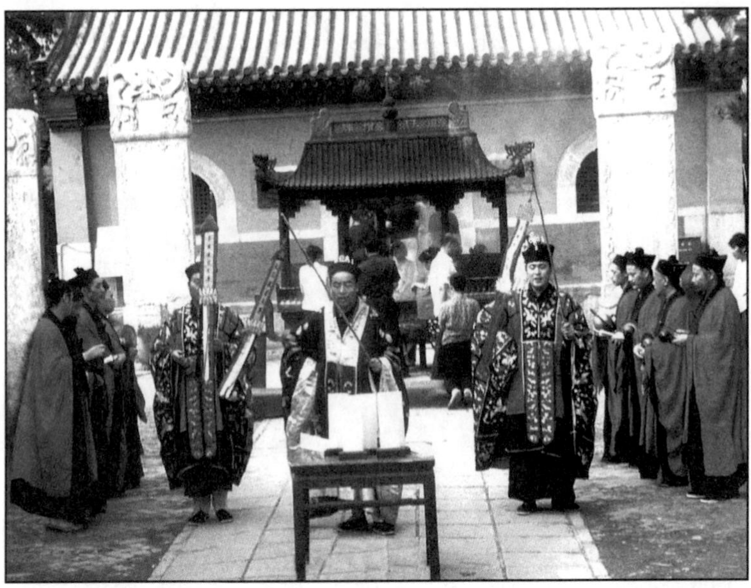

Photograph B. Turner, 2003

Taoist priest performing ritual of transformation at temple in Beijing,

the founding mother of alchemy in the early fifth century CE in Hellenic Egypt, Maria Prophetissa reported receiving the secrets of alchemy directly from God. Prophetissa's alchemy bore the flavor of Gnostic dualism, which paired the spiritual against the human. She ascribed masculine and feminine qualities to the metals of her laboratory and emphasized oppositional pairs in her work, such as wet and dry, earth and air, water and fire and cold and hot. Jung (1953/1977) was taken with the opposing pairs of Maria Prophetissa's work, recognizing in them the process of psychic transformation. Jung quoted Prophetissa's most famous words,

> One becomes two, two becomes three, and by means of the third the fourth achieves unity; thus two are but one. ...Join the male and the female, and you will find what you seek (Jung 1953/1977, p.23).

In Prophetissa's early writings, Jung (1953/1977) recognized the principle of *antonymy*. By this term he was referring to the dual pairing of opposites that appears in all of manifest reality, which has its source and its goal in the wholeness of the Self. Jung thus saw alchemy as the projection of inner psychic experience onto matter for the purpose of individuation and return to the Self.

The Process and Symbols of Alchemy

Across cultures, the alchemical transformation of base matter into the pure elixir progresses through similar definable stages. The Arab-Islamic alchemists described the sequence of change in metals as lead, copper, tin and then gold. The Hindu tradition posed the sequence as lead, tin, copper, silver and then gold. Antiochus of Athens, the Greek alchemist, depicted the progress from body to spirit to soul as the progression of lead, to silver and then to gold, and with the colors black, white, and yellow. Egyptian Gnostic, Valentinus, defined a process that begins with *pneuma*, the product of sublimation. This is followed by the *ebullient*, or boiling up that occurs to separate the impure from the pure. The resulting and final stage is *sperma*, the seed of gnosis.

In the West, alchemists agreed on a color progression from black to white to red, but had variations in the hierarchy of metals as they changed from base to pure (Edinger, 1991). They did agree that the product of their alchemy was the mysterious *philosopher's stone*, which had the capacity to make the impure pure. The color progression was correlated to stages in transformation. Black is the first stage in which the base substances are burned or killed. This is called *calcination*. The white stage, known as *separation*, is the part of the change process in which refinement and purification of the residue of what has been destroyed by fire takes place. This is a purification and the release of the soul, or spirit from the matter. This makes possible the final red stage, known as *fermentation* and *projection*, where the pure spirit is solidified in matter into the philosopher's stone. The purified matter then has the power to transform other impure matter.

Alchemy in Sandplay

We have devoted some time to the exploration of alchemy as a model that symbolically tracks the transformation process. Of course, this model, as with all others, may appeal to some sandplay therapists more than others. It is important to be versed in the stages and processes of alchemy, as this knowledge may provide a helpful tool in tracking the client's movement through transformation in some sandplay cases. It is essential to understand, for example, that deep-order change begins with burning and death. It is critical to understand what this is about intrapsychically, and why it is followed by a sorting out and purification, before the new qualities emerge. To have a firm grasp of the nature of this under-going is an indispensable component of witnessing the process as the therapist.

Symbols and indicators of the alchemical transformation in sandplay may be seen in themes of burning and death, followed by sorting out and surrendering of what is no longer necessary. A sanctification, or purification, occurs, and the Self manifests. In sandplay this stage of transformation is followed by an integration of the new psychic product. The client's ego, or sense of self, is informed by the transformed quality, and he or she returns to ordinary life.

An alchemical process can appear as story themes. For example, themes of burning and death frequently appear as skeletons and graveyards. Death may appear as the destruction of something in the tray. The color black may be a significant feature in the beginning stage of transformation, as may crude or base metal objects.

Purification and separation may appear as story themes of baptism, immersion in water, or sprinkling with sand or water. This stage in transformation may be held in the sandplay by angels or wizards or fairy godmothers who wield magic. Purification may be evident in the prominent use of the color white, or with the progression to a more refined metal such as silver.

The manifestation of the Self is equivalent to the alchemist's sanctification by the philosopher's stone. The Self, the source of all being, is experienced. In contrast to the alchemical process that tends to overemphasize the holy and the light, the experience of Self in sandplay also embraces the dark as a feature of wholeness. We will usually find some darkness in a Self tray. Perhaps it will appear as a dark jewel, or an otherwise threatening figure brought to witness the wholeness and interrelatedness of all being.

As we mentioned above, the Self manifestation is followed by a reintegration into daily life. This may appear as real people engaged in ordinary relationships, normal towns and villages. Whether or not it manifests as identifiable symbols of alchemy, in some ways the entire sandplay process is alchemical, as it is a process of transformation that bridges human life with the divine.

The Transformational Paradigm of the Elements

The elements may also indicate the process of transformation in sandplay. Various combinations of earth, air, fire, water and sometimes metal or ether may characterize qualities of psychic balance or imbalance and may indicate the progression through a change process.

The Elements and the Quaternity

Descriptions of the elements as reflections of the divine, or the undifferentiated wholeness that underlies the manifest world, are found across cultures throughout the world. The elements, whether four or five, are frequently identified with what is known as the *quaternity*, the four-fold structure that constitutes the basic template of material existence. The basic elements of manifestation—earth, air, fire, water, and/or metal and ether—are correlated with the four cardinal directions and in some traditions, a center. The elements are thus perceived as informing, or giving character to, the *stuff* of life. It is this matter that interacts on the horizontal plane of the earth that makes up what we see as the real world. Although the elements constitute material reality, they are considered reflections of that which is beyond the concrete world. The elements are also correlated with the four seasons, and the passage of time, characteristic of embodied existence. Thus, the elements are the workings of what is within the dimensions of time and space.

The Elements in Asian Traditions

Evidence of the concept of the four elements appears in the ancient Indian civilization of Mohenjo-Daro, located in present day Pakistan. Said to date from 2,500 BCE, scholars presume that the concept of the elements first appeared here at the birthplace of Hinduism (Rao, 1914/1985). In the Hindu tradition, the god-head consists of a triumvirate of three gods, Brahma, Vishnu and Siva. Brahma is the creator, and Siva is the destroyer. The god Vishnu maintains the balance between these polarities of birth and death as the sustainer of life. Vishnu has four arms, representing his authority over the four directions. In one hand he holds a conch shell, a symbol of the five elements in the Hindu tradition. As life grows and evolves in the progressive chambers of the conch, so Vishnu maintains dominion over the comings and goings of manifest reality. Vishnu also bears an arc and a lotus, symbolizing the changing nature of the universe. The Hindu tradition holds that the elements are not things, but processes. They carry the changeable universe. The goal of life in this tradition is to strip away the falsehoods of the ever-changing elements and to reveal the absolute wholeness that lay behind them. The way to the divine is thus through the elements.

Early Taoist Chinese traditions, circa 500 BCE, described five elements or phases, that constitute the ordering qualities of the material universe. Derived from the fundamental properties, yin and yang, (feminine and masculine) the elements wood, fire, earth, metal and water were seen as inter-related qualities of phenomena that are in constant motion (Major, 1995; Baldrian, 1995). In the fourth century BCE the Chinese observed that the *wu-sing*, the five elements, or phases, move in regular and predictable courses of change. The patterns of movement are complex, based upon the extensive variations in the relationships between them. These cycles of change are fully described in one of the revered Five Classics of China, the *I Ching*, the *Book of Changes*, stemming from the early Zhou dynasty, dated to approximately 1000 BCE (Ebrey, 1993).

The progression of the changing relationships among the five phases followed two basic courses. One was that of overcoming, or decay. The other was that of production and generation. These cycles account for and denote the process of change. Some of the primary correlations of the elements are to the planets, numbers, colors, cardinal directions, the seasons, animals, bodily organs, and tastes.

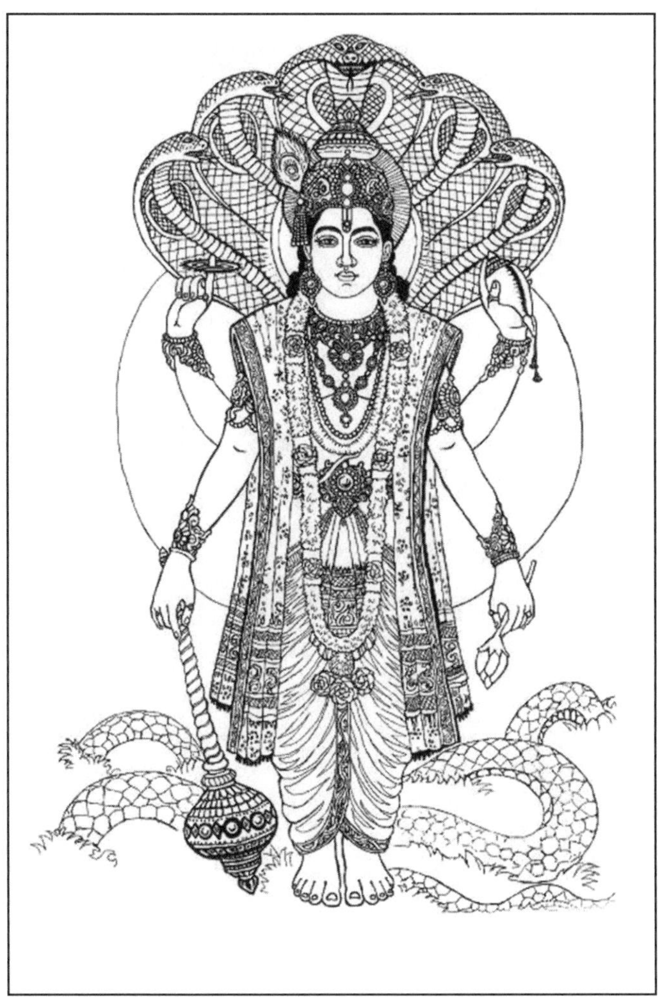

Vishnu, Hindu deity, *The Sustainer*, symbolizes the transformational processes of the elements and the changing nature of the universe.

Taoist Tradition ~ Five Elements
Correlation of Qualities of Being

Phase	+/−	Direction	Season	Planet	Color	Number	Animal	Organ	Taste
Wood	Yang	East	Spring	Jupiter	Green	3	Dragon	Liver	Sour
Fire	Yang	South	Summer	Mars	Red	2	Red Bird	Heart	Bitter
Earth	Balanced	Center	Mid-Summer	Saturn	Yellow	5	None	Stomach/Spleen	Sweet
Metal	Yin	West	Autumn	Venus	White	4	White Tiger	Lungs	Acrid
Water	Yin	North	Winter	Mercury	Black	1	Tortoise w/Snake	Kidneys	Salty

The elements in the Chinese tradition are thus concerned with qualities of being in time and space, and not simply with reducible elements of material manifestation.

In the Buddhist traditions, which originally developed in India, the four elements are considered properties or qualities of matter. For the Buddhists, matter does not exist in and of itself, but is described in terms of its function and appearance. As in the Hindu tradition, the workings of the four elements are always in flux.

The Pali Canon, the sacred text of the Theravada school of Buddhism, which contains the teachings of the Buddha, was committed to writing during the first century BCE, 500 years following the Buddha's death. It speaks of six elements (Collins, 1995). To the four elements of earth, water, fire, and wind, they added space and understanding. This concept was carried over by the Japanese Shingonshu school of Buddhism, established during the period 794 to 1185 CE. The Shingonshu recognized five components of the material universe, earth, water, fire, wind and space, called the *known*, and a sixth, observing element, referred to as the *knower*. Inherent in this tradition is the inseparable nature of the knowing and the known.

The Elements in the Western World

In the Western world, mention of the elements is found in many traditions. The Zoroastrians held that the divine is mirrored in the five elements of manifestation. In the Gnostic Christian tradition, during the late second century CE, Clement of Alexandria taught that angels controlled the movements of the stars and other celestial bodies, along with their earthly constituents, the four elements. Clement of Alexandria thus drew a correlation between divine destiny and its manifestation in the material world.

The Greeks also considered the four elements as the basic aspects of matter. Like the Chinese, in the fifth century BCE, Empedocles observed that nothing in the material universe was ever created or destroyed. Rather, it undergoes change as a consequence of the relationships between the four elements, earth, air, fire and water. Aristotle defined the fundamental properties of matter in masculine and feminine categories in his theory of sulfur and mercury. Sulfur, the masculine, was hot and dry and corresponded to the elements fire and earth. Mercury, the feminine, was cold and moist and corresponded to air and water.

A very interesting correlation was drawn by later Greeks in the fifth century CE between the elements and the alphabet. The Greeks surmised a mystical relationship between words or letters and material manifestation and destiny. The adoption of the Ionian alphabet around this time must have indeed seemed to hold powerful qualities. To be able to spell out words, to write and communicate complex immaterial thoughts, must have appeared very like the workings of the unseen gods and spirits. It is understandable how the Greeks correlated the seven vowels and 17 consonants of their alphabet with the divine and earthly spheres. To the Greeks and some Egyptians, as well, the vowels were considered to hold tremendous power. This power was so great that some Greek and Coptic writings indicated that their use could not only invoke the gods, but could create them. The seven vowels were likened to the seven planets and were thought to have come from the Fates. Vowels thus had bearing on a person's destiny, as did the planets. The consonants were thought to hold the twelve signs of the zodiac and the five elements air, water, fire, ether and earth, in which they manifest. The 24 letters corresponded to the 24 hours of the day and night and were twice the 12 months that marked a year. In this system of thought, we see the divine working through matter in time.

The Elements in the Native American Traditions

In the Native American traditions the four elements, earth, air, fire, and water, are correlated with the four directions. They are graphically represented by what is called the *medicine wheel,* consisting of a circle centrally intersected by two perpendicular crossing lines (Storm, 1972; Thomas, et al, 1993). The individual's heart, or the home hearth, is at the center.

The medicine wheel is a reflection of all manifest reality. All things on the medicine wheel are in dynamic relationship to each other. The medicine wheel is thus a paradigm of qualitative change and transformation. The healthy and whole person strives for a harmonious balance of the medicine wheel qualities. Each person is born at a particular location on the wheel, and thus has certain qualities of strength and particular deficits. In this way, the medicine wheel indicates the path of growth and change for the individual's life. Each node on the medicine wheel is characterized by an animal spirit and a color.

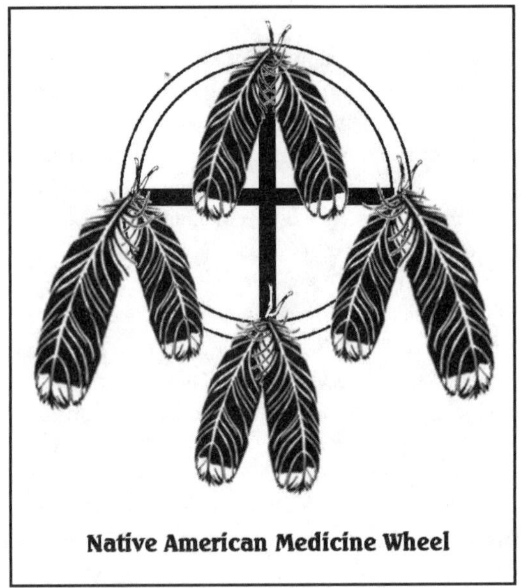

Native American Medicine Wheel

Native American Tradition ~ Four Elements				
Direction	Element	Color	Quality	Animal Spirit
North	Air	White	Wisdom	Buffalo
East	Fire	Yellow	Illumination	Eagle
South	Water	Green	Innocence	Mouse
West	Earth	Black	Introspection	Bear

water element, they also involve the earth, which holds and carries the water. Water wheels, buckets, cups and containers may hold water in the tray, but not be in relationship to the earth. We need to consider the significance of the subtle differences between water that is captured in a vessel, spilled upon the earth, or that floods the earth. We need to consider the psychic processes carried by the relative relationships of these elements. In other instances, trays that have no qualities of water or earth may indicate a need for these elements in order to catalyze the changes being undergone in the process.

Air may appear as birds, wind mills, flags, incense and so on. Its absence is felt in a tray that feels smothered, underground, closed or sealed off. When air is present in the sand tray, notice to which elements it relates. When it, or any other element, is absent, take note of which elements *are* present. Perhaps the lack of relationship between what is present and what is absent will lend greater understanding to the process.

Fire is held by flames and smoke, by the sun, by ovens in cooking. We feel its absence as a coldness or lack of vitality. Sand trays with too little or too much fire can point the way to what is required to balance the psyche. As an example, uncontained flames and burning buildings are very different than campfires ringed with stones, or bread coming out of the oven. As with the other elements, pay attention to how fire behaves and how it interacts with the other elements. If fire is absent in a cold and foreboding sandplay, we can gently and silently hold this awareness and the need of fire to warm things up. This awareness can greatly strengthen the quiet containment of the sandplay process.

We must bear in mind the metal element in cases that carry prominent metal figures. As an element, metal can be firm and powerful. In the absence of relationship to the other elements, it can be cold and rigid. The sudden appearance of metal in a case that has been confused or unclear may indicate the beginnings of a much needed firmness. On the other hand, if metal appears frequently without the tempering qualities of the other elements, we may become aware that the client has reached a part of the psyche that has rigidly isolated itself. To silently hold this rigid defense with tenderness, as well as with respect for the terror experienced in surrendering it, may significantly support and facilitate the client's movement through this difficult phase of the work.

As with the other transformational themes in sandplay, using the elements as a means of understanding may or may not apply to a sandplay case. However, our awareness of the elements, their inter-relationships and movement in the sandplay process may lend another perspective for comprehending and holding the work as the witness.

CARY Tracking the elemental qualities through **Cary's** sandplay process provides an illuminating example of the movement from an imbalance of elements to its more balanced rectification. In its early phases, **Cary's** process is predominantly characterized by the elements of water and earth. **Trays 1** through **4** feel sad and lonely. An indication of some fiery energy appears as lions and tigers in **Tray 5**. This is followed by the first indicators of air in the golden celestial figures of the angel and sea star, as the broken heart appears in the front left corner of **Tray 6**.

Water transforms into solid crystals in **Tray 7**, which initiates a deep, spiral decent into earth and water in **Tray 8**. The under ground journey is long and terrifying, until glimmers of new possibility appear atop the mountain arising from the sea in **Tray 15**. A fiery sun rises from the earth, which supports a whole, mended heart. **Tray 21** is a bare earth surface, readied for what is new. In **Tray 21** airy angels circle around a crystal ring, while figures from the underground look on. In **Tray 23** the fiery cats pace around the watery, damp earth, as angels encircle a hand which cradles the broken heart. All elements are present to support **Cary's** profound grief. Following this phase of her process, **Cary** begins to find and secure the jewels of the Self in **Tray 24**.

Cary's sandplay work does not end here, but continues on through a rich and challenging process of healing and transformation. While we have overlooked many vital aspects of this sandplay process, tracking the presence and movement of the elements through this first phase of **Cary's** psychic journey lends a sense of how valuable it can be to examine sandplay work through this lens.

The Chakras—Energy Centers as Content

> ***Note:*** *In our discussion of the vertical dimension in sandplay, we examine the seven chakras, or energy centers, as a paradigm of psychic development and transformation in some detail. It may be helpful to refer to that material for purposes of our discussion of the chakras as sandplay content below.*

Tracking movement through the chakras in sandplay may appear as a spatial ascent with or without clearly marked steps or stages. The awakening of kundalini energy may appear as a powerful coiled snake which is about to move. A powerful example of awakening energy appears in the work of ten year-old **Annie**.

> **ANNIE** **Annie's Tray 4** is a striking example of kundalini movement in her transformation process. The discovery of her core value in the rich centering of **Tray 3** clears the way for the vertical ascent of new psychic energy in **Tray 4**. Under the watchful eyes of a good fairy, Annie harnesses her dragon energy, putting it to use for her new development in the churning water wheel. As she does so serpents ascend a central, vertical tower.
>
> **Annie's** new energies are released in the beautiful horses of **Tray 5**. Here the psychic energy pairs off into oppositional polarities, as **Annie** readies for the ascent of more new inner riches in **Tray 6**. Sadly my work with **Annie** ended at this point and we were not able to see her sandplay process through to a more consciously integrated stage. As I review her work, I like to hope that **Annie** was able to continue her psychic integration process subsequent to this powerful beginning she experienced in her sandplay.

While **Annie's** work is a remarkably graphic example of the rise of energy through the chakras, the movement of kundalini energy more commonly manifests symbolically as the characteristic qualities of each chakra. For example, tents, food, huts and campfires frequently appear as the basic elements of survival upon activation of the first chakra.

While these are the basics of bodily and earthly survival, awareness of the chakras attunes us to the fact that the fundamental requirements for the psyche's survival and development are also being put in place by the sandplay client.

When the survival theme is later followed by sand trays with creative and reproductive themes characteristic of the second chakra, our knowledge of psychic development through the chakras alerts us to the client's further intrapsychic development. Cooking symbolism, fires, babies and baby animals, for example, may hold the energy of the awakening of the second chakra.

Third chakra symbolism has to do with power that is properly contained and used. This may appear as a beneficent protector, a good king or a warrior-hero. It may be the sturdy old oak tree, which is both solid and protective. The quality of power of the third chakra is that which is available for use. It is not power that is in the middle of horrific conflict.

The fourth chakra is the heart, the Self, the center of all that is. Fourth chakra symbolism may follow the first three chakras in sequence and manifest as the constellation of the Self. It may appear in a variety of ways as symbolism of the center. This may be a mandala formation or a single, central figure. The quality of a sandplay that holds fourth chakra energy is the meaningful interrelatedness of all things. It is peaceful, at the same time it is very powerful. It may have the numinous, or mystical quality that Dora Kalff (1980/2003) described as occurring when the Self manifests.

The energetic awakening of the fifth chakra may follow the fourth, manifesting as putting truth into action. This may appear in any number of ways in sandplay. It might be a simple, but powerful dispatching of a duty that needed to be attended to, as in the ritual removal of what is impure. A dignified and solemn funeral procession, or the delivery of something true to its rightful place are examples of ways the fifth chakra might manifest.

ELIZABETH An example of fifth chakra energy in sandplay is **Elizabeth's Tray 11**, where she fully accepts the value of her words and her voice. Here she emerges from the gates of a sacred place. In a basket at her side she carries her own words, written on a tiny

> book she crafted herself during the construction of the tray. In the basket rest several tiny babies, indicating the potential potency of these newly owned qualities in her. Mirroring this powerful possibility are several piglets, herded along by a mother pig that carries a bright-eyed, expectant little girl on her back. The parade is directed by a beautiful goldfish, who clearly sees its way in the depths of things.

The sixth chakra is the opening of conscious awareness to the immediacy of the divine. Although it is not a frequent event in sandplay, movement through this psychic center may manifest in sandplay. When properly grounded by the development of the underlying five chakras, the quality of this energy center is that of deep contemplation of the oneness of all being. This is a profoundly focused, meditative energy that consciously contemplates the Self as the ultimate source and goal of all being. Which particular figures it manifests as in sandplay are irrelevant, because the opening of this chakra concerns the divine in all things. What is significant in its appearance in sandplay is the quality of serene stillness and the conscious awareness of the presence of the divine in and through all that is.

As with the sixth chakra, the appearance of the seventh chakra in sandplay is rare indeed. I do not believe I have ever seen this in sandplay. The energy of this chakra is that of total absorption in the Self and it is beyond all duality. While this quality is touched in the Self, its grounding in the material world is necessary for individuation and continued development. The seventh chakra connotes a point of completion, wherein the individual no longer requires feedback and lessons from the material world. At this level of development the person abides in a timeless condition of the divine. In the Hindu and Buddhist traditions, the awakening of the highest chakra is the goal of yogis and monks. Known as *sannyasins* to Hindus, and *boddhisattvas* to Buddhists, these are people who seek the full enlightenment consciousness of the seventh chakra, but remain in the ordinary world for divine service to human kind.

Our awareness of the sequential development of psychic energy through the chakras is another guide for tracking and understanding the process of sandplay therapy. The application of this model of psychic development depends upon the unique characteristics of the individual case. It may or may not apply to a particular case, but nonetheless remains a valuable tool for understanding intrapsychic development.

Our familiarity with all of the allegorical content themes we have discussed opens many doors through which we can come into relationship with our client's work in the sand. Each theme provides us with a different means of experiencing sandplay. Each allegorical theme offers subtle language skills with which we can initiate contact and establish a relationship in the sandplay with the client.

As sandplay therapists, it is important that we become well-versed in all of the allegorical possibilities we have discussed. Myth, fairy tale, story, alchemy, the elements and the chakras are each worlds unto themselves. Each has its own language and meaning system. Yet each of these templates of transformation deals with the journey of the human body, mind and spirit to wholeness. To understand the culture of each transformational theme gives us entry into its unique context. And in so doing we are able to join the client's work with a deep and meaningful immediacy, which would be impossible without a solid working familiarity with these languages of change.

Sand as Content In Sandplay

Continuing our examination of the contents of sandplay, in this section we take a close look at the sand, itself. Sand is the core content of sandplay therapy. Brought together and held by the containing limits of the tray, the sand is a richly significant component of sandplay process.

In the material that follows we will examine some of the factors that have a bearing on the movement of the psyche in sand, as well as the underlying components that influence its capacity to promote change. Particularly, we will consider some of the myriad combinations of the psyche that manifest in the sand tray in this inimitable relationship of client, sand and water. We will look first at the general nature of sand, then to sand as dry and wet. Following this we will examine the client's manipulation of the sand, land formations and the places where sand and water meet.

The Nature of Sand

As an earthly element, sand has a fascinating career. In nature sand is formed by the weathering and disintegration of rock. Over time the forces of wind, rain, ice, heat and cold break rock apart into its components parts. Spontaneous forces of nature and chemical weathering, such as the growth of plant matter, transform the rocky components into minerals and nutrients, iron and alumina oxides, silica, silt and quartz sand. These components combine to form clay. The clay combines with the silt and sand to form loamy soil. Over the course of time soil is eroded by water and washes downhill, eventually being sorted and deposited along the way according to the weight of its ingredients. Being the heaviest, sand is eventually transported toward the coastal region.

Rocks themselves are ancient and enduring. Sand evolves from the wearing down of rocks over time. But before it reaches the beaches, sand serves as soil, in and upon which life lives and dies. It is when its career as soil is done, that these tiny pieces of quartz wash to the beach as grains of sand.

Sand is ancient. In her penetrating reflections on sand, author Annie Dillard (1999) observed that that it takes approximately one million years for a grain of sand to move one hundred miles down a river.

The sand in our trays is so ancient as to be timeless. To enter the sand in the ritual of sandplay is to engage in the timeless. To engage with the sand in the free and protected containment of sandplay is to exit ordinary time and space and to enter sacred time. The place where the sacred manifests is the center. The center is whole, and what is whole purifies.

Sand as Sacred

The image of the pearl as a symbol of the Self is intimately associated with sand. In nature the pearl is formed when a tiny grain of sand from the ocean floor works its way into the flesh of particular mollusks. Irritated by the piece of sand, the mollusk releases a protective agent known as nacre, or mother of pearl, to surround and coat the irritant. It is this layer upon layer of nacre that creates the precious, lustrous pearl. The allegory to the individuation process of the continual working with the irritant in the development of the pearl is evident. I am struck with the parallels between the center of the pearl as Self being a grain of sand and our trays of sand, as the medium or context for deepening connection to the Self. From the standpoint of pearls, the thousands of grains of sand in the sand tray hold infinite potential for psychic wholeness.

The cleansing and purifying qualities of sand are recognized across a wide variety of traditions. In Islam, washing is required before prayer. The Qur'an (Trans. 1996) instructs believers who are ill, traveling, or ritually unclean, to use sand to cleanse before prayer.

> O ye who believe!
> Approach not prayers
> With a mind befogged,
> Until ye can understand
> All that ye say –
> Nor in a state
> Of ceremonial impurity
> (Except when traveling on the road),
> Until after washing
> Your whole body.
> If ye are ill,
> Or on a journey,
> Or one of you cometh

> From offices of nature,
> Or ye have been,
> In contact with women,
> And ye find no water,
> Then take for yourselves
> Clean sand or earth,
> And rub therewith
> Your faces and hands.
> For Allah doth blot out sins
> And forgive again and again.
> (Surah 4:43)

Foregoing the need to discuss the cultural reference to women, in this context the important consideration is the use of sand for cleansing.

Traditional Navajo sand painting is another form of ritual purification and healing through sand (Bahti & Bahti, 1997). Carried out between sunrise and sunset of a single day, sand painting consists of intricate depictions of deities and mythological motifs rendered on the ground with sand and mineral pigments. Corn meal and pollen may be used also. Ranging in size from one square foot up to 20, a sand painting may involve the work of many tribe members. When the sand painting is completed, the patient sits in its center, while the sand from its images is picked up and applied directly to the body. The powers of the deities invoked in the images are thus transferred directly to the patient for purification and healing. The patient takes in the holy energies and is thus transformed.

In the Tibetan Buddhist tradition, monks create intricate mandalas out of colorful sand. The act of creating the mandala is sacred and centering (Bryant, 1993). Careful attention is paid to the correct time and place in preparation for the mandala construction. The completed mandala assumes sacred qualities and acts as a source of healing and centering to all participants and to the world at large. At the ceremony's conclusion, the mandala is destroyed, and the sand is returned to a nearby water source.

The Chinese tradition of *fu shi*, or spirit writing, uses a tray of sand for oracular purposes (de Groot, 1910/1964). In this process, the medium and the person making the inquiry each hold an end of a Y-shaped divining stick. As they hold it together, the longer end of the stick makes automatic movements in the sand, revealing the intent of the divine.

More importantly, the marks in the sand are considered the sacred place where the divine reveals itself. The marks are then interpreted for the individual making the inquiry.

Another facet of the sacred quality of sand is seen in the Latvian goddess *Smilsu Mate*, the sand mother (Gimbutas, 1963). Smilsu Mate is a *chthonic* figure, that is to say, dwelling beneath the surface of the earth (OED, 1994). As the earth gives life, so she receives it back in death. The Smilsu Mate tradition arose from the Latvian custom of burial of the dead in sandy hills surrounding the farming fields. In this tradition it is the sacred and purifying properties of sand that are drawn upon to receive the dead. As in the examples above, the sand absorbs and transforms what is no longer of use. The sand is the sacred place where this transformation takes place.

It is clear that the sand we use in our trays was not chosen as a medium to work in simply because it is readily available. Rather, sand has profound properties that the psyche recognizes. Sand is cleansing, healing, sacred, and oracular. In minuscule material form it holds the eternal. We have sand trays in our offices to create a place for the transformative properties of sand to occur. We can be grateful for the wisdom of experience that guided Margaret Lowenfeld (1950b) to include a box of sand in her clinic, and even more thankful for the innate wisdom of her children who knew how to put it to its proper use.

The Nature of Dry and Wet Sand

Dry Sand

Dry and wet sand both hold the qualities discussed above. Dry sand exists, however, without the element of water. It is fluid in the sense that we are not as able to control its shape, as we can with sand that is wet. It does not hold shapes in a firm way, but with soft edges and a wispy finish. Dry sand cannot be built very high. It is soft to the touch and easily moved. It can be moved with air, or wind, and is thus subject to the subtle movements of spirit.

In sandplay we must examine the quality of place in the dry tray. A dry tray—absent of water—does not automatically imply that the client is working at a shallow level of the psyche. While it is true that a wet or watery sand tray is engaged with the watery depths of the psyche, it does not necessarily mean, by contrast, that the dry tray is not.

A dry sandplay can be serene and elegant, almost rarified, particularly when the client engages with the sand to move and shape it. A dry tray can assume a sacred, spiritual quality. Using a vertical axis as a reference, a serene, dry tray such as we are describing may have an upward, heavenly quality about it. It may be ethereal in nature. This type of dry tray is concerned with ascent, rather than descent. As we will learn from our discussion of spatial dimensions in sandplay, an ascending movement has to do with raising something to a higher level. An important consideration in a sandplay process where such a dry tray occurs might be whether the apparent upward movement is grounded on a substantial psychic base. A high degree of personality integration is required to support such an ascension.

ELIZABETH Elizabeth's Tray 5 provides a good example of a dry tray with serene, spiritual qualities. In it a tiny statue of Tara, Buddhist savior and fierce defender of the faith, rests under a golden tree. She is embraced by seven glowing candles. Three fish swim toward the left in water, suggested by four jewels. Although the tray is completely dry, it has an intimate and sacred quality. This is not a bleak or arid location; rather, it is a very special and intimate place in the psyche.

The dry sand tray can be bleak and empty. It may be a place of very low energy, or vitality. It may be stark or depressed. These qualities are more likely to occur when the dry sand remains untouched. In this situation, the sand acts like a platform for what might sit atop it.

As the therapist, it is difficult to witness a bleak, devitalized tray. It can be draining, hopeless, or frightening. Initially, we must take into account where the bleak, devitalized sand tray fits in the overall sandplay process. The occurrence of such a sand tray in an otherwise energized sandplay process is entirely different than a similar tray in a consistently bleak process. This reminds us that all sand trays can only be properly understood within the context of the entire sandplay process. It is important to keep this in mind, even though in the context of our learning we are viewing many sand trays outside of their process context as illustrations and examples.

In an otherwise energized sandplay process it is important to hold the bleak tray within the context of the process movement. A tray that appears uncharacteristically empty in this context may have to do with grief and a reflection back to past losses. It may be clearing a place for something new to arise. In the latter instance, the affect associated with the sand tray is also important to consider. We will talk more about the feeling content of sandplay in our section on affect.

In a case where devitalized sandplays are an ongoing condition, we must look for any signs of vitality, however small. If we are able to detect some indications of energy, we must be mindful of them and hold them tenderly. These tiny possibilities for growth are very fragile. At the same time, it is of great significance that they are present and manifested in the sand. As therapists, our proper containment of them nurtures them with hope. Our recognition of them, our mirroring, very literally fuels their growth. The power of the therapist's recognition of what transpires in sandplay materially influences and stimulates development in all situations. This aspect of the therapist-sand tray-client equation seems so much more poignant in the cases that appear so bleak.

In a bleak, dry tray, the therapist must also consider where the client may have lost his or her energy. Perhaps it is something we can see in the sandplay process. Perhaps it results from a legacy of abuse and deprivation. Perhaps it is a chronic physical condition that may require the assistance of medical intervention. Medical research has verified direct links between chronic histories of environmental trauma and neuroendocrine dysfunction, resulting in chronic states of anxiety and depression (Nestler, Hyman & Malenka, 2001). In such cases, referral for medical evaluation and appropriate psychotropic medications may be necessary for the client to garner sufficient energy to do his or her psychic work in the sand tray.

Wet Sand

Water figures prominently in sandplay therapy. As the unconscious, or what is un-manifest, the watery blue bottom of the tray holds and supports the material component of the sand. As in life, everything we consciously acknowledge as existing, or being manifest, emerges from and is supported by all that is unconscious, or not manifest. In this way the construction of the sand tray mirrors the fundamental constituents of material manifestation.

In addition, the design of the sand tray *facilitates* access to the underlying, deeper aspects of being through the easy movement of the sand, which rests on the unconscious blue below. The water element may also be incorporated in sandplay by pouring or mixing real water into the sand. Adding water to the dry sand and opening the sand to the blue water are two common means of working with water in sandplay.

In this section we will examine the symbolic nature of water in order to deepen our understanding of this critical element of the sandplay process. We will explore the act of adding water to the sand, the significance of immersion in water, and the presence of mud.

The Nature of Water

As an element, water flows. It finds and follows the lowest places on the surface. It washes and penetrates, and over time, reconfigures the surface of things. When frozen, water becomes ice. As frozen water, ice arrests life in its movement. Also a formidable force of its own, ice has power enough to alter the face of the earth.

Water never fully takes form. Even as ice, it eventually melts. In this sense water never moves beyond its quality of potential. As in the sand tray, all form sits on top of it, or emerges, out of it. The sand, like consciousness, sits atop the waters of the unconscious. Yet when something does emerge, or manifest, from what is below, it is by nature inherently limited. It can only be a piece of, or a reflection, of the full potential of the waters from which it came. This is not to imply that sand equals consciousness. Rather that the elements of the sand and the water in sandplay interact, as do their psychic counterparts of consciousness and the unconscious. They are related to one another in ways similar to the ways consciousness is related to the unconscious.

The earth produces forms. It is the domain of time and place. The water in contrast is timeless. It precedes creation and is eternal. As the unconscious fount of all possibility, water holds an auspicious power of wisdom and prophecy. Eliade (1996) noted that mythic water gods tend to abide outside of time and history. Like the watery element in which they reside, they do not function by the common rules of the dimension of time. Considered this way, water is timeless. It is before time and outside of time. It is eternal.

Every contact with water holds regenerative potential. It fertilizes and feeds, for as the unconscious, it always holds more than the limits of our ego awareness. As the keeper of all possibility, water holds the qualities we require to be nurtured on the journey to the Self.

As the boundless potential of the unconscious, water restores life. Ultimately as the Self, the waters of the unconscious confer eternal life. That is, in the conscious return to the Self, we surpass the bounds of time and space and come to live in the eternal present. However, as with any approach to the Self, the water of life is not easy to penetrate. This requires substantial tests and trials. Frequently it is guarded by monsters with which we must contend in order to prove our worthiness.

Opening to the Blue

In sandplay, to open the sand and expose the blue water below is the act of moving through what is known to that which is unknown. However unaware the client may be when penetrating the sand, the act is one of intent. We recall from our discussion of Jung's personality theory that the conscious ego is torn between two opposing goals. The ego, while it holds dearly to what it knows, is driven to align itself with the Self. When we witness the client's hand open to the blue, we are in the presence of the ego's release of its rigid hold on its reality and its move into its life-giving counter part.

This remarkable act of transformation occurs within the context of the relationship of the holding environment. In the free and protected space of sandplay, the ego is able to exercise this drive toward wholeness.

Adding Water

Adding water to the sand is another act of intention by the ego. To add water to the sand is too engage with the unconscious in an immediate and intimate way. In the process of adding water, the sand absorbs it. Water, the element of what is deeper, is assimilated into the ground of being. It is held among and between the tiny grains of sand. The choice to pick up a container of water and add it to the sand demonstrates significant intention. In this action there is a willful movement to receive the unknown and to let it work from within. It is an act of absorption, one of ultimate trust.

I do not believe that we can conclude that opening to, or adding water in sandplay is necessarily more important than the work that occurs without the presence of water in the tray. It is significant. That is true. However, what transpires in dry sand is also significant. Neither can we assume that the dry tray is more conscious than the wet, as everything that takes place in sandplay entails some unconscious process. The presence or absence of water must be considered within the unique context of the individual sandplay process.

Water is present in sandplay when the unconscious is being directly accessed, or engaged in a noteworthy way. What is important to recognize with the wet tray is the relationship of the client and sand to the water. With the water, or *in the water*, if you will, the psyche moves, or transports, qualities from the depths. These previously unknown aspects of ourselves become available to us for exploration. Precisely how this takes place at any given moment for a client may vary widely. For example, the client's relationship to the water might have to do with exploration. To open to the blue in this way may have to do with looking into a deep reflecting pool to see what lay below. The relationship to the water may entail absorption and the letting in of new qualities. Or it may be a preparation to dive under water and to be submerged in the depths of the unknown. The relationship to the water may be concerned with transporting. Water fluidly carries qualities along. It floats away the old ways of being that no longer serve us and it brings in what is new from far off places in the Self. The client may relate to the water as an ablution. Water washes away the unclean and it sanctifies. The client may be in the water in the manner of inundation, or flooding. We will examine these important aspects of water in more depth later on.

A key tool in witnessing sandplay with water, as with all other aspects of the process, is to experience not only *what is happening*, but also *how it is happening*. The qualitative, indefinable aspects of sandplay often carry more significance in our containment of psychic movement than do those that are more apparent.

Water as Ablution

In sandplay, water may function as a means of ablution. In this sense, it is not a full immersion that occurs, but the use of water in a purifying and cleansing manner. We may see this in sandplay, for example, when a client ritually washes each figure, or pours water over figures. Ablutions are ritual actions that remove what is unclean. When this occurs in sandplay we may, or may not know what it is that is being removed. We can certainly know that very important psychic movement is taking place. For the therapist to hold it well, it is important to consider what has been happening in prior trays in the series. This may give us more awareness of this significant piece of the client's work. Even if we do not become consciously aware of what the ablution concerns, a review of the process will strengthen our lesser conscious containment of the overall process.

Immersion in Water

In the symbolic realm we understand that water precedes form. An immersion in water is thus a return to or regression to a state of being that comes before form. In sandplay, immersion takes many forms. In general, we consider that immersion occurs when the client is somehow in the water. As we discussed above, this may take place as a dive or a submersion. The client may venture to the bottom of the sea, or fashion an overall watery environment.

The ways that immersion may occur are varied. When immersion occurs in sandplay, the client is returning to a pre-formal mode of being. To go down into the waters in this way is to release the hold on form as it is known and to merge with the formless. Psychologically, the immersion in water is a dissolution of identity as it is known. The ego's hold on what it considers real goes into solution and enters a state of possibility, or pre-existence. As with all aspects of sandplay, it is essential to realize that this *is occurring as the client shapes the sandplay.* It happens at that very moment in the sandplay room, in the relationship of client and therapist.

Immersion in the water is a death. Eliade (1996) likened immersion in water to orgy, noting that it destroys creation while, at the same time, reconstitutes it. Entry into the water in this manner is an immersion in primeval chaos. It amounts to a regression to the undifferentiated state that precedes material existence. Immersion is the dissolution of form. To enter the water is to enter the underworld. It is an entry into the potential of the Self. Viewed this way, immersion can be understood as an entry to the center, the place where the planes of being intersect.

Entry into the water in sandplay is understandably a gravely serious undergoing. In the water, the ego must release its hold on identity. Going into solution in this way is terrifying. However, in order to open to the greater potentials of the Self, it is absolutely necessary.

Immersion in water purifies, in that prior forms dissolve and the past is surrendered. In this way, immersion re-configures the moment of creation. The past is done away with and time begins again. As in baptism and countless religious rituals involving water, contact with the water is a new beginning. It marks the surrender of what is old and unneeded and the emergence of what is new and life-giving.

To re-emerge from the water is a new birth. It recapitulates the moment of creation when new form arises out of the formless. Psychologically speaking, re-emergence from the water is the re-birth of the ego, which has transcended its own prior limits and is more ordered to the Self.

In sandplay, we can understand how immersion in the water confers hope in the greatest sense of potential for wholeness. At the same time, we must fully appreciate the unimaginable hazards of such a dissolution. As therapists, we must be sufficiently prepared to securely and mindfully hold the precarious reality of immersion.

Mud and the Flooded Tray

While adding water to the sand is a penetrating participation in the body of the sand, there are times in sandplay when the client adds more water to the tray than the sand is able to absorb. The excess water floods the sand, creating mud. Putting aside for now the issue of how we are going to contend with this mess after the client has left, there are important issues to consider with the muddy tray. As we discussed above, the water dissolves boundaries. In sandplay, the therapist must be prepared to discern whether the flooded tray is in the interest of transformation, or disintegration.

Eliade (1996) emphasized the creative forces of water that are indicated in mud. In mud, the potential of the waters of the unconscious stirs the earth, the material of form. In this way mud holds the potential for new birth. New form may emerge from the fusion of these elemental forces. However, while in the mud, the client is in the deepest darkness. This is the place where no form exists and there is no light to find direction. In mud there is no direction, no time, no space. No definition of any kind exists in the darkness of muddy waters. This is utterly terrifying.

In sandplay, we need to consider if the client is in relationship to the mud in such a way that supports its creative potential, or if the client is sinking and drowning. The question to hold is whether the client's level of individuation is sufficient to undergo the dissolution and see it through to its creative ends. This is a terrifically hazardous condition in sandplay.

As therapists we must take into account the overall psychic development of the client, his or her centeredness in the Self and the relationship of ego to Self. The client who has some relationship to the center of the Self is far more likely to successfully emerge from these treacherous waters than is the client who lacks the touchstone of the psychic center. Without the organizing principle of the center, the client is close to, or in psychotic process. In such a case, sandplay is far too evocative. It is dangerous and can be highly destructive to the client, if the therapist is unprepared to work with psychosis in the sand. There is however, some exciting work being done with schizophrenic clients in the sand by sandplay therapists who are highly trained in work with this population (Baum, 2002).

Flooding can also occur in sandplay with an excess of figures and confusion in the tray. Such a tray may have objects spilling over the boundaries of the tray. In lieu of an excess of water, the muddy darkness may appear through the use of dark, demonic-like figures. A tray flooded in this manner will feel ominous and highly discomforting. Of course, there are countless cases where clients use large numbers of dark figures and we do not consider the tray flooded. The important distinctions appear to be the respect for the boundaries of the sand tray, as well as the degree of relatedness among the figures in the tray. Boundaries and relationship inherently issue from a sense of order that has its root in the center. A lack of relationship and the lack of edges are the conditions of uncontained primordial darkness. Further discussion regarding the flooded tray can be found in the section on relationship in sandplay.

In large measure, it is the quality of the therapist's preparation as container of the sandplay process that influences the appearance of flooding in the sand tray, as well as its creative or destructive outcomes. However, even the most experienced sandplay therapist can misjudge a client's stability and be surprised. For the most part however, the qualified sandplay therapist senses when sandplay is not suitable for a client. He or she is fully aware of the indeterminate nature of psychic transformation in the sand. The highly trained sandplay therapist assesses the client's psychic stability and recognizes when the client is ready for sandplay work. There is no formula for making these determinations. The strongest advice to therapists interested in sandplay is to fully appreciate the profound nature of sandplay and to seek thorough training and experience. In the hands of the unprepared, sandplay can be very dangerous.

Manipulation of the Sand as Content

The sand in our trays is formless until the client engages with it. The manner of manipulation of the sand is a significant component of sandplay content. In the same way, sand that is untouched holds critical elements of the client's process. In this section, we will examine various aspects of sand manipulation and its role in healing and transformation in sandplay.

Touching the Sand

To touch or move the sand in the tray is an intentional act to engage with and to re-configure matter. The sand is an elemental form of matter that provides a simple, unsullied format for the appearance and movement of the inner psychic constituents that fashion mind and behavior. Touching and moving the sand validates our existence. It is a fundamental form of mirroring the Self and its myriad manifestations in us. Touching and moving the sand in the safe presence of the therapist *establishes relationship of Self to other.* The significance of this act must not be underestimated. In the simple gesture of putting his or her hands in the sand, the client *affirms his or her existence.* Doing this in relationship to the therapist *establishes the right to belong.* To touch the sand in the free and protected space of sandplay is a gesture of intent *to take a place, to be*. Undertaken under the protective witnessing of the therapist, the movement of sand establishes the client's fundamental value as a human being. Moving the sand in the watchful presence of the therapist affirms, "I am here. I belong, and I am of value."

In addition, touching or moving the sand initiates the possibility for change and transformation through the intention to move matter. For example, aggressive hole poking may have to do with the individual's capacity to penetrate the layers, to probe deeper or go beyond the surface. Slapping, chopping or digging at the sand may be concerned with the client's developing sense of empowerment or anger. Gentle combing and smoothing may indicate a tenderness or reverence. Touching the sand is healing in whatever form it occurs. As the earth reclaims all living things in death, touching the sand initiates the release of troubles and ills into the earth. In this way the sand, as earth, receives and transforms what is no longer needed.

In her discourse on sand and body, Markell (2002) spoke of the intimate connection where sand and body merge to create a transformational dialogue between what is inner and what is outer. Blurring the distinction between psyche and matter, the hands in the sand function simultaneously to effect change in body and mind.

> The energies that are carried by the hands as the images are shaped become enfolded by the body, by matter itself. Simultaneously the inner image imbued with meaning is transformed by the hands into a concrete, external image and in this way becomes part of the unfolded order. That is, it becomes an image of a lived experience in the time-space dimension of the inner as well as the external world (p. 62).

In the *temenos*, or sacred space, of sandplay, the intentional movement of sand, this most fundamental matter, constitutes a direct engagement in the shape of being. Guided by deep, inner, unseen forces of the Self, moving the sand literally and immediately moves and re-orders the psyche. In sandplay we step outside of time and space to enter that place without time, where what is disordered within us may safely appear and transform. In the process, the Self of the therapist mirrors the Self of the client. The discordant elements of the client are thus pulled toward alignment with the Self. In the process, the psychic elements that are no longer needed are eliminated and new contents that are in greater Self-accord arise from the unconscious.

Moving through the sand may create a path, a direction, a place for psyche to move. Steinhardt (2000) observed that whether meandering or straight, paths indicate direction. The psyche has somewhere to go. Paths may take us back, as in a horizontal regression, or visit past events. Paths may lead us forward to the discovery and incorporation of new and deeper aspects of the Self. Paths may also bridge, or connect, previously isolated or unknown parts of our experience and possibility. Paths may be blocked and reveal obstacles that must be surmounted on the journey to Self.

Touching sand may occur by impressing a handprint in the sand. The handprint is a personal stamp or signature. The client makes a similar statement by writing his or her name in the sand. It affirms *I am here*. It is the conscious acknowledgement and ownership of personhood. With the gesture of the handprint, the embodiment of Self is acknowledged. As a stamp of presence, the handprint affirms the capacity to consciously participate in the journey to the Self and it acknowledges personal responsibility for the passage. Although the seminal developmental significance of this gesture may not be fully conscious to the client at the time, it is firmly and irrevocably set in the psyche. When words are written in the sand they also become symbolic elements and must be considered both for the general meaning of the word and its significance for the particular client.

Impressing an object into the sand is similar to the handprint, but with a less developed affirmation of presence and intentional capacity. While pressing an object into the sand and removing it to reveal its imprint does affirm autonomy and initiative, it does not have the personal acknowledgement of Self of the handprint. I recall the work of a three-year-old boy, who witnessed violent domestic abuse. Midway in his process, he marked his growing ability to deal with his fears by impressing the form of Batman in the sand. His powerful hero was not fully present at this phase of the work, but his strength and centrality were taking their position. Three-year-old **Billy** uses an impression in a similar manner.

BILLY In his **Tray 4, Billy** overcomes the terrors that resulted from his witnessing the violence between his mother and father. Formerly afraid of even touching the scary monster figures, **Billy** is now able to handle them without the therapist's assistance. Proudly, **Billy** impresses the large skeleton monster firmly in the sand, announcing, *...I pressed him in the sand!* In this example, **Billy** makes his mark of victory over his terrors.

The sand can be used as a plastic medium for the creation of countless marks and designs. When presented with impressions in the sand, it is important to consider both the quality of the client's contact with the sand and the character of the marks made as symbolic elements. As there are countless possibilities for designs in sand, the therapist must reflect on each occurrence within the context of the individual sandplay process.

As we can see, touching and moving the sand is one of the most fundamental aspects of sandplay therapy. The ways of touching or moving the sand are diverse. How and when the client moves the sand is a critical and formative aspect of the sandplay process that deserves our attention and full consideration.

Untouched Sand

To be able to engage with the sand through touch, the client must feel sufficiently strong and capable. Many clients who begin the sandplay process have histories of wounding, which have stunted the developmental capacities that touching and moving the sand require. In these cases, a client may touch the sand in very limited ways, or not at all. In our discussion of untouched sand we are concerned with a process in which the sand remains habitually untouched. We are not referring to the appearance of the anomalous untouched trays in an otherwise sand-engaged series. As an element of content, recurrent untouched sand is as significant as sand that is heavily worked.

Why it is that a client is not able to engage directly with the sand will vary depending upon the particular case. Untouched sand may result from an underlying depression. Depending upon the nature of the depression, the sandplay work may, or may not be sufficient to move through and overcome it. In cases of endogenous depression arising from a hereditary condition or chronic trauma that has severely impacted neurotransmitter functioning, a referral for a medical evaluation is in order. The depression may be so deep as to make meaningful work in the sand tray impossible. In severe cases, properly administered medication may restore the client's ability to engage with the sandplay.

Untouched sand may also be indicative of early developmental deficits. These are deficits of trust and initiative and may best be understood as the absence, or arrest of, the fundamental psychic accomplishments that are required to make gestures in the sand, as we discussed above.

It is essential to weigh the inability to touch the sand in its unique context. Some of the possible implications of untouched sand may have to do with fear of contact or relationship. This client may have had to withdraw as a means of survival. An acute withdrawal such as this may result from experiences of severe deprivation or violation during early, formative psychic development. Lacking sufficient early experience of healthy, safe contact, this client may suffer serious wounding of the fundamental developmental tasks that ensure a right to exist and a sense of belonging. To be unable to touch the sand may even be connected to the most fundamental assurance of one's existence. This client may suffer wounding and doubts about being, or existing, or may suffer disassociative tendencies. Deprivations and wounding in early bonding experiences may manifest as the inability to be in relationship. Touching and moving the sand in the presence of the therapist is a motive demonstration of the client's existence in relationship to other. Early bonding deficits may seriously impair the client's capacity to manipulate the sand.

Hesitation and inhibition about touching the sand may also be related to a lack of initiative and a learned powerlessness. This may stem from early experiences of disempowerment in overly controlling environments. In these cases the therapist's witnessing attitude of permission and acceptance can be an immeasurable support in the sandplay. On a very deep level, the client's Self will recognize the freedom and safety of the sandplay container. In its own time, the client's psyche may gain sufficient trust to risk initiating authentic presence in the sand.

We will explore the issues of healing early developmental deficits in greater detail in our chapter on developmental norms and patterns in sandplay. What we need to understand regarding untouched sand is that the client's work may be concerned with early issues of trust, safety and contact. These fundamental developmental building blocks must be established before further development can take place.

We must be cautious about assuming that untouched sand necessarily indicates early developmental deficits. This characteristic in a sandplay series may have a unique connotation for the individual client. At the same time we must be alert that early wounding may not appear in so evident a manner as untouched sand. It may be well-masked by acquired personae that allow the client to survive by *appearing* to belong.

> **RACHEL** Fifteen year-old **Rachel's** work in the sand poses an interesting example of a highly developed persona, which masks a profound underlying emptiness. **Rachel's** sandplays all consist of exquisitely constructed intricate villages, laced by streams and bridges. Tiny people, all proportionate to the size of houses and trees relate properly to each other throughout. The doctor and nurse talk in front of the hospital and children play together under some trees. Delicate paths connect the houses and town buildings to common transportation routes, and so on.

To look at these sandplays, one would immediately have the impression that this is a well-developed youngster with a defined sense of belonging and relationship. It appears that her ego functioning is strong and clear. In this particular case however, this orderly village with everything as it should be is a façade that shields a vast inner emptiness. It is obvious that this child is gifted with a genuine artistic sensibility. She employs it to lend a nice outer dressing to a severely wounded sense of self. This child is like a chameleon that assumes the roles she anticipates people expect. Born into a large family, her birth parents suffered multiple mental handicaps that resulted in minimal, if no parenting. She lived in filth and chaos. When they had anything to eat, it was mostly consumed directly out of cans with no cutlery. As a fifteen-year-old suffering attachment disorder with well-habituated survival patterns, the road to healing and transformation will be long, if it is even possible. In **Rachel's** work we would hope to see a movement through the façade, as trust and safety become established. We would also hope for the establishment of the fundamental mother-child unity and a re-building of authentic personality rooted in the Self.

Sculptural Formations in Sand

As a plastic, malleable medium, sand lends itself to shaping and sculpting. Wet sand, in particular, can assume a wide variety of forms in the sand tray. Although it has its own physical limitations, wet sand can be built up, carved, poked, textured and so on. When the client actively and intently engages with the sand, identifiable figures and land formations that carry significant psychic energy may emerge. In this section we will examine the possible significance of landscape and land formations. We will examine the appearance of unique sculptural shapes and body parts in sandplay and the nature of the places where sand and water meet.

Land Formations

The elements of earth and water in the sand tray frequently lend themselves to the creation of a landscape. Chinese tradition reminds us that all of manifestation is a reflection of the Tao. The Chinese belief is that the landscape is tangible evidence of the divine in the material world. For this reason, landscape painting holds a revered place in Chinese culture.

Sandplay as a landscape may also be regarded as the manifestation of the workings of the Tao. Caves, mountains, and tunnels are significant features of this psychic scenery that hold notably concentrated energies concerning the relationship of consciousness to the unconscious. Let us take a closer look at some of the elements that frequently appear in the landscape of sandplay and their implications in the sandplay process.

Caves in Sandplay

Caves are entrances to the body of the earth. To enter a cave is to enter into the earth. To create a cave in the sand tray is the psyche's acknowledgment of the means and the necessity to go under ground. Eliade (1959) observed that all caves are sacred. They are the earth's navel from which all being manifests. As such they are the center and are holy.

Many cultures carry out sacred rituals in caves and consider caves oracular sanctuaries. I remember visiting many Hindu temples located in caves in travels through India and Sri Lanka. One day in South India, I recall that several of us ventured to have our fortunes told by a holy man, who dwelt high on a hill in the depths of a cave. Whether his predictions and advice were of merit or not, I cannot say. His location and the pilgrimage-like effort it took to reach him certainly lent an air of mystery. Time ran out before my turn came, but the experience of the trek into the cave was itself memorable.

The cave is the place of potential. As an earth womb, new life can emerge from the cave. The cave in sandplay is the place that gives birth to what is new. As a womb, however, proper gestation must take place. To enter the cave is to enter the center. The center is the place where the divine manifests. To enter the cave in sandplay is to be psychically fertilized by the Self in order to give birth to new possibilities from deep within.

To meet the Self is to venture into the unconscious. In this way the cave is the entrance to the underworld. To enter the underworld is a vertical descent and is concerned with matters of the spirit. To move downward is a critically important factor of sandplay that we carefully explore in our discussion of spatial direction.

The act of hiding in a cave, or of secreting treasures in its recesses is an entry into the earth and the underground. While it protects, it is at the same time a place of mystery, set apart from the ordinary world. In this sense, any venture into a cave is transformative.

The underworld is also the realm of the dead. Many cultures have used caves for the burial of the dead. The catacombs of Rome, as well as the sewers of Paris are both examples of man-made funerary caves. Instead of interring the dead directly in the earth, the Romans and Parisians put their dead in underground chambers. Another example of funerary caves are those constructed by the Etruscans, the Roman predecessors. In the Italian regions of Cerveteri and Tarquinia, these early peoples constructed rounded caves that emerged out of the earth. They furnished the caves with household and religious objects their departed might need in the afterlife and placed them on tidy benches surrounding the interior walls. After death, the Etruscans returned their dead to the earth to live in the under ground.

To enter the cave in sandplay is to be in the darkness. It is treacherous and terrifying, because any encounter with the Self demands that some aspects of the ego must die. Many cultures carry out rites of passage in cave sanctuaries. The initiate enters in one form and emerges from the cave reborn.

The Sumerian myth of Innana colorfully depicts the transformation journey undergone in the belly of mother earth (Meador, 1994). In this ancient tale, Innana, goddess of the upper world, descends to the underworld where Ereshkigal, the mad goddess of the underworld, holds her captive and threatens her with death. Two little demons share her grief and rage, eventually causing Ereshkigal to release her. Innana and her brother, Dumuzi, must each agree to spend half of every year in the underworld.

Innana's ventures in the cave illustrate that a proper balance between masculine and feminine energies is maintained by devoting significant attention to the unconscious. For Innana and Dumuzi, this was to last for half of their lives. Additionally, the myth well illustrates how subject we are to unconscious forces when we encounter them. In the cave, this force transforms us according to the agenda of the Self. From the conscious position we have no say over how or what is to take place.

To enter the cave in sandplay can be a tremendous undergoing. In all instances, the cave is concerned with transformation directed by the Self. To enter the cave in sandplay is to submit the ego to its own extinction with faith and hope that new and more vital qualities will emerge.

Mountains in Sandplay

Mountains assume a variety of symbolic values in the growth and development of the psyche. As the highest places on earth, they are frequently associated with the divine. To reach the top of a mountain requires a vertical ascent. To ascend is to reach that which is higher. What is high is frequently associated with heaven and the divine. Because upward and downward movements are of great significance in sandplay, we discuss the significance of psychic ascent and descent in detail in our section on the spatial dimensions of sandplay. In this section we will consider the significance of the mountain itself.

Although mountains generally carry positive associations, there was a period of time during the sixteenth and seventeenth centuries when Luther and other Western thinkers considered mountains the scarred remains of the great flood (Nicholson, 1959/1997). Peaks and valleys were thought to disrupt the tranquility of earthly symmetry with their massive imposition. Luther preached that mountains were pockmarks upon the face of the earth that foretold chaos and decay. Fortunately, this line of thinking was replaced by a greater appreciation for nature in the early eighteenth century. Apart from this curious departure in Western thinking, mountains are considered places of divine revelation. Their peaks house the gods and their massive size is sometimes considered a manifestation of the divine.

In cultures around the world, the topography of large mountains configures both earthly and spiritual dimensions. Mountains are considered sacred links between heaven and earth. Their size anchors a culture as to direction. That is to say that space and frequently time as well, is measured in relationship to the mountain. In this sense the mountain is considered central and functions as the sacred center of the world. The four cardinal directions ensue from the mountain and the mountain serves as the *axis mundi* or world axis.

Just as temporal space can be defined in relationship to the geography of the mountain, the psyche is similarly oriented to the center. We discuss these issues in greater detail in our exploration of the spatial dimensions of sandplay. What is important here is that the mountain is the center. The mountain is the Self. The mountain is the hub that compels what is around it to move toward the center.

Because it is of the earth, the mountain is rooted deep in the underworld. In this way, the earthly mountain is rooted in the netherworld of the unconscious. It is both material and immaterial. The mountain is the place where both the manifest and the un-manifest meet and emerge out of one another.

Mountains around the globe have divine attributions. Mount Hara was sacred to the Zoroastrians. The Atlas range is referred to by the Moroccans as a *pillar of heaven*. The Japanese regard Mount Fuji as a link between heaven and earth. Tradition holds that Mount Ararat in Turkey is the place where Noah sought refuge from the great flood. In East Africa Mount Kilimanjaro stands for all that endures and that is honorable.

Mount Meru is a mythical mountain sacred to Buddhists, Hindus and Jains. A variety of tales from these three traditions describes how all of life emerges from the heavenly Mount Meru. The island of Bali has its central mountain, known as Gunung Agung. Shrouded in cool mist, Gunung Agung is a place of holy pilgrimage to Balinese Hindus. It is interesting that temples throughout Bali assume the shape of Gunung Agung, and are called *merus*, after their heavenly prototype.

Hindu temples in India frequently take the shape of mountains. The temple as mountain is found in quintessential form in the Buddhist *stupa*. The stupa originated in India as a burial mound, called a *caitya*. Buddha requested that his cremated remains be buried beneath a stupa. Buddha specified that this stupa would be the only devotional object commemorating his life, death and enlightenment. Under King Asoka in the third century BCE Buddhism was given national sanction and many stupas were built around India. Each contains a relic of the Buddha or that of another holy being.

While they were originally conceived as funeral mounds, stupas became places of pilgrimage and worship (Reyna, 1993). The stupa is a large dome-shaped mound several stories tall, generally encircled by a railing or colonnade, which separates it off from the ordinary world. The five elements of what is *known*, or what is material, go into the construction of the stupa. In addition, it holds a sixth element, which is the *knower*, the un-manifest underpinnings of all manifestation. Pilgrims circumambulate the stupa as a ritual form of worship, entering and exiting through prescribed portals in the railing.

The appearance of the rounded hill or mound in sandplay may well function in a way that is similar to the ritual centering place of the Buddhist stupa. In one sense, every mountain fashioned in sandplay is made by hand and carries the sacred connotations of a stupa.

Mountains are considered the place of the dead in other cultures, as well. The Shoshoni peoples of Wyoming regard the Teton Range as the foreboding home of the dead. Some Japanese literature refers to the mountain as the place where the souls of the dead reside. In fact, coffins are referred to as *mountain boxes*, and dying is called *going to the mountain* (Nicholson, 1959/1997/1997).

Given the nature of symbols, the opposite is also true of mountains. As they are the place of the dead, they can also be the source of the waters of life. The Nile and the Ganges rivers have their sources high in sacred mountains and are attributed with mysterious and divine beginnings. As the arteries of life that have fed these lands since ancient times, these waters are literally the bringers of life. For thousands of years, and to this day, all Hindus attempt a pilgrimage to the holy water of the river Ganges. Many pilgrims go to the Ganges as their last mortal gesture, dying in her sacred embrace.

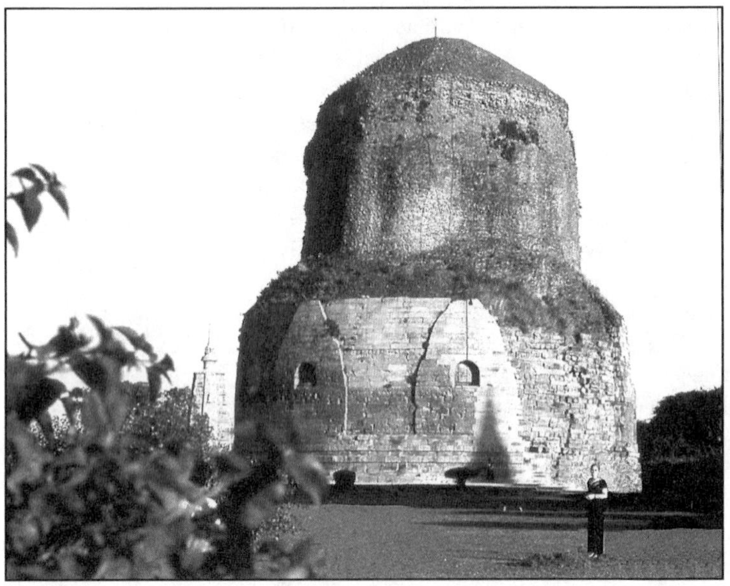

Photograph B. Turner, 1976

The stupa at Sarnath, Northern India, where Buddha is said to have given his first sermon upon attaining enlightenment. The author stands front right.

Mountain tops are often considered places of revelation and clear vision. Many traditions account for the receipt of divine disclosure from high mountain peaks. Moses met Yahweh on Mount Sinai (Nicholson, 1959/1997). The Deuteronomic tradition recounts that Yahweh appeared to Moses on Mount Horeb. The transfiguration of Jesus also took place on a mountain. To the Hebrews, the dwelling place of God was not Sinai, but Mount Zion in Jerusalem, where God could live among the people.

In the Native American tradition, the mountain top is associated with vision and power. The tribal member on a vision quest will frequently travel to the mountain top to acquire the powers and insights of spirit. The Japanese yamabushi mountain ascetics undertake a similar quest.

One of the oldest known traditions of mountain sanctuaries is found on the island of Crete. Occupied between 2100 and 1900 BCE, both cave and mountain peak shrines devoted to the goddess have been located on Mount Dikte, Mount Juktas and Mount Ida. The mythical mountain of Olympus was also home to the gods and goddesses of ancient Greece.

In India, Lord Siva is known as *the lord of the mountains*, who dwells on Mount Kailasa in the Himalayas. His consort, Parvathi is called the *daughter of the mountain*, as *parvat* means mountain.

Chinese tradition links four mountains with the four cardinal directions. A sacred bodhisattva, or being destined for enlightenment, is associated with each direction. Mount Wu-t'ai Shan is in the north and is associated with Manjusri, the bodhisattva of wisdom. To the south is Mount Chiu-hua. Mount O-mei is in the west and the isle of P'u-t'o Shan is off of the eastern coast.

Dora Kalff (1980/2003) spoke about the Japanese figure, *Ta No kami*, who appeared in her sandplay work. A *kami* is a spirit being from the Shinto folk tradition. Spirits called Yama No kami dwell up in the mountains during the fall and winter and descend into the rice paddies in the spring when they become *Ta No kami*, the overseers of rice cultivation and harvest. Significantly, Japanese thought makes no distinction between the place where the kami dwell and the kami themselves. When Yama No kami is on the mountain, Yama No kami *is the mountain*. When Yama No kami descends in the spring, to become Ta No kami, it is the mountain itself that descends to fructify the earth below. That which is high descends to what is below bringing about new growth. Yama No kami embodies the psychic potential for the union of opposites in the meeting of mountain and earth.

The unification of the mountain with divine power is shared by Native American cultures as well. Mythic tales from the peoples of the Pacific Northwest frequently begin with the words, "…Long ago, when the mountains were people…" (Nicholson, 1959/1997). Mount Rainier, formerly known as *Tacoma*, is a tribal ancestor, as are the other great peaks. The Native peoples of Mexico and Meso America similarly regard Popocatepetl, Chimborazo and Mount Huanacauri as divine personifica-

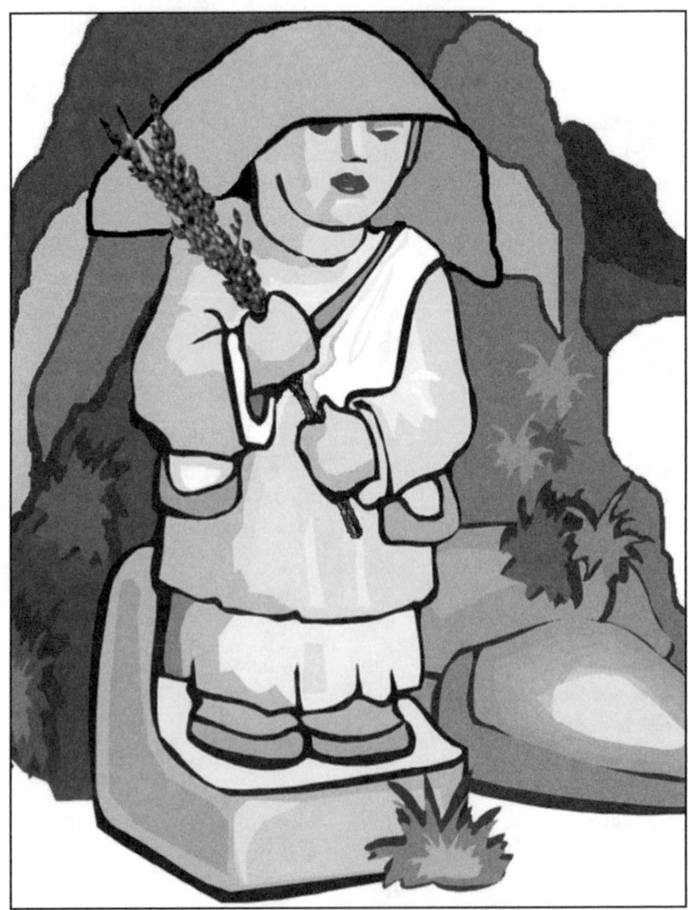

Ta No kami.

tions. When the mountain is inseparable from the sacred and *is the tribal ancestor*, the people live with and upon the earthly embodiment of their origins. Their connection to the earth is unquestioned and its ubiquitous presence defines life as being in the presence of the sacred. Mountains endure, as do stones. There is little, if any, perceptible change in a mountain over the course of a lifetime. Of great interest is that the sacred nature of the mountain also endures through time. There are many mountains that have been regarded as holy by successive cultures and mythologies throughout history. Mount Moriah in Jerusalem was an early place of worship in Canaanite traditions. Biblical tradition records that

Abraham took his son, Isaac, there for the sacrifice demanded by God. Solomon built his temple there, and Muhammad ascended to heaven from the same mountain. Catholic tradition records the appearance of the Holy Mother on mountains held holy by former Aztec peoples. Our Lady of Guadalupe manifested on Mount Tepeyac, the same hill considered the holy place of the Aztec goddess Tonantzin, and Our Lady of Remedios appeared at the mountain pyramid of Quetzalcoatl in Cholula.

Although the mountain may be regarded in a variety of symbolic contexts, its formation in sandplay is the material embodiment of the psyche's grounded connection to what is higher. There can be circumstances when an upward direction is inflated and not properly anchored. We discuss this in greater depth in the material on the spatial directions in sandplay. Here we are talking about the mountain as an upward ground swell that is based on a solid psychic foundation. In the sandplay process, the psyche of the client builds itself up from the two-dimensional plane of the sand's surface. What is underneath, unconscious, swells upward as new potential. This movement ensues from the center of the Self and is by its very nature sacred. The building of a mountain in the sand tray is the psyche's movement toward more of what it is in relation to the center. The mountain is formed up from and out of the sand, as the ground of being. In sandplay the building of a mountain is the psyche's intentional digging down for the purpose of building something new. What is on its surface is more readily accessible to consciousness. What lies underneath has yet to appear.

ARTIE Artie's Tray 30 contains an example of a stupa-like mountain arising out of the center of the tray. In his sandplay work, characterized primarily by land formations and shapes, **Artie's** stupa appears following a breakthrough and connection in a tunnel he constructed in **Tray 28** and the glowing warmth of 33 candles in **Tray 29**.

IVY **Ivy's** work is a good example of the many-sided values of the mountain in sandplay. While the mountains in these two trays reach to very high points, they concurrently arrive at great depths. Mountains appear frequently in **Ivy's** sandplay, where they take on a powerful transformative character. In **Ivy's Trays 4** and **5**, a tall mountain appears in the near center area of the tray. In both trays, **Ivy** calls these mountains *castles*. A castle is the place where royalty resides. In **Ivy's** sandplay process these castle mountains assume a profound significance, as they have to do with what is royal within her, the Self. The castle in **Tray 4** is surrounded by the fierce and frightening energies of serpents, monsters and mythical beasts. Touching this area of the psyche is fraught with danger and terror, as it threatens to destroy significant aspects of her ego structure. In **Tray 5** the castle transforms into a gold and glittering place that houses precious jewels. In this sandplay **Ivy** appears to have penetrated beyond the fearsome monsters that guard the sacred Self.

Holes and Tunnels in Sandplay

Holes and tunnels in sandplay are formed by a piercing movement of the psyche. In the case of a hole, the surface of the sand body is pierced in a downward direction. This is a gesture of the psyche's movement toward and into its less conscious dimensions. Holes are of various sizes and qualities. Holes so large as to create ponds or lakes are also openings to the unconscious waters below. The nature of this form of digging into the sand's surface is discussed in our section on water. Smaller holes, such as those formed with the fingers or small objects are of a different nature than clearly defined lakes or ponds.

It is important to consider the manner in which the holes are made. Holes through the surface of the sand that are resoundingly and firmly poked with a finger are different, for example, than holes tentatively dug with a stick. The significance of the gesture is the relationship of the conscious ego to the unconscious. This varies from sandplay to sandplay and must be regarded in its own context. However it is formed, the hole is a conscious engagement with the unconscious. It marks the ego as present, whether this is with confidence or apprehension.

The hole is a penetration through the surface to what is below (Steinhardt, 2000). When open to the water, it may function as a resource, such as a well. When a hole pierces through the sand to the bottom of the tray, the psyche accesses what is below. This access may function in a number of ways. As with the well, the psyche may draw upon that which is less conscious, providing a channel to the surface. The hole may provide the psyche a vent for the release of pressures from what is surging up from the underground. A hole may be a place of disposal, where the psyche can drain away what is excessive or no longer needed.

Creating a hole in sandplay may have to do with planting. In this way, holes may carry erotic energies, as in the fertilization rites performed by peoples since the Neolithic age (Eliade, 1991). In many cultures, penetrating the soil for agriculture is seen as a sexual act. The relationship of seeding the earth is viewed the same as the penetrating relationship of human procreation. In this way, holes in sandplay may be gestures of seeding or impregnating the earth for new growth. Their intentionality also carries capability or potency to engage with the unconscious.

Tunnels are more difficult to construct in the sand. While some tunnels come ready made and are included in the sandplay collection, those that are sculpted in the sand require greater effort to shape than do holes. Tunnels that are constructed by the client from the body of the sand may involve a more penetrating engagement with the element of earth, or a more urgent, compelling psychic need to shape the structure by hand. Generally speaking, both types of tunnels function in similar ways. The therapist must listen carefully to the individual process to discern differences, if any.

Ready made and hand sculpted tunnels both present highly interesting movements of psyche in sandplay. The bridge over the tunnel functions on the surface to connect two circumstances of psyche, as the passage below works underground to connect two places in space (Steinhardt, 2000). When a tunnel reaches underground to connect elements on both sides of a body of earth, it bridges components of the psyche that have been so separated as to be from different worlds. The tunnel horizontally penetrates the body of earth. It is psyche boring through. The tunnel is a deep form of penetration that opens new unconscious pathways, new connections and means of movement in the underworld. It is important to carefully observe what the tunnel connects on either side of its openings. On the other hand, the tunnel may not appear to bridge any elements, but serve solely as a new means of navigation in the under world.

In sandplay, the tunnel is the psychic means for the passage through dark, unknown, and frightening psychic material. To bore a tunnel in the sand is a precarious undertaking. The tunnel is always in danger of collapse. The presence of a tunnel in the tray indicates a preparation or readiness for what must be undergone. The tunnel is a way and the way is clear. To better contain the client's frightening undergoing, it is important to be as aware as possible of what the client may be in the process of connecting. In some cases, these psychic elements do appear at either end of the tunnel. In many cases, however, we must look back over several trays in order to discover what psychic elements the tunnel may connect.

In certain cases, the tunnel may have more to do with developing motility in the underworld than with making connections. When the client sculpts a tunnel and consciously touches fingers underground as the tunnel is completed, there is a more conscious awareness that the there is a new route or passage way available in the unconscious. It may also indicate that necessary underground journey can be accomplished. When a client's fingers touch in a tunnel, we may see visible evidence of a sense of accomplishment in the client's demeanor. Fashioning the tunnel does not eliminate the need to walk this underground path. While the psyche has accessed a new pathway, it must also be put to use.

ARTIE Eight-year-old **Artie** suffered from some learning difficulties that made his school life frustrating. In spite of a willing, happy attitude, this delightful boy was unable to make the mental connections necessary to stay on track with his learning. In addition, **Artie's** life suffered a second division when his parents divorced. **Artie's** sandplay process was primarily carried out in the movement and changes in land formations. Although he uses figures in most of his trays, the force of his process appears inherent in the corporal investment of his body in the sand. In most of his trays, **Artie** heavily kneads and works the sand between his fingers. An overview of his work highlights his use of the sand in the movement of his psyche and gives us a powerful example of how psyche can move and transform sandplay with limited use of figures and images.

In **Tray 12 Artie** uses a glass tube to form a deep cave in the hillside. Penetrating more deeply into the body of his psychic obstacles, he puts small wrestlers in the whale's mouth, and pushes the whale deep in the cave's interior. In the following **Tray 13, Artie** works the sand for nearly twenty minutes, then shapes a volcano. Having penetrated more deeply into his work via the cave in the prior tray, new potentials rise from the depths of the sea. In addition, the volcanic opening is a channel or passageway for new psychic material to come to the surface.

In **Tray 18, Artie's** psychic landscape assumes a well-integrated archetypal form, consisting of a bisected circle and a sphere. Clearly, this child's work is taking shape and progressing, although I had no conscious awareness of exactly as to where it was heading. After further sorting and ordering in the intervening trays, **Artie's** sandplay process nears completion in **Tray 41** with a large central mountain, penetrated completely through by an underground passage. Tiny black and gold knights battle in what he dubbed, *The Sand War*. **Artie's** work concluded with an ordinary playful game of racecars on a track he made in the sand. Reminiscent of the divided circle shape of **Tray 18**, **Tray 42** consists of a large ring, neatly divided vertically down the center, with an active racetrack on each half. Underscoring the completion of his process, **Artie** returned all of his vehicles to the shelves and smoothed over the tray. He was done.

Although I will never know exactly what was transpiring with **Artie** neuropsychologically over the course of his sandplay, he continued to do better in school, gained many friends with his affable personality and adjusted to his parents' separate lives.

Sculpted Shapes and Figures in the Sand

The plastic malleability of wet sand affords the possibility of sculpting identifiable or unidentifiable forms and objects. Such sculpted forms may emerge out of the surface of the sand or the blue water may surround them as islands. Sculpting an identifiable figure from the sand is a particularly significant moment in the symbolic process as a result of the intensity of focus between the client and the energies held by the symbol. The emergence of a symbolic figure in the sand is the birth of those budding energies in material form. It is certainly true that the psyche directs the selection and placement of figures from the sandplay collection. However, when the form is born directly from the sand as the ground of being, the immediacy between client, psyche and symbolic form is so great as to be inseparable. There is an intensified investment in the particular symbol that is created entirely by hand. The same can be said for figures made by the client and brought to the sand tray.

SANDER A good example of sculpted form is the giant tadpole that appears in seven-year-old **Sander's Tray 9**. The metamorphosis of the development of the frog holds powerful energies about psychic, as well as bodily development. **Sander** underscores the new potentials for growth available to him by burying a frog on the back of his tadpole. Set with amethyst eyes, **Sander's** transformative figure had keen vision for the journey that lay ahead.

In some instances, sculpted forms arising out of the sea as islands are more defined than are those that emerge from the earth itself. The edges of islands are clearly defined, and their presence is unquestionable. On the other hand, sometimes the forms appearing from out of the earth are more grounded. As with all aspects of sandplay, there are no formulae. Each case is unique and must be considered on its own merits.

Some sculpted forms are not immediately recognizable, as in the first tray of eight-year-old **Maizie**.

MAIZIE In **Tray 1, Maizie** carefully sculpts a mounded shape in a fairly central position. At the time I recall having no idea what this was about. Upon completion of the tray, when I inquired if there was a story or title for this work, she happily referred to the mound as *...the house*. In the context of the sand tray, it became clear that the issues **Maizie** addressed in her sandplay process would lead her to be at home in herself. Also bearing the rich archetypal significance of mountain, the mound and the stupa, discussed previously, **Maizie's** house was here, but unformed. Her work had to be undergone in order for it to materialize.

Body Parts

Designs or sculptures that resemble parts of the body may also appear in sandplay. What they signify in the particular sandplay case will vary widely. The appearance of a head or a face may hold energies similar to the impression of a handprint, or name in the sand. It may have to do with the growing security of the ego and the client's recognition of his or her unique identity. It might be an awareness of inflation or an overly rational approach to life.

Unconscious land formations and waterways frequently assume the shape of male and female genitalia in the sand trays of both adults and children. As the bodily region of reproduction, genital imagery is vitally creative. In sandplay this imagery may have to do with opening up to new creative potentials. It may be concerned with awakening new psychic capacities previously unknown to the client. Imagery of genitalia may have to do with the development of the contra-sexual elements of the personality, the anima or animus. In prepubescent children the appearance of genital imagery may be about the child's developing sexuality and all that is entailed in moving from the realm of childhood to that of an adolescent. Genital imagery may also appear in the healing processes of clients who were sexually abused or devitalized in some way.

Body parts in sandplay may have to do with illness in the body. As mentioned previously, in some ways we may consider the sand as an extension of the body. When the hands and body move and configure the sand, it is easy to understand how issues regarding the body may appear in the sand tray. Amatruda and Helm-Simpson (1997) correlated areas of bodily distress with the elements and chakras, sandplay imagery, therapeutic goals and presenting issues. Having had rich experience with critically ill patients, their work provides an informative integration of these factors in sandplay.

Attributes of afflicted bodily areas may be unconsciously depicted in the sandplay. It is interesting that the illness depicted may belong either to the client or to someone to whom they are closely attached. Perhaps we can infer from this that the client shares the field of psyche with their loved ones in much the same way that the psyche of the client and the therapist come together. As the psyche exists beyond the limits of time and space, matters of great concern such as illness are held concurrently by those to whom we are connected.

The psyche holds what is past, as well as what lies in the future. Even though we may experience a strong intuition about bodily affliction in a sandplay process, we can never be certain about what it is that appears in the sand tray without the client's conscious communication to us about an illness. The therapist may have a strong urge to talk with the client about his or her perceptions, however symbolic process does not support this level of certainty. As with all other facets of the symbolic process, I feel that the therapist's task is to simply hold the information as a possibility. It is essential that we hold a firm, compassionate container for the psyche's work and that we trust it will move as it needs to.

Many years ago I worked with a little boy of five, whose mother had been diagnosed with a serious, life-threatening illness. She elected not to tell her son. In spite of the mother's efforts to keep her many hospital and doctor visits a secret from her son, his sandplay work was filled with themes of illness, hospitals and care-taking. In this case, I felt it was important to tell the mother that her son carried all of this stressful information below conscious awareness. The concerns about the illness were in the family unconscious.

SHANNON Another interesting example of the shared field of awareness regarding physical health is the case of **Shannon**, a woman in her forties. Having suffered painful and difficult relationships with her parents, she was primarily attached to her older sister. In **Tray 8 Shannon** sculpts two islands, about which she said, *"It looks like two boobs or two eyes and is incredibly ugly!"* In **Tray 10 Shannon** repeats the two-mound breast pattern, this time with deep reverence, saying, *"It does not make any sense, but I like it. I like the colors."*

The manner with which she constructed the sandplay was profoundly ritualistic. After shaping the sand and positioning the house, trees and flowers, **Shannon** carefully intertwined the black and white ribbons, gently draping them across the mounds. She placed a bridge over the ribbons and between the mounds then put three blue horses in a circle on the right mound.

> At the time **Shannon** made **Tray 8,** I deeply felt its significance and intuited it had something to do with physical health or illness. Directly afterward her beloved sister was diagnosed with breast cancer. After a long, noble battle the illness took her life. Although this was the greatest loss **Shannon** had suffered, her work in the sandplay had cleared a path for her to come through her torment with dignity and wisdom.

In retrospect, we can see that it would have been meaningless, if not a serious interruption to her work to have said anything about illness being present in the sand tray. The appropriate action was to hold it and wait.

> **TARA** An example of wounding and bodily trauma can be seen in the first sand tray of Tara, a woman in her early thirties. In therapy, to address relationship difficulties stemming from her early history of sexual molest, **Tara's Tray 1** assumes the figure of a female torso. The land formation sculpted in the sand can be viewed as a reclining female figure, with neck and shoulders to the left. The area of the breasts, the primary region of her early abuse, is carved out as two depressions. **Tara** had no conscious awareness that she fashioned a wounded woman in the sand. I silently held this awareness, realizing the depth of the impact of her early abuse, now held in the very ground of her being.

As we can see, myriad formations can be made in the sand tray. At times we will have a clearer impression of what energies are held by the shapes, cavities, and convolutions than at other times. In all circumstances, we must consider the possible significance of these emerging forms, while we continue to carry their inevitable uncertainties.

Where Earth and Water Meet

The places where sand and water meet in the sand tray create a special type of relationship that deserves close attention. From one vantage point, the two fundamental contents of sandplay, the sand and the blue water, may be regarded as the two energetic poles of material being. Drawing from the Taoist tradition, we may think of sand as yang, the masculine, and of water as yin, the feminine. Each is defined in relationship to the other. In addition, each contains within itself, the possibility of its opposite. In the sand tray we may think of sand under water and of water underlying the sand, or earth. In the most fundamental way, the relationship of the sand and water reflects the essential constituents of how being is manifesting at that moment. This relationship holds the manner of the relationship between the conscious position and the unconscious.

In sandplay, take notice of where and how the sand and water meet. Very different psychic positions are present, for example, when a body of water is surrounded by land versus when the land is surrounded by the water. Water, as moist, feminine, unconscious energy is held very differently when surrounded by the body of sand than when it is open ended. In all cases we want to consider how the unconscious material is related to conscious awareness, and vice versa.

Another consideration has to do with the proportionate size of the body of water to the sand. A vast body of water with only the smallest indication of land around it may have very different symbolic significance than does a much smaller lake held by a larger body of land. In the former example, the emphasis would seem to be on the water and the quality of descent. In the latter, the opening to the depths is certainly present, but perhaps without the sense of urgency or possible trepidation indicated by the larger water opening. Similarly, a tentative opening to blue in a vast sandy landscape may indicate apprehension or a defensive conscious position.

LENAE Lenae's Tray 1 is an interesting example of the relationship of land and water. Here a body of land is clearly defined on the right side of the sand tray by its relationship to a large body of water on the left. This relationship of water to land carries a sense of the significance of the degree of unconsciousness operating in this child's inner and outer lives. When considered with the supine placement of the family of nesting dolls on the edge of the water and the addition of books covering the eyes of the two children, the theme of unconscious perception is strengthened.

Wells, Lakes, Ponds, and Streams

The formation of wells, lakes, ponds, and streams in the sand tray requires a certain amount of intention and conscious direction. As they are typically formed with distinct walls or edges, these types of openings to water are well contained by the body of the sand. Their boundaries and uses may be clearly defined. The sand surrounds these openings to the water and supports them. Wells will frequently have structures for drawing water placed above them. This is an indication that there is intention to draw upon what is below and that the means exists to access what is deeper.

Ponds and lakes may appear as places of reverie in the landscape. They may hold fish, turtles, ducks, and other water life, indicating that they are penetrated, fertile and accessible. Clearly defined ponds and lakes are very different in nature than are random openings or holes through the sand that seem unexplainable in the context of the sandplay. These may seem less defined, more unconscious, perhaps somewhat ominous.

Streams and rivers are horizontal channels cut through the landscape. The body of sand supports their sides and their shapes. Yet what moves through the channel is water. Streams and rivers are pathways for the flow and direction of unconscious material. They are channels for the transport and movement of psychic content.

Streams and rivers may divide the landscape into separate sections. In this way, rivers and streams may work to define and to initiate connection between heretofore ambiguous or isolated aspects of the psyche. In a sense they function as a bridge, but it is still an unconscious one. When functioning this way, rivers and streams define the gaps that must be bridged in a more conscious manner.

Beaches and Oceans

Beaches and oceans are of interest in sandplay, as they are the places where the conscious and the unconscious meet. The possible significance of how, when and where the body of the earth meets the vastness of the great ocean depths in a sandplay process may be better understood by considering some of the qualities specific to beaches and oceans. Previously, we examined the nature of water in some detail. In this section we explore the profundity of the ocean with particular attention to the significance of the beach as the touch point between surface and what is underneath.

Beneath the surface the great waters of the oceans hold the unknown, the unconscious. What is new, that which is born, emerges from the unknown. This is reflected in the creation myths of many cultures that recount tales of the seas as the great source of life (Eliade, 1996). The ocean is the source of the gods of the universe in the Western mythologies told by Homer, Virgil, the Orphic texts, Plato, and others. The Sumerian tradition of the ancient Near East tells of the mountain of heaven and earth arising from Nammu, the great sea. Some ancient Egyptian tales describe the earth as resting upon the source waters called *Nun.* The dais of the god Horus is a hill of sand that emerged out of the primeval waters when time began. Many ancient Indian tales speak of gods and life having emerged from the waters. Chinese mythology describes four seas that surround and hold the earth, each associated with a great dragon king. Some Mayan myths similarly describe the earth as held by four seas, each of a different color. Ancient Germanic myth describes a vast, foreboding sea that encircles the world (Sturluson, 1954/1984). It is surrounded by and is held together by a uroboric serpent that bites its tail.

These tales of the oceans as the source waters of being cross all cultural lines and are virtually endless. Said in Jungian terms, the essence of each of these water origin myths is the perennial recognition of the generative nature of the unconscious. Creation is the product of that which is quintessentially mysterious. The image of the uroborous in the Germanic tradition emphasizes the totality of the unconscious. Like the snake that bites its own tail, it holds all of time and space.

The ocean exists as a body. We are able to see it and are certain that it exists. However, we are never able to fully penetrate it and know all that is beneath its surface. When the client encounters the ocean in sandplay he or she meets the vast, abundant resources of the Self that exist below the surface of awareness. The possible treasures of psychic growth that exist beneath the waters are immeasurable. At the same time, what is below the surface is in the darkness and is treacherous. Psychologically speaking, we must engage with the ocean with great caution. To mine its treasures demands thorough readiness and deep respect. Its powers are great, and it can consume us.

Symbolically, the beach is the place where the psychic encounter with the unconscious possibility occurs. In nature, the beach functions to collect and purify natural debris that originates from both land and ocean (Smitter, 2002). Waste materials travel down to the beach from land and up to the beach by the wave action of the ocean. Those that are biodegradable are processed and recycled back into nature by the sun, waves, sand and wild life on the beach. In this way, the beach is both a place of disposal and of purification.

The concept of the beach as a place of disposal is reflected in a variety of cultural traditions. A highly interesting one is the annual ritual to expel evil spirits in the Nicobar Islands off of the coast of India (Frazer, 1922/2002). Once a year villagers carry a small wooden boat from house to house to gather all evils on board. After traveling to each home, they take it to the beach and launch it out to sea. In this way, they return what is dark to the darkness of the sea.

The treacherous nature of the beach as the place of surrender is reflected in the culture of Bali. The natives of this beautiful Indonesian island avoid the beaches, as they are considered the place where evil exists and are place of disposal for the remains of the dead. To the Balinese, virtually every aspect of ordinary life is accorded daily blessing. By imbuing everything with the sacred, the Balinese drive evils to the shores of the island where they can be eliminated or transformed.

The purifying aspects of the beach are also reflected in the tradition of the Ainu peoples of Japan. The Ainu hold the home hearth sacred and undertake rituals to assure its purity. After a death in the home, the ashes from the hearth are ritually removed to a special depository outside of the house and fresh sand from the beach is put in the hearth to purify the home. Whereas the Balinese drive the evils to the shore for purification, the Ainu people use the sand that the beach has processed and cleansed.

In sandplay, the beach is a place of arrival and departure of psychic qualities. In this way the beach may serve purposes of both disposal and purification during a transformational process. From our examination of change and transformation we know that a surrender of what is no longer needed is required in order to access new psychic possibilities from the unconscious. In sandplay the qualities of the beach may indicate the manner in which this transformational process occurs. An abrupt or rugged shoreline indicates a very different quality of passage than does a gentle, populated swimming beach.

The shape of the beach may also indicate the client's position in relationship to the change process. I recall the case of a young man whose sandplay process pictured many scenes of boats alternately venturing out to sea then returning to sheltered bays for safe harbor. This man's transformation was underway, but in a step-at-a-time fashion. His work proceeded in this way until his transformation was complete and the forays back and forth were no longer necessary.

A beach front in the shape of a promontory or peninsula indicates a psychic advance toward the transformation. A beach shaped in this way shows a readiness or anticipation of the coming changes. It is a penetration into the depths that fertilizes psychic possibility.

Although there is no formula for how sand and ocean meet, taking notice of the formation and nature of the beaches in sandplay may help us better contain the client's encounter with the new psychic qualities held by the deep waters of the unconscious.

Islands

Eliade (1996) gave striking attention to the psychic significance of the island. Observing that water precedes all of existence and that all of creation is sustained by water, he likened all of creation to an island that appears amidst the waters.

Islands are of particular interest in sandplay. By definition, an island is a body of land that is completely surrounded by water. In sandplay this tends to occur in two ways. One is the island that emerges out of the sea. The other is an *inland island* that is created in a body of land by a circular river or moat. Both types of islands are isolated. They are places set apart from the main body of things. In this way they are special, different, or new. An island that is set apart from the main body of land by a circle of water may be a place of refuge. This type of island offers a place for psychic retreat and reflection. Viewed in this way an island provides a place for the definition of Self that distinguishes it as central.

Islands point to centering, as they create a circular relationship to space and time. On an island, everything is in relationship to the water. On the flat plane of an expanse of land, coordinates along a horizontal grid conceptually define time and space. For example, we commonly think of the past as behind us and the future ahead. The spatial configuration of an island dictates a very different relationship to time and space. As the island is round, time and space relationships are defined in a radiate pattern that emanates from the center outward. The conceptual pattern of the island is concerned with what is inner to what is outer.

As a body of solid ground arising from the depths of the sea, an island is a place of creation. It is a birth of qualities arising from the depth of the Self into the light of consciousness. As archetypal points of creation, islands are considered the birth places of ancestral gods in several cultures. The Japanese, for example, attribute island births to the guardian deities, Izanagi and Izanami, later considered the parents of Amaterasu Omikami, the supreme deity and imperial ancestor. Polynesian tales of the ancestral island gods Hine and Tane account for the cycle of life and death. Western tradition describes the birth of Apollo on the holy island of Delos and tells of Aphrodite's birth directly from the sea. Having emerged from the sea, Aphrodite is an island goddess. Her erotic and sexual qualities are the same creative and transformational components archetypally attributed to the island. In this way Aphrodite might be thought of as a personification of island mythology. It is interesting that temples to Aphrodite were frequently located in transition places between land and sea, such as in marshy beaches, or on misty seaside cliffs. Her transformational properties encompass symbols of both island and beach.

Just as the island is regarded as a place of creation and birth, it is frequently associated with death. In early Greek culture the island god, Apollo was the patron of young men. He was associated with transitional rites of passage from boyhood to manhood that entailed the symbolic death of the initiate prior to rebirth as an adult member of the society. In the Trobriand Islands of Melanesia the souls of the dead travel to the island of Tuma, where they transform into souls of unborn children. Tradition holds that they enter the wombs of the women to await rebirth into the tribe. For these Aboriginal people the end is also the beginning and the transformation occurs on a sacred island. The Semang peoples of Malaysia combine island and cave symbolism with transition and renewal. After death, the Semang believe that the souls of the dead travel to an island in the west. A tall pillar stands on this island and on top of the pillar is the cave of the thunder god.

In sandplay, there may be symbolic representations on the island that indicate what the new, or changing psychic qualities are. In many cases the changing qualities are held in the broader context of the entire sandplay process. Whether we have indications of the particular nature of the transforming aspects of the psyche or not, what is significant is that something is coming to the surface that originates in the center of the Self and that the birth of the new psychic product follows the death of the old.

Island and cave symbolism is combined in the sacred island temples of India. One well-known island cave temple is on the island of Elephanta near Bombay, which holds the 5-8th century CE sculpture of Siva Trimurti. Hindu pilgrims from around the world travel to this sacred spot to make obeisance to the three aspects of Lord Siva, Rudra, the destroyer, Brahma, the creator, and Vishnu, the preserver. In a visit to Sri Lanka many years ago, I traveled to a sacred island cave temple off of the coast. The nerve-wracking journey was made on a large, old wooden ferryboat filled to at least three times its capacity with Indian pilgrims. As it is commonly known that the Indian people assiduously avoid the water and are notoriously poor swimmers, I assure you my prayers and devotions began the moment I boarded that rickety old craft. All was well however, when we safely arrived on the island some time later, greeted by ceremonial elephants, colorful umbrellas and the strains of haunting wind instruments. Now reflecting back on the experience I recognize that the crossing was as significant as, if not more important than the temple puja itself.

MALCOLM Eight-year-old **Malcolm's Trays 8** and **9** are a wonderful example of something new arising on an island in the sea. Although he lived in a sound and loving family setting with his father, **Malcolm's** identity was seriously compromised by his grief and conflict over his birth mother's severe mental illness. Through his sandplay, **Malcolm** was able to grieve the tragedies of his mom and to clarify and integrate his individual strength and character. **Malcolm** releases significant anger and sorrow early in his process, as seen in his **Trays 1** and **2**. In **Tray 8, Malcolm** clears the channel for his new psychic qualities to emerge with the central placement of a plunger. Following this, a powerful space shuttle readies for launch on a cubicle island in **Tray 9**. **Malcolm** was now free to explore the wonders of himself under his own power. Following an ardent process of construction and de-construction in his intervening work, in his final **Tray 27, Malcolm** soundly harnesses his inner fire and builds an Olympic style torch-like tower of sand. The delight of his victories, both psychic and sculptural, could not have been greater.

~ Conclusion ~

Chapter 1
Content Themes in Sandplay

This concludes our exploration of content themes in sandplay. To cultivate another means of entering into relationship with the symbolic process, we now turn our attention to spatial themes in sandplay.

Chapter 2

Spatial Themes in Sandplay

Introduction

Spatial themes are concerned with the spatial relationships between the components in a sandplay process. The pattern of the layout of the sand tray functions as an important part of the symbolic process. In some instances, the pattern *is* the symbolic content.

In the material that follows, we will explore the nature of the vertical and the horizontal axes. We will consider the nature of the center, as well as that of archetypal formations such as the circle, square, triangle, star, and radiate. We will also explore the issues of placement and relationship in the sand tray. Much of our discussion will focus on the archetypal or symbolic qualities of the spatial dimensions. Although the discussions may appear somewhat esoteric, a well-developed understanding of how spatial dimensions function in the movement of psyche is essential to the study of sandplay therapy. Together with the themes of content, motion, and affect, a firm grasp of spatial themes works to strengthen the therapist's containment of the sandplay process.

The Vertical Axis

The vertical dimension appears in a number of ways in sandplay. It may emerge as the sculpting of the sand into mountains or towers. Verticality may be indicated by traditionally tall figures such as trees, ladders, flagpoles, and so on. Objects hung above the tray certainly imply the vertical dimension, as do objects propelled up- or downward. The appearance of arrows and archers aiming decidedly up- or downward, or wells with water buckets that descend into the depths, are other means of showing the vertical axis in sandplay. Caves and volcanoes imply verticality in their connection to what is below. Opening the sand to the blue water is another indication of the vertical axis to the underworld.

In traditional symbolism, the vertical axis is indicative of the connection between heaven, consciousness, the masculine force above, and the unconscious, the underworld, the feminine force below (Eliade, 1958/1996). The vertical axis in sandplay may indicate a client's relative conscious or unconscious position in relation to what else is happening in the sand tray and the overall sandplay process.

Because the vertical axis connects heaven, earth and the underworld, it is the line, or direction along which an individual can travel intrapsychically to access other planes of being. Movement along the vertical axis may be up or down. Although the journey to heaven is very different than travel to the underworld, both are equally valuable. They are qualitatively different aspects of psychic travel along the same continuum. The process of individuation entails our having a reasonable degree of experience in both realms and the ability to move up or down as the situation demands.

Height and Ascent

Height is removed from profane space and is closer to the sky. Height thus assumes qualities of the sacred (Eliade, 1958/1996). Ascent, or movement to a higher place, is difficult to separate from the dimension of height itself. An ascent is a breakthrough to a new plane of being. It moves away from the limits of what is strictly profane and toward the sacred. Ascent is symbolic of moving toward the absolute reality. As one moves away from ordinary conscious awareness, ascent may invoke feelings of uncertainty and fear. The ego loses its hold on the definition of reality as it opens to new dimensions of experience. There is thus a link between ascent and death, because movement to a higher plane of being entails a transcendence, or relinquishment of former ways of being. Grief may be involved as the ego relinquishes its former identity.

Extremes in any dimension must be carefully considered for elements of inflation and deflation. It is important to observe the stability of the footing from which the movement is initiated. Ascent or height in a sandplay process that indicates solid ego functioning will more likely attest to the client's ability to undergo an opening to new planes of awareness, than does one with a less solid footing. Height and ascent in sandplay work that is not based on solid ego functioning may be inflated. It might be an attempt to escape. It may also be an attempt to get an overview. It may have to do with the pursuit of conscious awareness or the masculine energies. Each situation must be considered from the context of its own reality.

AARON Aaron's work provides beautiful examples of the use of the vertical axis. Over the course of his sandplay it became clear that, in addition to his more pragmatic nature, **Aaron** has a profound spiritual side. In eight of his fifteen trays, **Aaron** suspends items above the sand tray. One spectacular example is **Aaron's Tray 12,** where he hangs a one-pound crystal star on string from the ceiling.

Aaron had his feet firmly planted on the ground, but there was a part of him that yearned to explore higher planes of existence. In **Aaron's** case there is no fear associated with these vertical ascents. In fact it felt as though he was very comfortable with these higher planes of consciousness. A follow-up interview with **Aaron** many years after completing his sandplay indicated that he remains deeply religious.

Vertical Ascent As Shamanic

Vertical ascent in sandplay may be concerned with shamanic explorations of the various dimensions of being. Unlike the souls of the dead, which are thought to move to other realms of existence after life, the shaman is able to move between the planes of being while still living. As we examined in our discussion of Mimir's well, the shaman ascends and descends the various dimensions of being with conscious intent. Upon his or her return to profane existence, the shaman brings the gifts of insight and wisdom garnered on the higher planes.

In sandplay common indicators of ascension are drawn from shamanic practices, such as ropes, trees, vines, kites, arrows, wings, rainbows and ladders. The presence of any of these elements does not indicate that the client is necessarily engaged in a shamanic ascent. Again, every element of a sandplay process must be allowed to inform us from within the context of its unique reality.

JASON Following a long struggle to integrate his deeply spiritual nature into his life in a meaningful way, **Jason**, a man in his forties, confronts new psychic contents in **Tray 19**. They first appear as a variety of terrifying monsters atop an island, which has emerged from the sea. The tensions of this moment of transformation are great. It is noteworthy, that the first figure **Jason** placed in the tray is the figure of an elephant that he had carved from a stone he found at the beach. As terrifying as it is, the new psychic qualities are firmly anchored in something wise and solid.

In **Tray 20**, **Jason** undertakes the shaman's vertical ascent through the figure of a small troll doll, who has climbed to the top of a golden tree. His elephant is now more developed and patrols the depths, along with a large whale, on top of which stands a magnificent tropical butterfly. The black and white panda bear enters the scene, as if to foretell a new integration.

In his final **Tray 21**, **Jason** returns to the earth with his newly integrated qualities from the depths and the heights. A large black and white zebra assumes a central position, as a colorful marching band plays in celebration. His golden tree is now a part of his natural psychic landscape. The fishing boat and the camel hold his new capacities to travel the depths as well as on the earth.

The Vertical Axis and the Chakras

Eliade (1952/I991) observed that the shaman climbs seven steps on the ceremonial ladder in his or her ascent up the World Tree. In so doing the shaman passes through seven planes of reality. This mythic ascent to higher planes of being is perhaps drawn from its energetic corollary in the human body. The ritual ascent of the shaman parallels the rise of *kundalini* energy in the body and its movement through the seven *chakras* as detailed in the Hindu tradition.

Ancient Hindu and later Buddhist tantric traditions identify invisible energy centers located in the body along the region of the spine. They are said to be activated from the base upwards as human consciousness undergoes change and transformation (Reyna, 1993). Each chakra, or *wheel*, is identified with particular qualities of consciousness, which refine and expand in ascending order from the root chakra at the base of the spine, up through the crown chakra, located at the top of the head. With the energizing of each chakra, ancient tradition has it that the initiate awakens to its characteristic qualities of consciousness.

The chakras are the energetic embodiment of the human potential to move into and beyond the limits of rationality. They are subtle energy centers that process the psychic energy that runs through each individual. We might liken them to electrical transformers, which receive current in one form and emit it in a transformed way. The forms of awareness experienced as the kundalini energy progresses up the spine range from the most fundamental conscious awareness of survival at the base, to the supreme union with cosmic being at the top. In this way the chakras may be regarded as developmental. There is a qualitative order to *psychic* development as the individual progresses through the chakras. For this reason, and because of the potential depths accessed during sandplay, it is important to be aware of the progression and qualities of psychic energy as it moves through the chakras. In his classic work, *Philosophies of India*, Heinrich Zimmer (1971) provided an authoritative account of the progression of psychic energy, or kundalini, through the various energy centers. Following are their names and qualities:

The First Chakra

The first chakra is known as *muladhara*. It is said to be located at the base of the spine and is known as the seat of the earth. The quality of energy at this chakra has to do with survival. As with the energy of any of the first three chakras, it may manifest either light or shadow qualities.

The Second Chakra

The second chakra is called *svadhisthana*. It is located at the level of the genital area and is associated with the element water. Energy at this level is concerned with generativity, or creativity. It may be expressed in any number of ways from raw sexuality to refined forms of creative expression.

The Third Chakra

The third chakra, located at the level of the navel, is called *manipura*. It is associated with the element of fire. This energy center has to do with power. Energy at the third chakra may develop as firm, steady empowerment. It may also run to warring aggression and violence.

Most people live their lives from these first three energy centers. The qualities of these energies manifest as concerns for survival, reproduction, aggression, and gain. Development of the energies of the four higher chakras is based upon the development in the lower three. Again we see that a firm grounding in the body and the world is a necessary prerequisite to development of higher levels of awareness.

The Fourth Chakra

The fourth chakra, known as *anahata*, is located at the level of the heart. It is at this level of energy that the individual becomes aware of the presence of the divine in the world. It is associated with the element of air.

In Jungian terms, we may say that the fourth chakra is the awareness of the Self. Thus, the psycho-physiological corollary to the constellation of the Self is the activation of the fourth chakra. When the Self is constellated, the individual becomes aware that all of life is divine and that there is an essential connection between all people and things. The fourth chakra is initially awakened at about age three and can be made the conscious center of life with subsequent individuation. When the fourth chakra is opened the individual becomes aware of his or her purpose in life as a return to the Self, or wholeness. For this reason, the three upper chakras are not generally considered to manifest shadow qualities. There are people, however, who forcibly open the upper chakras through specific yogic exercises, without having opened the underlying lower chakras and the heart. Instead of progressing in their psychic development up through the chakras in sequence, it is possible to bypass essential phases of development. In these cases, the qualities of the upper three chakras will manifest shadow qualities. The fifth chakra will manifest as energy given to wrong voice. An example of this is the compelling, though misguided religious orator, or political leader. The sixth chakra may manifest in what are known as *siddhis*, psychic and spiritual powers that permit movement and knowledge outside of the normal limits of body and space. Examples of such people are misdirected visionaries with selfish motivations. The crown chakra may open prematurely, providing the individual with a brief look at the possibilities of conscious awareness that may be developed with thorough grounding in work through all of the chakras. Yoga practitioners concur that the forcible premature opening of the crown chakra results in death (Yogiraj Sri Swami Satchidananda, personal communication, November 17, 1977).

The Fifth Chakra

The fifth chakra is known as *visuddha*. It is located at the level of the throat and is associated with the element ether. The energy of this chakra is said to be purified. Like its energetic counterpart in the third chakra, the fifth chakra has to do with the enacting of truth, of giving it voice. This is the center of conscious embodiment of the Self in thought and action.

The Sixth Chakra

The sixth chakra is called *ajna*, and is located at the point between the eyebrows. When one's energy reaches this level, the mind is said to be beyond the limits of the five elements and the senses. It is free to experience the immediacy of the divine. This is the center of divine contemplation. It is the seat of the meditative exploration of the Self as source and goal of being.

The Seventh Chakra

The seventh and top chakra is the *sahasrara*. It is located at the crown of the head. When consciousness emanates from this chakra it is said to be beyond all limits of duality. At this level of awareness, the individual experiences complete absorption, or oneness with the divine. From this place, one is fully absorbed in the Self.

The shaman and other enlightened beings are able to energetically travel up and back down these planes of consciousness.

There is certainly far more to know about the chakras than we have outlined here, and further study of Indian philosophy may appeal to some sandplay therapists. We have introduced the movement of kundalini through the chakras to provide a structural model for understanding the growth and development of human consciousness. This is one model among many and may appeal to some more than others. What concerns us as sandplay therapists is that we be able to track and contain the client's movement through these various qualities of experience in the sandplay process.

Depth and Descent

A descent, or going down, is concerned with the lower regions of the psyche and with the underworld. Eliade (1958/1996) observed that likening descent to a visit to the realm of the dead comes from the natural observation of the daily descent of the sun in the west. It is not a final death in that it returns each morning. Looked at from a psychological perspective, this is a descent into the dark regions of the unconscious. It can be terrifying, as we do not have the light of conscious awareness to find our way around. It is, by nature, unknown and shadowy.

A descent in sandplay can be evidenced in many ways. Digging down through the sand to the underlying blue water is a common form of descent. Movement of figures to a lower position might indicate a descent. Images and figures indicative of the shadowy unknown is another. Its content may be dark and chaotic. With a descent, there is a feeling of apprehension, of unknowing or even horror about the tray. The presence of caves or prominent trees in the sand tray may be indicators of descent. Shamanic tales frequently portray the shaman as descending into hell through a cavern, as well as along the axis of the World Tree (Eliade, 1952/1991). A tray that evidences depth indicates a descent into the unconscious. It may be concerned with the development of the feminine energies and the activation of the unconscious. Extremes of depth or descent may have to do with flooding and being overwhelmed by the unconscious.

The Marketplace

As we have previously discussed, a sandplay series may evidence a pattern of descent to the unconscious dimensions followed by ascent or a return to a more commonplace, ordinary world. We typically refer to this ordinary world as the *marketplace*. It may appear as an ordinary town or village scene with or without people going about daily tasks. The marketplace sandplay may assume any number of forms, but it always makes a striking contrast to its more archetypal precedents. It looks and feels normal and worldly.

In the processes of healing and transformation, a pattern of descent and return may occur several times. This may indicate that the client is accessing unconscious material and bringing it up to a more conscious position as the ego is enhanced and develops greater conscious awareness of the Self. This pattern of descent and return may also function to give the ego a rest as it relinquishes its hold on conscious awareness and confronts unconscious material.

The Horizontal Axis

The horizontal axis is traditionally symbolic of the earthly plane (Eliade, 1952/1991). It has to do with the circumstantial field, or the environmental challenges confronted by each person. The horizontal axis is concerned with the individual human being's passage through time and space. In this section, we will be concerned with the various ways the horizontal axis appears in sandplay as another thematic element to assist in our understanding of the sandplay process.

Diagonal Opposition

Diagonal configurations appear as figures facing each other from opposing corners of the tray. The appearance of figures on the horizontal plane along diagonals frequently carries insight into the nature of a primary conflict being addressed in the sandplay process. Diagonals represent the greatest distance available in the horizontal plane of the sand tray and can thus accommodate the full continuum of the negative and positive poles of a symbol. Additionally, diagonals are thought to be dynamic lines. These are places of movement and change.

Examining the symbolic qualities at both ends of a diagonal can lend great insight into the nature of the client's work that will be undergone in the sandplay process. Diagonal opposition often manifests early in the process in the first two or three trays, as the client's psyche settles on the work it needs to undertake in the sandplay.

Opposition on the horizontal dimension is concerned with the conscious reckoning of the polar antagonism in a symbol. This is the oppositional standstill we explored in our discussion of symbolic process. We recall that becoming conscious of both poles of the symbol results in the standstill of the ego, which is the precondition for the transcendent function.

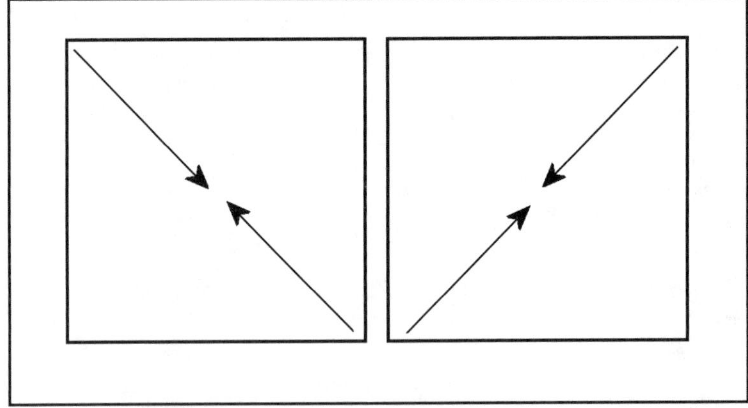

Diagonal Opposition in the Sandtray

When the conscious position, the ego, recognizes that it is unable to identify with both extremes of the opposition at the same time, the swing of conscious identification from one side to the other comes to a halt. The ego is paralyzed, as it no longer *knows* what it is. The paralysis of the polar antagonism in the symbol forces the psychic energy down into the unconscious. This brings new, and as yet unknown qualities to consciousness, which resolve the current dilemma. The new material is drawn from the archetypal core of the symbolic material currently undergoing transformation. The result is psychic growth and development. In Jungian terms this reconciliation of opposites is known as the *coniunctio.*

Parallel Confrontation

Parallel confrontations appear as lines of figures facing one another across the plane of the sand tray. Such horizontal confrontation in sandplay is the squaring off of balanced energies. This rivalry can appear as armies, monsters, animals, vehicles, and so on. Characteristically the sides are about equal and face each other in parallel formation.

The character of a parallel confrontation in the sandplay may be determined by the nature of the archetype that is activated in the client's

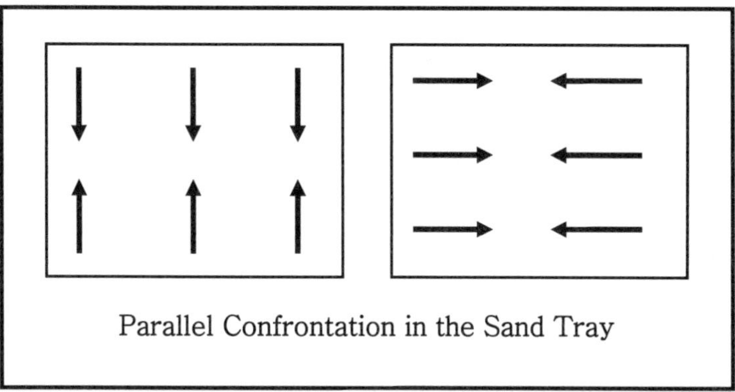
Parallel Confrontation in the Sand Tray

process. At times it is clear which archetype is held in the state of confrontation. More often, however, confrontations assume a more generic character.

The nature of the opposition is not necessarily clear from the appearance of the figures used in the confrontation. At times of confrontation, it is the opposition itself that is of greatest significance in the symbolic process. Whatever the nature of the work in process, ultimately this point of standstill between the opposites is itself archetypal.

AARON Diagonal configurations appear in **Aaron's Tray 1**, defining the nature of the work that lay ahead in his sandplay process. In the far left corner, a raging wild tiger roars at a lion tamer. On the diagonal in the near right corner, Batman poses over an angry, unruly bad guy, who attempts to escape in a red boat. Both ends of the diagonal hold uncontrolled rage and an ordering principle, the negative and positive poles of a core issue in **Aaron's** process. New positive potentials sit at the terminal lengths of the intersecting diagonal in the form of Asian wise men and artful, balanced skiers. A rigidly encased knight stands prominently at the intersection of the two diagonals. The dynamic energies of these diagonal configurations carry **Aaron's** uncontrolled rage and the need and possibility for order. They also hold his profound spiritual nature, the manner of its balance in his life and the rigid psychic defense in which he finds himself at the time of **Tray 1**.

In **Tray 6,** two armies line up for battle, facing each other across the plane of the sand tray. Mirroring the confrontation, a soldier representing each side confronts his opponent in the center. **Aaron's** conflicting psychic energies held in the diagonals of **Tray 1** equally square off in this tray, readied for the transformation ahead.

Lines in the Sand

Lines of figures moving in the same direction in the sand may relate to the client's history. As the horizontal dimension is concerned with movement through time and space, the lineage of the client may appear in a horizontal form. It is important to examine the character of the content of the lines that appear in the tray to develop an understanding of the intrapsychic components of the particular lineage. Lines may be about a family lineage, ethnicity, traditions and people here or gone. Lines may involve the client's intrapsychic lineage in the sense of defining a story or history, or they may have to do with both inner and outer history.

The movement of energy along the horizontal dimension of the sand tray is concerned with material, worldly embodiment. The appearance of lines of movement may have to do with the mobilization of energies regarding the symbolic work at hand. Significant blockages may similarly have to do with places of arrest or fixation that will require the client's deeper probing. It is important to notice in which direction the lines appear to move, where they are coming from, where they. We investigate the direction or movement of energy in greater detail in our examination of motion themes in sandplay

KAILEGH Seven-year-old **Kaileigh's Tray 5** features two lines of jewels, which create a brilliant pathway for the princess to follow. Organizing and transforming her formerly chaotic energies in **Trays 1 – 4**, these lines define a clear, hopeful future for **Kaileigh**.

ELIZABETH Lines of movement frequently appear in the work of **Elizabeth**. The inner and outer transformational passage that is ahead of her is delineated in her **Tray 1**, as a small frog begins the journey along a well-defined pathway. A small bell sits at the threshold of the pathway, which is marked by seven crystal stones. Although mirrors reflecting the truth of the Self define the path, **Elizabeth's** line of travel must first pass a line of horrors, consisting of four dark angels and three skulls. **Elizabeth** has to confront the demons of her past. Her line of travel necessarily requires that she pass by each one in an orderly fashion. The position of the demons at the beginnings of the journey suggests events from her history that require a systematic review and acceptance before further growth can take place.

In her final **Tray 11,** another line of travelers prepares to exit the transformational central area and to enter the outer world. This time the procession consists of a large-eyed gold fish who leads the way by seeing in the depths and a Native woman, securely mounted on her white horse of spirit and instincts. In her basket the woman carries babies and books. A bright-eyed baby girl, riding on top of a sow that shepherds her piglets along the path, follows up the procession. By confronting and integrating the demons from her history in her sandplay process, **Elizabeth** is now able to carry her own voice and to give it birth in her world.

Horizontal Use of the Sand Surface

Sometimes the sand is used as a format for a two-dimensional presentation, such as a drawing, handprints or a picture. When this occurs, it is important to consider if the sand tray has the quality of a statement of the client's firm presence in the horizontal plane. It may feel like a resounding affirmation of the client's being. In this way, the horizontal surface of the sand tray is employed as a firm ground upon which to stand, as an individual who is worthy and who belongs. By contrast, a two-dimensional presentation may feel tentative and unformed. This may be something that the client is not yet able to manifest, or make three-dimensionally concrete. It is significant in any case that it did make its appearance in the sand tray, however fragile or uncertain.

ISAAC Near the end of his sandplay process, young **Isaac** salutes his acceptance of a highly disturbing family event that he found devastating and confusing. In **Tray 23** he draws a simple happy face on the horizontal surface of the sand. The element of fire, which figures prominently throughout his process, now illuminates the smiling face. Referring to the fire, **Isaac** playfully remarks, *"It's in the middle of the forehead, instead of the middle of the forest!"*

Isaac comments that the golden soldier standing on the far right edge of the tray salutes the big, colorful flag he proudly plants in the far left corner of the tray. In this tray, the surface drawing functions as a base upon which the figures are grounded. The qualities of the surface and the figurative elements in **Isaac's Tray 23** work together symbolically in an eloquent integration of healing from grief and loss.

The Vertical and Horizontal Axes in Sandplay

To better understand the function of these two very important spatial themes in sandplay, we must look back to some of the dynamics of symbolic process we have already explored. We have learned from Jung (1960/1981) that symbols are creations of the psyche that arise to reveal a whole, complete reality that is currently unknown to consciousness. What is revealed in the symbol is unavailable in all other ways of knowing. The coincidence of opposites is held in symbols. Eliade (1952/1991) observed that this coexistence of polarities is found nowhere else in the experience of human kind. What is held by the symbol is not available to the rational thinking of humans. It is beyond duality.

Eliade (1952/1991) observed that the transformative power of the symbol can be understood when we recognize that the symbol becomes sacred, while it remains the same as it is. In other words, the outer form of the symbol is ordinary. It is of this world. It suffers the comings and goings of duality. At the same time however, the active, charged, alive aspect of the symbol encompasses the totality of duality. It surpasses duality. This aspect of the symbol transcends time and space. It abides in the dimension of the eternal and is sacred.

Matters of transcendence involve both the horizontal and the vertical planes of existence. Time and space, on the horizontal dimension, are necessarily involved in transition to the eternal, on the vertical dimension. While transcendence is ultimately concerned with moving beyond time and entering the eternal via the vertical axis, the transcend-*ing*, the vertical movement between planes, occurs in the embodied dimension of time and space on the horizontal axis.

In our work in sandplay, the horizontal dimension is necessarily involved as psychic movement occurs along the vertical axis. Sandplay literally embodies the symbolic process that seeks to move beyond the limits of time and space. The sand tray functions as the horizontal axis that gives substance and form to the symbolic process that moves along the vertical axis in the eternal. In this way sandplay might be thought to assume the symbol of the cross. Just as the vertical and horizontal dimensions of the cross intersect in their archetypal form, so the process of sandplay functions as a point of intersection of the eternal with the material field. It is at this point of intersection that change or transformation occurs.

The Center

The center and the act of centering are of great significance in sandplay as they are concerned with the archetype of the Self. Because of this, the symbol of the center is associated with the cosmic axis. The center is likened to the archetypal center of the world and is the place at which ascent to other planes of existence is possible (Eliade 1952/1991). As we learned from the Yggdrasil myth, the cosmic tree stands in the center of the world as an axis that connects the planes of heaven, earth and the underworld.

The central mountain is a frequent construction in sandplay. The mountain is considered sacred because it reaches toward the higher planes. Eliade (1958/1996) observed that the mountain assumes the role of the sacred center because it serves as a temple in nature. It is the highest point of the universe and is thus where the earth is thought to be closest to heaven. Likewise, the center may be thought of as an earth navel, the *omphalos* and thus the point that joins the earth with the lower regions of the underworld.

The Sand Tray and the Center

Eliade (1952/1991) observed that any place where the sacred has manifested is regarded as a center. Any spatial locality where someone has broken through the plane of commonly observed reality similarly becomes a sacred place or center. In this sense sandplay functions as a cosmic center. The sand tray and its attendant field of reverence repeatedly function as the locus of movement through the planes of reality. Sandplay works as the spatial location of the manifestation of the sacred and doing sandplay is a sacred ritual.

The design of the sand tray pulls the psyche toward centering. The physical dimensions of the tray are designed to fill the visual field of the individual without requiring eye movement. This facilitates a relaxation of the hold on conscious awareness and allows access to less conscious perceptions, which emanate from the central archetype of the Self. The motility of the sand allows the client to give form to the archetypal energies that are ready to become manifest from the regions below conscious awareness.

Just as engagement in the ritual of sandplay promotes access to sacred space, it also facilitates entry into sacred time. To enter sacred time is to enter timelessness. It is outside of the profane and is by nature without time, or eternal. Sacred time is *now*. Eliade (1958/1996) observed that the mythic enactment of ritual functions to reinstate the original sacred event being represented. The ritual enactment is not an *as if* it were happening now; rather, it recreates the *original mythic act in the present moment.*

This has critical bearing on sandplay when we begin to appreciate that the mythic presentations rendered in the sand tray by the client are *actually occurring in the client's psyche at that very moment.* There is *no separation* between the client's movements of the sand and figures and the very real movement of his or her psyche. The ritual engagement in the sacred time and space of the sand tray concurrently moves the psyche.

When working in the sand tray, the client exits profane time and space.

He or she enters a highly charged and powerful place where the sacred makes itself manifest and time stands still. All that the sandplay holds for the client, whether it is worldly memory, collective memory, or mythic archetypes of unconscious patterns and potentials, is occurring for the client *at that very moment.*

Constellation of the Self in Sandplay

Ultimately life is a journey to the center. It is a return to the source of one's being and a passage out of un-truth. This accurately describes sandplay. As the Self is the source of all being, it may be said that all creations in the sand tray are manifestations of various aspects of the underlying archetype of the Self.

It is common to see work on various issues in the sand tray, only to see the same issues later brought to the center. This is not a constellation of the archetype of the Self, but rather a re-ordering of previously disconnected elements to the central wholeness.

Eliade observed that raising the question of the center, or simply becoming conscious of the existence of the center is sufficient, "...for the life of the cosmos to be for ever renewed (1952/1991, pg. 56)."

Psychologically, to raise the question of the center initiates the journey and re-orders worldly passage to the Self. It does not however, necessitate its discovery. The life quest is ultimately about approaching the central truth of the Self and embodying centeredness in action. Symbolically the center is the point of what is most sacred and the place where one attains to immortality. Being what is most precious, it is frequently guarded by a serpent or a dragon.

ELIZABETH A tiny green dragon guards a golden egg beneath the crown at the center of **Elizabeth's Tray 2**. At the terminus of an inward-turning spiral of pearls originating in the uroborous, it is clear that **Elizabeth's** process will demand considerable sacrifice. The colorful jester carries the voice of truth and submits to sacrifice to protect the king when necessary. A crucifix mirrors the sacrifice that is necessary to abide in the center. While this tray is not a constellation of the Self, it clearly indicates movement toward what is central.

The constellation of the Self in sandplay is a momentous event. In the experience of this sand tray, the client has the nascent realization of the oneness of the deepest Self. He or she is profoundly and irrevocably changed. With the constellation of the Self dawns an awareness of the deepest connection to being. With this awareness comes meaning and purpose to life. And with the constellation of the Self comes a palpable awareness of the inter-connection of all of life and one's own participation in this profound, living relationship.

The constellation of the Self is shared and witnessed by the therapist. The certainty of the reality of the Self as the core of being is firmly established in this mutual experience of client and therapist. The client's participation in this wholeness is real and undeniable.

With the constellation of the Self, the client's entire life begins to re-order to the central archetype of the Self. Dora Kalff (1980/2003) described the constellation of the Self as the *beginning* of the healthy development of the ego. Kalff observed that with the awareness of the Self, choices can be made with resonance to the callings of the deepest truth. Actions can be taken in accord with ultimate meaning. The ego, the conscious position in the psyche, becomes aware that it does not function as an independent choice maker. Rather, the ego acquiesces to the service of the Self for greater purpose.

The energy attending the constellation of the Self in sandplay is breath-taking. Dora Kalff (1980/2003) described it as *numinous*. What is numinous is defined as, "revealing or suggesting the presence of god" (OED, 1994). It inspires awe and reverence. What is numinous is, by definition, an active event. It is an occurrence of the presence of the divine happening in that sandplay at that moment in time and space. At the same time, it is eternal and transcends time and space. The experience of the constellation of the Self in sandplay is unforgettable. The room fills with numinosity and the relationship between the client and the therapist is suffused with the awareness of a mutual participation in the sacred. Even years after witnessing a constellation of the Self, observing a photo of the sand tray can re-activate the numinous event. This re-experience of the numinosity from the artifact of a photograph gives us a sense of the manner in which contact with the Self, with the center, transcends all time and space.

The constellation of the Self in the sand tray assumes any number of forms. It generally appears in circular or radiate form because of its nature as the central archetype. However there are no rules or formulae to the presentation of the Self in the sand tray. It is primarily identified by its numinous qualities.

The constellation of the Self does not occur in all sandplay cases. Some processes may be marked with a distinct *shift* instead of a full constellation of the Self. After such a shift, the sandplay process may evidence dramatic healing or transformation. We saw a wonderful example of such a shift in nine-year-old **Ivy's Tray 10** in our discussion of the archetype of the Self. In lieu of a full constellation of the Self, **Ivy's** work took a dramatic turn after she tapped the central source of being through her village well.

Why the constellation of the Self does or does not occur in a particular case is difficult to say. Perhaps the client is not prepared for a full constellation of the Self. Perhaps the client's psyche is already centered in the Self archetype. Perhaps the client lives in an abiding awareness of the Self. Again, we must be careful not to exercise any judgments. Each case must be honored in its own uniqueness.

The constellation of the Self generally occurs in the middle of a sandplay process. As the Self is the central and deepest archetype, its constellation is the deepest part of a process. This fact implies that some preliminary work in the sand tray takes place that facilitates movement toward the Self. It also assumes that there is work subsequent to the Self constellation in the return to an ordinary level of awareness. However, the Self constellation may appear closer to the beginning of a process or more toward the end. Even with these general considerations, it is clear that there is no way of knowing if and when the Self may constellate in a particular process. Each case must be considered in its own unique manner of presentation.

Although the client certainly has the sense of the sacred nature of the Self constellation, its full integration into conscious awareness is not complete at the time the tray is made. As with any other work done in the sand, its integration into consciousness lags behind its appearance in the tray. Importantly, the constellation of the Self demarcates the central point for re-ordering subsequent and prior life attitudes and experiences. We should not expect it to be fully understood or fully integrated into conscious awareness. The constellation of the Self is an embodied experience of the archetype of the center. It is a deep level of knowing of which the individual becomes increasingly conscious with accumulated experience and in concert with a specific intention to understand.

With the constellation of the Self, the client experiences an opening to vast resources of energy. The therapist must be alert to the proper containment of these newly found energies coursing through the client. The client's behavior can change dramatically. Without proper containment it is even possible for the client to get carried away with overwhelming projects in an almost manic-like frenzy. Sandplay pioneer Estelle Weinrib provided a memorable account of her sudden flight into a huge remodeling project in *Images of the Self* (1983/2004) after the Self constellation in her own sandplay process. It may be important to talk with the client, or parents of child clients, about the possible release of great energies and the need to be aware of them. This is a perfect time to encourage both child and adult clients to engage in art work and movement, or perhaps meditation for adults.

As the source of all being, the constellation of the Self in sandplay will necessarily include some acknowledgement or reference to darkness. Recall the dark orb and the attendance of naughty Pinocchio in the Self tray of **Lenae's Tray 14**. The reason for the presence of some form of darkness is that the completeness of being also encompasses the underworld. The authority of the Self becomes central, and all of life's experiences are seen as emanating from and returning to this center.

Manifestation of the Self in Sandplay

In my work I have observed subtle differences between a *constellation* of the Self and a *manifestation* of the Self. My experience indicates that the manifestation of the Self is the appearance, or touching of the Self in the casework of clients who have already had the experience of the Self constellation. In some cases, the client's psyche has centered in the Self in their course of normal development. In some cases, the constellation of the Self has occurred visibly in prior sandplay work.

While not common, it does happen that the client has an abiding awareness of the Self as center before beginning the sandplay process. This type of work is the way of wisdom or shamanic engagement that we described earlier in our discussion of the differing processes of sandplay therapy. Eliade (1964/1974, 1952/1991) stated that to be conscious of the center is the shamanic way of change. Such clients are conscious of the adaptation of their life experience to a deeper purpose. This is evident in their sandplay, where the Self is felt as an abiding presence, or is frequently alluded to as an organizing principle.

Mindful of this, I distinguish between the constellation of the Self as the initial numinous realization of the oneness of the deepest Self and the manifestation of the Self as the subsequent appearances or references to the Self in the work of people whose lives and sandplay inherently acknowledge the central organizing purpose of the Self. The constellation of the Self is characterized by numinosity, the *active* revealing of the presence of the divine. The numinosity is born of the divine presence being manifest in the moment. The manifestation of the Self on the other hand, might be described as *mystical*. It has the quality of a sacred mystery. It is a known spiritual truth that has been revealed through divine revelation. It is known because it has already been revealed.

Other Fundamental Spatial Configurations in Sandplay: Squares, Circles, Triangles, Stars, Radiate Patterns, and Spirals

In the language of symbols, we view basic geometric shapes as the psyche's earliest and quintessentially archetypal manifestations of being in material form. Simple shapes such as the circle, the square, the triangle, and so on, are the rudimentary indications of oneness, or the embodiment of non-manifest being. To better understand the significance of the various geometric shapes, we first need to return to the psychic threshold through which what is non-manifest enters embodied manifestation.

The Buddhist tradition describes the dimension of being immediately before material manifestation as comprised of five *skandhas*, or essences that come together to form differing shapes. It is thought that the *skandhas* are effervescent qualities that give rise to shape and form by moving in and out of contact with each other. This concept may lend understanding to sandplay when we consider the combined qualities of the plasticity of the sand and the suspension of time and outer reality that are inherent in the method. Perhaps the basic geometric configurations that appear so frequently in the sand tray are the very earliest fashioning of new reality. Like the movement of the *skandhas,* perhaps the nascent character of sandplay provides a venue for the manifestation of new embodied possibility.

The Hindus have a similar concept that describes what we call "reality" as *maya,* or "illusion." All phenomena that exist in *maya* are referred to as *samsara,* the flux and flow that give rise to form. Of particular interest to us as sandplay therapists is the Hindu observation that *play,* or *lila,* is the essential nature of the comings and goings of *maya.* Play *is* the essence of change, and all that exists is forever changing. This concept has corollaries in the Chinese *I Ching,* or *Book of Changes,* where the only unchanging constant is thought to be change, itself (I Ching, 1950/1971).

It was no accident that Dora Kalff (1980/2003) gave the name *play* to her method of working in the sand tray. Sandplay establishes the environment in which the psyche moves to restructure our reality. The sandplay client's movement of sand and figures in the tray in the safe and respectful presence of the witnessing therapist provides the material environment for an analogous movement and reordering of first inner and later, outer reality. The relatively unrestricted possibility of the sand provides the material format for this play of change, for the movement and re-ordering of psyche.

Time is suspended in the dimension of play. The client engages with the immediacy and total receptivity of the sand, giving form to new reality. This psychic movement and change may emerge in the sand as fundamental structures, such as circles, spirals, stars, and so on. These basic shapes serve to define space. They create an order and a means of orientation. A means of orientation supports the growth of meaning and purpose. With this in mind, the common appearance of basic geometric shapes and forms in the sand tray becomes understandable.

The various geometric shapes embody particular characteristics that are well articulated in symbol dictionaries and reference materials. As with all material of a symbolic nature, it is never possible to fully understand the breadth and fullness of any geometric shape. Although we cannot fully abstract the meaning held by the shape occurring in a sand tray from its particular context, we generally ascribe common archetypal qualities to the basic geometric forms. We will not attempt a complete discussion of each shape, but will concern ourselves briefly with their general traits. When geometric configurations do appear in sandplay, the therapist must bear in mind the following along with many other possible symbolic potentials. The two most important considerations are to be mindful of the essential emergent nature of geometric shapes and to avoid reductionism.

The Square and the Circle

Given its four equal sides and right angles the square is thought to hold qualities of stability, grounded-ness, embodiment, temporal existence and materiality. By contrast, the circle is considered the eternal. The circle holds the quality of perfection, in the sense of ultimate Oneness (De Vries, 1984).

Dora Kalff (1980/2003) gave particular attention to the circle and the square. Kalff maintained that in the course of normal development at about age three, "...the center of the Self is stabilized in the unconscious of the child and begins to manifest itself in symbols of wholeness" (p.2). Kalff observed that squares, or units of four, appear in sand trays as psychic wholeness develops in the client. It is soon after, or in conjunction with the square that the circle emerges in the sandplay. Kalff observed that the appearance of the square and the circle are the budding material manifestation of the psyche's drive toward order. Kalff recognized the fundamental geometric shapes as powerful symbols that work on the psyche to establish order and wholeness. In her classic work, *Sandplay: A Psychotherapeutic Approach to the Psyche*, she commented,

> The circle is not only a geometrical form; it is also a symbol that brings to light something which lives invisibly in man. Symbols speak for the inner, energy-laden pictures, of the innate potentials of the human being which, when they are manifested, continue to influence the development of man. (p. 6)

Martin Kalff (1993) distinguished between curvilinear and angular shapes in the sand tray. While round, curving shapes are commonly thought to reflect a more feminine energy and are associated with feeling and the body, Kalff observed that angular shapes, by contrast, are considered to carry a more masculine energy. They reflect rationality and the mind.

Martin Kalff's consideration of the energetic difference in line quality gives me to wonder about possible differences in line quality between the sandplays of clients with a predominant thinking function and those with strong features in the other functions, sensation, intuition and feeling. This will no doubt prove a rich area of future research.

> **SHANNON** Angular and geometric shapes are characteristic of **Shannon's** sandplay. **Shannon** is a strong thinking type person. Her trays are supported by angular configurations. **Shannon** frequently began her work in the sand with sharp designs she sculpted with the sides of her hands. The repeated geometric structures in **Shannon's** sandplay process lend support to Kalff's observations. **Trays 1, 6** and **8** all carry this dramatic sculptural foundation. The sculptural angularity softens in **Trays 15** and **17**, where **Shannon's** psyche opens to new qualities of being. While **Shannon's** sandplay work maintains its overall sculptural quality, her new relationship to her inner and outer worlds is borne by the subtler, perhaps softer relationship to the form of the sand.

Triangles and Stars

The triangle may be seen as the division of a square into two halves. In this sense the two halves refer to the two poles of material manifestation, the masculine and the feminine. When pointed upward, the triangle holds the masculine principle. When it points down, it is the feminine. When the upward and downward triangles interlace, they form the Star of David, the conjunction of opposites. The equal-sided triangle is stable, as it sits on a firm base. Its three sides also allude to the trinity, or the interface of spirit between earth and heaven (De Vries, 1984).

> **IVY** **Ivy's Tray 1** begins her series with a dramatic triangular pond. Generally pointing downward, this triangle foretells the exploration of her feminine nature that her sandplay work would undertake.

Stars are complex figures, with particular attributes based on the number of points. In the heavens, the stars reflect the light of the sun and illuminate the night sky. The energy held by star symbolism is rich and bears thorough consideration when stars appear prominently in sandplay. As a geometric figure, the five-pointed star is interesting. Upon creating the initial line, it is formed by bisecting the opposite line (De Vries, 1984). The five-pointed star is likened to the complete human being, the *anthropos*, with two arms, two legs and a head.

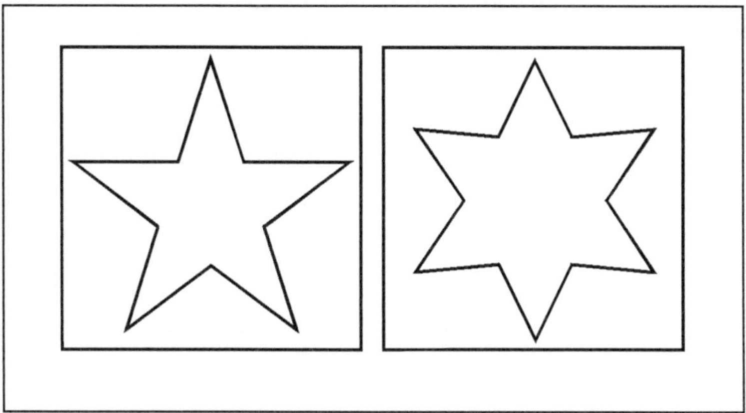

Five- and six-pointed stars.

ELIZABETH Elizabeth's Tray 10 is an interesting use of the five-pointed star. Centrally located, the sparkling star carries wholeness. At the same time however, it forms a cage for the dead doctor, who is held captive inside. Acknowledging that her esteemed career must end in order for her growth to continue, this central star holds both death and the promise of fullness.

Radiate and Spiral Figures

Radiate and spiral figures are concerned with the center, which we have discussed above. Both figures bear the movement of energy either from the center outward, or from an outer to a center point.

Radiate figures function primarily in the horizontal plane, while spirals may integrate movement in both horizontal and vertical directions. Radiate forms consist of many lines of energy centrally connected. Psychologically speaking, a radiate pattern is an emanation from the center. In some instances, the lines of radiation may also indicate a return to the center, perhaps as an acknowledgment of the centrality of the Self.

The spiral is a single linear path that travels in a curvilinear direction upon itself. The spiral may be flat upon a horizontal surface, or it may extend vertically. When operating along the vertical axis, the spiral may hold energy that moves either to the right or to the left from a lower outer place to a central high point or the reverse higher to lower movement. Conversely, the energy may travel in a right or left direction from a higher, outer place to a lower central point, as well as from a lower, inner point to a higher outer one. The spiral is a rich and complex psychic form. The spiral bears all facets of manifestation from the source. Concurrently, the spiral holds all facets of destruction and return to the source. The spiral holds this movement of energy for the individual as destiny and for each moment in time. The spiral carries the perennial truth of the cosmos for all of time and beyond time in eternity. The spiral also holds the complete history, or lineage of the significance of each moment in the passage of the individual and for all of human kind.

The archetypal significance of each figure and the directions of their energetic movements are both important in sandplay. Attention to these considerations may strengthen the containment of the client's emerging development and lend some understanding to these early manifestations of newness in the sand.

Considerations of Placement in Sandplay

The spatial location of the sandplay figure or sand formation may lend particular significance to the symbolic process undergone in the tray. We have previously discussed the important spatial dimensions in sandplay. As we recall, both horizontal and vertical dimensions bear great significance and consideration in the containment of sandplay process. Given this foundational understanding, in this section we will examine some details of placement in the tray.

Prominent Figures and Forms

Although we recognize that the entire sandplay process functions in a symbolic manner, it is clear that prominent figures or formations carry added significance in the process. These may appear in individual trays, or be seen throughout the sandplay series in various forms. A wonderful example of a prominent figure is the large mental-encased knight in the first tray of **Aaron**.

> **AARON** The size and the central location of the knight in **Aaron's Tray 1** gives the observer the definite impression that the symbolic content held by this figure is a prominent aspect of this client's work. In **Aaron's** final sandplay the metal figure returns, now transformed into a silver loving cup. Standing beside it is a small fighter who faces the enemies he overcame during his work. Behind him, on the other side of a small stream, lies the new, peaceful life that has opened up to him. In this example, it is the size and central placement of the figure that indicates its prominence. In addition, the energy of the large knight is dark and heavy. Its reappearance in a variety of forms throughout the case also underscores its significance.

There are certainly no formulae to determine what if anything is prominent in sandplay. Prominence may be indicated by extremes in the spectrum of possibilities. It may be awfully large, or very small, incredibly near or especially far. It may be up high, or exceptionally deep. It may be particularly bright or colorful, or profoundly dark. It may have a particular emotional impact. To observe what is prominent provides the therapist another means for coming into relationship with the greater symbolic process of sandplay.

Hidden and Buried Figures

The flexibility of the sand creates the possibility of hiding or burying figures in the tray. Figures may be secreted away in caves, locked in chests, tucked carefully behind something else or craftily hidden behind foliage in a tree or shrub. It is a common experience to see figures placed in the tray, then buried. Sometimes they are repeatedly buried, exhumed, re-buried, and so on.

In one of her many studies of the Lowenfeld World Technique, researcher Ruth Bowyer Pickford (1956) observed that burying figures in the sand can be an aggressive or hostile gesture. However, she quoted Eve Lewis from the Exeter Child Guidance Clinic, saying,

> I have observed the careful burying of some toy to indicate, not aggression, but acceptance of that which the toy symbolized in the collective unconscious (p. 162).

What Lewis described is the child's thoughtful acceptance of the symbol into the body of the child's being via its incorporation into the corpus of the sand. In this example, it is the gesture of the burying that lends its particular meaning.

All gestures of burial are not so clear, and we can only speculate as to what their significance might be. Again, they are uniquely relevant to their own context. What seems important is the intent of the gestures undertaken with the objects being hidden, buried and otherwise concealed.

Not only is *what* is being hidden significant psychically and symbolically, but the very fact *that it is being hidden* is of equal importance. If we remember that all aspects of the sandplay are faces of the overriding drive toward wholeness, we must consider the role this gesture of hiding plays in the movement toward integration.

Where the hiding place is located may be an important consideration. Some factors to take into account might be whether the hiding place is at a distance from, very near, above or below other significant features in the tray. What the hiding place consists of may also be an important consideration. The symbolic content held by the hiding and by what is hidden will be different if it is, for example, a weapon, a person, or a golden egg.

In the case of buried figures it is important to consider whether the figure might be going down or coming up. Figures that are going down may be issues that are repressed. These might be issues that were once known to conscious awareness, but have been pushed back into the personal unconscious, into the shadows. Perhaps these are qualities or events that the client is developmentally unequipped to deal with, so must repress for the time being. However their presence in the sandplay indicates that they figure prominently in the growth and transformation being undertaken by the client.

If what is buried is coming up, it may be an unconscious quality that is emerging. Similarly, it may be a shadow feature that is re-emerging. The nascent emergence of figures in sandplay is a budding acknowledgement of their symbolic content. Because they are present, albeit deep down, we do know that they are becoming available to the client. For example, when we see a hidden or buried treasure that has not fully emerged in the sand tray, we share in the client's dawning awareness of the treasure of his or her wholeness.

What is buried may also be something fully conscious that is being given a proper funeral. This may be a quality that is no longer needed. Maybe it is a wounding or self-concept that is undergoing transformation and is being released from the ego's grasp.

Perhaps the burying is a return to the earth of what is dead, as a participation in the cycle of birth and death. Like the dead, who are buried in the earth in anticipation of transformed life ahead, burial in sandplay may be concerned with the end of particular identities and ways of being. Such a burial in the sand may foretell transformation that is fed by the riches of the underworld.

To enter the earth is to enter the darkness and to release the hold of consciousness. A burial parallels the planting of a seed. In the chaos of the unformed darkness of the underworld, the original form of the seed disintegrates and gives rise to new form. In this sense, burial is like an entry into the underworld as a means of being fertilized for new growth. When burial manifests as planting and new growth in sandplay, it is important to pay attention to what might eventually gestate and reemerge from the womb of the earth. It would impede the symbolic process to assume that we know what will emerge, but it is critical that we hold the *possibility* for transformed being.

Relationship of Figures in Sandplay

The degree of relationship between figures and elements in the sand tray is another important feature of the spatial dimension of sandplay. The relationship between elements in sandplay may range from chaos at one end of the spectrum to rigidity at the other.

High Levels of Relatedness in Sandplay

The extent to which the figures within the tray are meaningfully related can indicate the extent to which the psyche is organizing what were previously confused, or unconscious elements. Generally speaking, greater relatedness indicates a higher degree of differentiation. We recall from our discussion of Jungian personality theory that the differentiation of the four functions into distinct activities of psychic experience plays a major part in individuation, or the development of the individual personality. A fundamental component of individuation is the person's growing ability to maintain a clear sense of personal identity *in relationship to* other people and things.

Take careful note of the quality, or the nature of the relationships within the tray. When the relationships among objects and scenes appear fluid and relaxed, it may indicate that the client is safe and at peace with this phase of psychic movement or development. If the relationship between the figures and activity seems rigid and tense, it may indicate fear from within the client. Such rigidity may also allude to real outer world threats to development or personal safety. Rigidly controlled configurations may include both inner and outer threats. Alternations between rigid and fluid relational patterns in a sandplay, or from tray to tray might embody movement in and out of areas of threat.

An important consideration is the significance of relationship and unrelatedness in sandplay in the overall context of the symbolic presentation. For example, if the case evidences a predominant quality of strong relationship and differentiation, a tray in the series with an unrelated, more chaotic presentation might indicate a temporary dissolution of ego boundaries in the service of growth and transformation. When this occurs, a deconstruction may be underway prior to the emergence of new, creative elements from the unconscious.

KAILEIGH Seven-year-old **Kaileigh's** sandplay is a beautiful study of the changes in the element of relationship over the course of the work. **Kaileigh's Tray 1** holds an almost random distribution of fantasy people and animals around a table, which is set for tea. While the elements around it are scattered and hold little relationship to one another, the central table does provide a relational anchor point. Everything is going on around it.

In addition, the placement of the well and the jeweled house on the near left-far right diagonal and the praying girl and the beautiful rearing horse on the opposite diagonal provide a form of archetypal relationship. From the structural container of the corner figures and the table and the symbolic energies they hold, **Kaileigh's** sandplay process carries the prospect of the truth of Self to be found in her depths (the jeweled house and the well), grounded in a balance of instinct (the horse) and self-awareness (the praying girl). These symbolic qualities cross in the round tea table, which promises nurturing and comfort.

As she places figures in the sand in **Tray 2, Kaileigh** verbalizes a story that concerns her pain and loss. The characters in her story bear more advanced relationship than the items in **Tray 1**. When the symbolic content of the emerging story becomes very painful, **Kaileigh** buries the evidence beneath a flood of objects poured from baskets. My session notes read:

(Figure placement is followed by verbalizations in *italics*)

Golden eagle
Silver bird
His wife.
Large white bear
The doctor. The doctor said, "I'm sorry, you cannot have your baby, because it is dead in your stomach."
Prince
Hedge hog
Poor pup. He took him to the doctor and said, "Someone shot him in the leg. He wants to find his mother."
Mermaid
He asked if she was his mother. "No!"
Batman
Him? "No!"
Zeus
Him? "No, but I live in the sky and will make your life special."

Jewels (poured into tray)
(Speaking to therapist) *What if I took everything and made a big mess and never cleaned it up?*
Therapist: Would you want to do that?
No, but I could!
Gold (poured baskets of the following)
Whales
Gold
Jewels
Pigs
Food
Umbrellas
Musical Instruments
Music!
Yarn and string
Body Parts
Poured in more baskets of items
People said it was a piece of junk, but they came up and stole the money.
Therapist: Is there a title for this one?
"The Night of the Witches, Gold, and the Poor Animal"

Kaileigh's flooding in **Tray 2** reflects her emerging recognition of her painful history. At the same time, it serves as the deconstruction of the false sense of self that is necessary to re-order her ego to the Self for a healthy growth process. In **Kaileigh's Tray 2**, the figure placement prior to the flooding shows movement toward greater relatedness. This is reflected in the symbolic content of the story, which dives into the well of her depths to symbolically reveal her pain and loss.

The relationship of the figures continues to evolve as **Kaileigh's** process moves forward. At the same time, the thematic content of her impromptu fairy tales progresses. By **Tray 6,** the spatial placement of the characters in **Kaileigh's** personal version of the story of *Rapunzel,* is coherent. The figures move into a meaningful relationship to one another, as the story she tells reflects a painful history of loss, deprivation and needs that were beyond her control.

Bridges as Relational Connection

Bridges may appear as conduits of relationship, which bring together formerly discreet, or unrelated psychic elements in the sandplay. In sandplay the transcendence of opposites concerns the appearance of the opposition, as well as the places where the opposites are able to come together. It is about the gateways, the portals, the narrow places and interstices where the polarities meet. It is at this point of coming together that the center of the Self is tapped. It is at this place of coming together that rich unconscious material is accessed and made available to consciousness. Ultimately, it is in this reconciliation of the opposites that the reality of the Self is attained.

When bridges appear it is important to observe what is being connected. Bridging may occur in any number of ways in sandplay. Bradway and McCoard (1997) observed that elements that appear between opposites may serve to reconcile them. They may function to bridge the polar conflict held by the symbolic process. This may appear in the literal form of bridges, or as any variety of figures that serve as linking devices in the symbolic work.

When bridges appear to make no apparent connection, or seem to aimlessly float in the sand tray, they may evidence a disorientation of the psyche. When this occurs, the presence of the bridge holds the awareness that connecting is needed. The bridge is, after all, selected and is in the sand tray. The psyche has not yet moved to a place that clarifies what is to be connected or how the integration will be accomplished. The elements to be connected may be present in the same tray with the bridge, or may have appeared in an earlier tray. In the case of these *floating* bridges, it is important to examine the process for what appears to be fragmented, or split off. This may facilitate containment of the later bridging.

When a bridge does connect two elements, it is equally important to examine what it is that is being bridged. Martin Kalff (1993) emphasized the qualities on either end of a bridge. Kalff observed that a more energetic connection is formed when the bridge connects distinctly different scenes or qualities. He commented that connections bridged between very similar scenes may indicate low energy or a lack of decisiveness.

LEELA A striking example of the use of a bridge as a point of psychic synthesis occurs in six-year-old **Leela's Trays 11** and **12. Leela's** work revolves around her attempts to resolve the profound intrapsychic disparities resulting from her warring parents' divorce dispute. Not since she was two years old had her parents even spoken. Only silently and from the safe distance of the street had they exchanged the child for weekly visitations.

Leela's psyche was so divided she often found it necessary to construct two separate worlds in two separate sand trays. In **Trays 11 – 12**, done on the same day, **Leela** builds her two worlds then carefully places a bridge to connect them in the far right corner of **Tray 11**. While the bridge does not physically yet reach **Tray 12**, which sits beyond and below **Tray 11**, the psychic bridging required to re-connect the severed aspects of her inner world is now in place. Although it appeared impossible that the two parents would ever come together peacefully, the appearance of the bridge between her two worlds indicates that **Leela** is able to repair the severe fissure in her internal world.

Happily, **Leela's** bridge was also prescient regarding her parents' relationship. A follow up many years after her sandplay bore the good news that Mom and Dad were able to work kindly and cooperatively to raise their beautiful child.

Low Levels of Relatedness in Sandplay

Tentative Relationship

Tentative relationship among figures in the sand tray appears when figure placement indicates some degree of association, but not an evident or clear affiliation. For example, animal or human figures may be near one another, yet not clearly doing something together, walking side by side, looking at each other, and so on. Tentative figure relationship may occur in the course of a process when psychic contents are re-ordering.

Tentative relationship among figures in what is otherwise more relational work is likely concerned with the characteristic de-construction or re-construction of transformation and is a meaningful and understandable aspect of psychic development. Disjointed or unrelated groups or elements in sandplay may evidence a fragmented psyche. This may reflect conditions of severe wounding or of developmental deprivation. The fragmented groups or figures also indicate the psychic elements that seek a cohesive organization. Over the course of the sandplay process we hope to see the disparate elements move into meaningful relationship to one another, leading toward the client's more integrated personality. These normal process components are very different from sandplay work that holds a predominantly tentative character, which is our current concern.

The tentative quality of the sandplay may indicate the client's resistance to the process. Perhaps sandplay is threatening, or too evocative to the client and thus it may not be wise to engage in a sandplay process.

A serious consideration in tentative sandplay presentations is whether the therapist is adequately prepared to hold what may emerge in the course of a sandplay process. Perhaps, whether consciously or unconsciously, the client does not feel secure with the therapist. Frequently when therapists attempt to do sandplay work without the proper training and experience, they report that their clients do not seem interested in doing sandplay after the initial one or two trays. Although the transference between client and therapist might otherwise be strong, the necessary *co-transference*, described by Katherine Bradway (Bradway & McCoard, 1997) is not sufficiently in place to engage in sandplay. For the client to feel safe enough to agree to engage in the depths of psyche evoked by work in the sand tray, it is essential that the therapist embody a very sound grasp of sandplay and that he or she undergo extensive preparation. The co-transference of sandplay holds not only the mutually shared field of psyche of the therapist and the client, it simultaneously holds the sandy medium in which the client's psyche is invited to move and venture freely. For the therapist to be unfamiliar, or uncertain of the possibilities of sandplay is to invite harm, if not disaster. We thoroughly explore the issue of sandplay therapist training and preparation in the material on sandplay procedures.

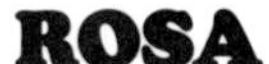

Twelve-year-old **Rosa's** sandplay is a good

example of work that progresses from a tentative to more stable state of relatedness. **Tray 1** reflects a highly tentative condition. **Rosa** began her brief work in the sand in a highly fearful manner. As we saw in our discussion of the ego, **Rosa** stood, touching the sand for a period of ten to fifteen minutes. Her touch was light, but hesitant. I recall watching and holding her uncertainty, wondering if her reticence might move into more certainty. In lieu of the anticipated affective shift, there was a building atmosphere of fear. It was at that point I quietly inquired if it was too scary and she stopped.

One month later in **Tray 2, Rosa** spontaneously placed three origami figures she made during our session into the sand tray, and scored her fingers confidently along the right border of the tray. The figures, two paper ducks and a box bear a much greater quality of relationship than was evident in **Tray 1**. The two ducks sit side by side, facing forward and to the right. The brightly colored pink box is to the left and behind them. **Rosa** took it upon herself to dig a nest-like hole for it to sit in, then soundly patted sand up along the sides of the box. In this tray, **Rosa's** initiative and gestures in the sand carry a significantly greater degree of relationship to the process than was experienced in **Tray 1**. Additionally, the alignment of the pair of ducks and their placement facing the direction where I was standing at the time demonstrate a growing level of the spatial relationship factor.

Four weeks later, I asked **Rosa** if she would like to do a sandplay. She willingly agreed, actively shaping the sand into a prominent rectangular island and a rounded landform in the far left corner. **Rosa** carved a significant depression in the center of the main island. After doing this, she promptly sat down with an expectant look on her face. I said, "You know, you can use any of these figures on the shelves in your sand trays, if you like." No sooner did the words cross my lips and **Rosa** bounded up and began gathering figures for her tray. **Rosa's Tray 3** continues to show growth in relationship on many dimensions. This is evident in her delightful energetic relationship to the sand and the figures, in her growing alertness and responsiveness to my presence and in the spatial relationships among the figures in the tray.

The swan and her baby cygnets are the first figures **Rosa** places in the tray. The swans carry the relationship of the protective and loving mother to her children. **Rosa** positions the swans at the far left corner of the central volcano-like island, between it and the remote location where the magical horses and rabbits are positioned. A transformational turtle is poised to enter the waters, which separate this place of hope and potential from the central activity on the main island. Three dogs guard the perimeter of the crater as cats stand beside a red crystal heart.

Rosa's red heart feels so sad. I feel the sorrow as I sit with her tray now, fifteen years hence. **Rosa's Tray 3** is filled with the grief of her extensive losses and deprivations, yet it is clearly held in relationship to the safe anchor point of a center and the guardian instincts of the dog triad. The activation of the mother-child unity sets this remarkable transformation in motion.

The promise of new development and growth of spirit stands ready in the far corner, as the little turtle enters the depths. Mirroring the square and the circle of the predominant landforms in **Tray 3** on its shell, the turtle also functions as a bridging element between the wholeness of spirit and the misery of **Rosa's** unfortunate life experiences. Culminating her newly developing level of intrapsychic integration of what were formerly terrifying and chaotic psychic contents, **Rosa** moves the heart and kittens to its center position and lightly sprinkles everything with sand.

Unfortunately, this was **Rosa's** last tray. The forces of family dysfunction and chaos abruptly ended her work. **Rosa** made significant psychic development in her three sandplays. We can only hope that the work she accomplished was able to aid her in her journey.

Chaos

Chaos may appear as an acute level of disconnection and disorder that emerges in the holding container of the sand tray. In each unique situation, the therapist must carefully consider what the particular chaotic process concerns and also understand the archetypal significance of chaos in general.

Initially, we must consider the age of the client. If the child is a three-year-old, chaotic sandplay may be developmentally normal. With the very young child, random, unrelated figure placement may have more to do with the child's level of cognitive and motor development than with chaotic psychic content. However, chaotic sandplays in even young children may hold normal developmental limitations *and* chaotic psychic content, as we see in the work of **Billy**, discussed below.

Chaos can be understood as the formless condition that precedes creation. In this sense, chaos has a regenerative capacity. Primeval chaos, like orgiastic ritual, functions to break down boundaries. Eliade (1958/1996) emphasized that chaos eliminates the clear, conscious definitions that we take for granted and forces the issue of re-defining who we are and how we see things. Chaos is sacred because it unleashes the abundant regenerative powers of the unconscious. Understood in this way, chaos is extremely fertile ground for psychic movement. However, holding and containing the client's chaotic disintegration in sandplay is a subject to be taken seriously and soberly.

Frequently in sandplay, the journey into chaos is a sudden tumbling brought on by pressures of the transcendent function. The polar opposites may make a rapid appearance in the course of sandplay. As we know from our exploration of the dynamics of symbols, the failure of the conscious mind to deal with the opposing poles of the symbol builds a tremendous pressure that plunges psychic energy into the depths of the unconscious where it taps new and expanded psychic resources. Said in the language of Norse myth, this is the plunge into Nidhogg's well in Hel's realm of the underworld.

It is possible to visit chaos with conscious awareness. To enter chaos with awareness is the shaman's journey. With awareness, he or she moves between the planes of being, suspending the comings and goings of time and space. Just as chaos works to dissolve boundaries and to bring about a state of disintegration, it affords the possibility of re-entering the unified condition of undifferentiated being that prefigures manifestation. With the dissolution of the bounds of normalcy, chaos takes place outside of ordinary time and space. It is in sacred time. Chaos is cyclic in the mythic sense that every entry into chaos eliminates the past. It is thus a new beginning that regenerates time (Eliade, 1958/1996).

Chaos in sandplay may be about a profound need to bring meaning into life and to live in sacred time. It may be about the urgency of infusing life with meaning and being willing to let go of all known comforts and securities to do so. It can be comforting to remember this when we experience chaos in sandplay. However, the regenerative capacity of chaos in no way obviates its extraordinarily hazardous qualities. The degree of differentiation of the client along with the added holding power of the therapist always factor into the sandplay client's ability to re-emerge safely and transformed from the descent into chaos. In chaotic, unrelated presentations in the tray we must make an effort to look for primitive indications of order. Any early signs of order may hold the direction of later organization and development. The therapist's conscious awareness of budding indications of organization will greatly strengthen the containment of the undergoing.

Chaotic sandplays may appear in the work of clients who have suffered disordered lives with little or no structure and consistency. The chaos and un-relatedness of such sandplays are indicative of the clients' psychic deprivation. On the other hand, a client who has suffered severe developmental deprivation may be overwhelmed by the choices available in the sandplay room. Sandplay may not be suitable until significant development has taken place outside the tray.

The Flooded Tray

What is commonly referred to as a *flooded* sand tray may be inundated with figures or literally flooded with water. It is distinct from the condition of chaos in that it is characterized by un-channeled, overpowering psychic energy. The flooded tray may be chaotic, but not necessarily. It may contain simple figurative content, but overwhelming emotional impact. A primary consideration with the flooded tray is about containment and whether or not the sandplay process can adequately and safely hold the overwhelming psychic energies that manifest in the client's work. Each flooded tray must be considered in its unique context.

The flooded tray may indicate a psychosis. There are no specific indicators of psychotic process in sandplay. The clinician must remain acutely attuned to his or her sense or feelings about the work. One important consideration is if the material is not completely within the boundaries of the sand tray. The walls of the sand tray create a boundary that provides a physical form of containment. Whether this boundary and the overall containment of the process by the therapist will be adequate to hold a client's psychic tumult is the primary concern. When a sandplay feels psychotic and is spilling out of the tray there is less certainty of containment.

Sandplay is generally contraindicated in cases of psychosis. However some specialists do use sandplay for treatment of psychotic clients (Baum, 2002). These highly experienced clinicians employ sandplay during the reintegration phases following psychotic episodes and in cases of disassociation. Very serious caution is advised in these clinical presentations, as they demand specific training, experience and consultation with experts in this area. My experience indicates that clients with very fragile psyches or those experiencing psychosis steer away from sandplay. I have consulted on cases where this is not the case and clients effusively flood their sand trays. As we repeatedly stress, clinician preparedness and containment are the overriding considerations in how or if sandplay should be used.

Occasionally, a flooded sand tray may appear in the work of a client experiencing a serious crises. If the previous sandplay work of the client indicates adequate stability and differentiation, sandplay may provide the perfect medium for processing, healing and integrating the situational loss. The therapist must listen carefully to his or her inner direction in order to decide if this client should proceed with sandplay at this time, or take a temporary break. The therapist must listen carefully to the direction of the client as well.

BILLY Three-year-old **Billy** was initially overwhelmed with the sandplay process. **Billy** experienced domestic violence between his parents and was traumatized. In addition, his father as the perpetrator, had been removed from the home by the police and little **Billy** had not been able to see him for some time. His trauma was compounded by loss. Understandably, **Billy** was scared and confused. Although **Billy** eagerly entered the sandplay room, he entered a mixed state of near-panic and fascination when he abruptly stopped in front of the shelf of monsters and hero figures. Three- year-old, **Billy** had not fully developed the capacity for pretend play. His psyche was on the threshold, drifting between perceiving the monsters as real and *playing as if.* **Billy's** terror was palpable, yet his attention was rapt. As the therapist I made a moment-to-moment assessment of whether he appeared to profit from his mastery of the terror held in the symbolic energies of the monsters, or if he might be lapsing into a flooded condition of being overwhelmed.

Billy begins **Tray 1** by fearfully pointing at the monsters while instructing me to pick them up for him. I did as he directed and set the figures randomly in the sand tray. To begin with he refused to touch them and averted his gaze from the ones he selected. **Billy** continued issuing instructions, until he had a number of monsters sitting in the tray. At this point, he announced he had to go to the bathroom and dashed away. After taking care of this need, **Billy** returned to the sand tray and began tentatively touching the monsters one at a time with his tiny index finger. His confidence gradually built and he began to smile. Soon **Billy** was deep in interactive play, with monsters threatening and attacking each other. **Billy** assured me that the "strong guy" beat up the others. He then returned all of the figures to the shelf and asked when his mommy was coming.

Billy begins his work in a near condition of flooding. In fact, it appears that he rides the crest of this wave through the course of **Tray 1**. His level of development and the severity of the traumas he experienced compounded to test the limits of his psychic capacity. The atmosphere of **Billy's** work was intense, yet there was a shared knowing between us that we were in it together. I knew that we were working on the edge of being overwhelmed, but we were still on this side of the boundary.

Billy unconsciously knew he could trust that I was patrolling the borders for him and proceeded ahead with some remarkable work. As Billy's work progressed, he gradually handled the monsters by himself until he was able to do it entirely on his own in Tray 4. While his work maintains an air of intensity, the sense that he was precipitously on the edge of flooding subsides as it advances. In addition, Billy contains his interactive battle of bad guys and good guys within the boundaries of the sand tray. Although his finished products appear rather chaotic, the interactive thematic play is symbolically coherent.

In his final sandplay Tray 5, Billy handles all figures himself. In this tray he buries several figures, demonstrating his growing capacity to manage the losses and the accompanying fear and grief. As his final gesture, Billy asked me if he could place some things around on the floor. Making a large circle of snakes and bugs, Billy proudly stepped into the center and grinned triumphantly. Billy and I shared that glorious unspoken celebration of the rich dimensions of his many private victories.

Rigid Configurations in Sandplay

Rigid configurations appear in sandplay when the relationship of the figures appears rigid and overly controlled, as if placed in systematic, resolute uniformity that feels tense or stiff. When this occurs the ego may be unstable or threatened and require additional external support or defense. The source of the client's threat may originate in the outer or the inner world. The rigid sandplay presentation may carry the client's need to hold tightly onto boundaries to guard against incursion or violation in outer life, or from becoming overwhelmed by psychic eruptions.

Another manifestation of a rigid configuration in sandplay is the phenomenon of double fencing, or double boundaries. Duplicating boundaries calls attention to the need to insure division. It is important to consider what is under siege, or what is so fragile as to require rigid protection. Equally important is to observe what psychic forces pose a threat to the enclosed elements. If the threat is something present in the tray, it is visible and held, or contained, by the tray and the holding environment.

When the entire tray is fenced, as when fences surround the inner walls of the tray, what poses the threat is unseen. Perhaps the entirety of the sandplay process is a fragile, emergent newness that must be particularly protected and delicately held. Perhaps what is emerging in the sandplay is the only experience of individual authenticity the client has ever been allowed. In this case, it is very much in need of protection.

Clusters and Groups of Figures

The assembly of figures into clusters and groups raises important considerations about spatial relationship in the sandplay. Of fundamental concern is what it might be about that elements of psychic process are organized into separate units.

Lowenfeld (1993/1979) observed that children organize their experiences by grouping them into what she termed *clusters*, based upon, "*...the quality of the personal experience the child has of the thing and event in question* (p. 21)." In this early manner of making sense of his or her world, Lowenfeld observed that the children group clusters of awareness according to their subjective sensory experience of objects and events. Importantly, Lowenfeld noticed that the clusters are not simply associated incidents and objects, but that they *coalesce together as unified components* of the psyche. In the course of normal, healthy development, children later separate and reorganize these clusters of psychic contents using their more developed cognitive abilities. Although ideas similarly assemble around a feeling-toned center in Jung's theory of complexes, what Lowenfeld observed in the children's clusters is a developmentally earlier means of organizing experience. Lowenfeld observed that clusters frequently appear in the early protosystem form of consciousness characteristic of sand tray worlds. Lowenfeld's observations about the elemental organization of experience in sensory, feeling-laden clusters is a valuable tool for coming into relationship with the sandplay client's efforts to differentiate various aspects of their inner and outer experience into coherent meaning systems.

As there is no certain way to identify how a group or cluster functions in a sand tray, we must be careful to remain open to a variety of possibilities. To better understand groups and clusters in sandplay, it may be helpful to consider what is related in the groupings and what is isolated. The differences between clusters may also lend insight into the client's process. We might look for significant contrasts between figure groupings in the tray, or between various areas of the tray. The content, size, energy, organization and relationship of the clusters may also provide insight into the process occurring in the tray. A close study of the clusters may indicate a direction of movement, either toward integration or toward disintegration. These considerations may indicate the psychic elements that are beginning to coalesce in the client's work. On the other hand, examining the content and feeling nature of groups and clusters in a sandplay may facilitate understanding of the qualities of experience that have inappropriately coalesced in the client's psychic development. This may lend understanding to what it is that is attempting to differentiate in the client's sandplay work.

AARON **Aaron's Tray 1** is an example of clustered groupings of the psychic work he would undergo in his sandplay. Around the highly-defended and imprisoned metal knight in the center are the various faces of **Aaron's** inner and outer world, which the guiding force of the Self pulls to integrate in a meaningful way. We see the police in pursuit of a speeding car and a lion tamer, who has subdued the wild beast. The playful cartoon figures mirror the need to restore balance in their colorful portrayal of villains and heroes. In addition, **Aaron's** deep religious and spiritual potential is held by the Asian wise men, who gaze into the crystal ball knowing what lay ahead. The quiet beauty of the skiers holds the balance and freedom inherent in the successful integration of these clustered aspects of **Aaron's** psyche.

Figures on the Edge of the Sand Tray

Figures placed on the edge of the sand tray may carry a variety of psychic energies. Perhaps the particular figure sitting on the edge provides a view from the outside of what transpires in the tray. In this way, it gives an overview. Figures on the edge may be a vehicle that carries what is going on in the sand tray to the outside world. Figures used this way serve as a bridge to real life. Like some figures that are buried in the sand, figures on the edge may also indicate pieces of the process that are not fully contained within the body of what is going on in the sand tray. These figures may be isolated elements of the process that are entering, or moving toward integration. On the other hand, they may be psychic contents that are no longer needed. In this way, a figure on the edge might be thought of as leaving the sand tray. A figure on the edge may stand as a sentry, or guard, to protect what is taking place in the sand tray. In some cases a figure is placed on the edge of the tray as a way of placing it above the scene in the sandplay. We listen carefully to what the client might say about the figure on the edge, if anything.

AARON A beautiful example of a figure on the edge is a Native American girl reverently positioned on the far edge in **Aaron's Tray 4**. After completing the sandplay, **Aaron** quietly said,

She was the first Indian, who is now dead. She is a spirit, who hangs above the fire [watching as] *they have an Indian ceremony.*

In this example, the Native princess on the edge of the tray is a spiritual over seer, who views from above.

LENAE Near the end of her sandplay process in **Tray 41**, **Lenae** reaches new levels of understanding of the losses resulting from her family discord, as she taps her own ability to establish a safe relationship with her much needed inner masculine energies. In so doing, she is able to safely corral her instinctual energy in **Tray 42**. This evokes a celebration of the more conscious, grounded embodiment of the jewels of the Self in **Tray 43**. Four dancing girls form a square, which stands on end, like a diamond, as the treasures of the Self are now readily available in the far right corner of the tray. **Tray 44** begins with a central mountain upon which **Lenae** scores the figure of a cross. Ritually running her finger first from top to bottom vertically, then from left to right horizontally, she comments, *I'm going to make it have a crack up on the mountain.*

Lenae archetypally marks her own crucifixion with the integration of her worldly strife made meaningful in terms of her inner wholeness. She then wipes it away and happily states, *I'm going to make a face out of this, as if it was a pumpkin.* The resulting happy smiling face reflects her newly integrated sense of presence and safety.

This hard-won integration prepares **Lenae** for the plunge that takes place in **Tray 45**. On the far center edge of the tray, a mermaid dives into the depths of the sea below. The unknown nature of the sea and what lay ahead is reflected in the alien-like red headed troll doll on the right. Referring to the mermaid, **Lenae** says,

She is taking diving lessons.
Therapist: Who is teaching her?
Her father.
Therapist: Is she scared?
No.

After this **Lenae** asked to quickly look through her file at the instant pictures of her sandplay work. Flipping through them quickly, when she came to the photo of **Tray 14** the constellation of the Self, she spontaneously said, *I used thirty-two figures in that one!* I was stunned by this remark and by the perspicuity of the psyche to automatically separate this sandplay out as special and to be aware of how many figures it contains. We had never discussed the number of figures, nor had she seen my count, as the picture was affixed to the reverse side of my notes! **Lenae** is ready to face her issues on an even deeper level and she touches the Self as an anchor point as she makes the dive. She is ready and confident. Now she is guided by her own inner father. She also alludes to her newfound ability to be receptive to her outer world father, while remaining safe and true to herself.

In **Tray 46, Lenae's** psyche presents another figure on the edge of the tray. This time it is a dark witch on the front of the tray, who faces an assembly of figures from her **Tray 14**, the centering of the Self. **Lenae** comments that the wicked witch is telling them something scary, but they are safe. The dark feminine characteristics held by the witch stand apart from the central assembly and on a different level. She is present and to be contended with, however the strength of **Lenae's** developing psychic structure is held in her centered wholeness. It is her anchoring in the Self that allows the darker feminine qualities to remain a part of her functioning without the danger of her being consumed by them. **Lenae's** positioning of the figures on the edge of the tray in both of these examples holds new psychic qualities that **Lenae** is beginning to integrate.

The Client's Relationship to the Sand Tray

The relationship between where the client stands and the figures and activity in the tray can also aid our understanding of the sandplay process. The rectangular shape of the tray is an important component of sandplay. Thus, based upon his or her stance in relationship to the rectangular shape the client's position at the tray functions as an element of the psychic process.

The Shape of the Sand Tray

Being rectangular the sand tray is square-ish. Archetypally, the sand tray is reflective of the square, the grounded, material world. It has four corners, which anchor it in the material dimension. It is not, however square, but it is intentionally rectangular. In the Jungian sandplay method, there are several factors we take into consideration. We want to have a free and protected space in which the psyche can move to depths beyond consciousness. We must have a place in which the central archetype of the Self can manifest. That is to say, the Self needs to appear in a material, three-dimensional form. The sandplay arena must also facilitate the integration of inner world, unmanifest archetypal content into consciousness.

If the sand tray were to be square or round, the pull toward grounded conscious awareness would be absent. Squares and circular formats are archetypal configurations. They pull for archetypal process, but fail to facilitate its integration into material world conscious awareness. The side-to-side breadth of the four corners of the rectangular sand tray exerts a psychic pull along the horizontal axis. What emerges from the center of the depths is thus, energetically impelled toward conscious integration.

Work From the Front of the Sand Tray

In most instances, the client makes the sandplay by standing or sitting at the long side of the tray. From this position, the client sees the tray as a rectangle whose shorter dimension extends away from him or her, and whose longer dimension extends from side to side. From this vantage point, the size and shape of the tray fills the client's field of vision, but is not so large as to require much head movement from side to side. The sand tray thus, facilitates the client's concentration and deepening by embodying a holding environment for the psyche. At the same time, the horizontal breadth facilitates the conscious embodiment of the work of the sandplay process.

Work From the Side of the Sand Tray

A very different condition exists when the client works from the narrow side of the tray. By electing to work from the end of the tray, we see that the client's psyche is manifesting a specific need to work, or manipulate the *material body* of the tray. From this vantage point, the physical area of the sand tray no longer functions to fill the client's visual field, but presents itself as something to be worked with or upon. It becomes a field, an extension of the client, if you will, that can be moved and altered with sand and figures. A length-wise relationship to the sand tray is thus frequently concerned with the client's physical body. A length-wise tray may have to do with physical illness. It may be about wounding, or physical intrusion and trauma that the client has experienced in the body. The sudden appearance of a length-wise tray in a process may also have to do with qualities that the client is embodying in a new way.

Movement Around the Sand Tray

While movement around the sand tray is common for the very young child, circumambulating, or changing position presents some interesting considerations in older clients. In the deeply wounded, or less differentiated client, circumambulating the sand tray may indicate that the client has no clear vantage point. This may be a client who is uncertain about whom he or she is and has poor ego development. In this case, the client's relationship to the process in the tray is uncertain.

Dora Kalff (1980/2003) observed that circumambulating figures and scenes within the sandplay are concerned with the center. Kalff saw that clockwise movement indicates a movement toward consciousness, and that counterclockwise movement is toward the unconscious. A client's movement around the sand tray may similarly be concerned with centering, as a ritual movement around a center.

Movement around the tray during a process that otherwise indicates adequate and developmentally appropriate differentiation, might also have to do with the movement of psyche in a new direction. It may be a bodily and kinesthetic means of seeking, or arriving at a new vantage point. We want to notice if the client moves consistently in one direction, or if the relationship to the tray seems random and haphazard.

Relationship of Figure Placement to Client and Therapist

In some sand trays, the placement of figures and scenes in relationship to the client or therapist is a significant aspect of the sandplay process. Figures that are placed directly in front of the client's position, may reflect aspects of the process that are nearer the client's awareness. In the same way, far away figures may be parts of the work that are more distant to the client's awareness. A figure placed near the client may be an immediate threat, or possibility, whereas the same figures placed at greater distance may hold looming threats or vague possibilities. When the figures or scenes appear to be moving away from the client's position, they may hold energies that he or she is ready to manifest and move out into the world. If the symbolic material appears to move toward the client, it may hold new qualities that are entering the field of awareness. Depending upon the content, figures moving toward the client may also be imminent confrontations the client must face in the inner and outer world.

The placement of figures near the position of the therapist may reflect transference. I do recall my alarm a few years ago when I spotted a single, crouched rifle-bearing soldier on the edge of the tray pointing directly at me! As therapists we need to take these things seriously and do some soul searching. It is important that we study the sandplay case to attempt to become more conscious of what might be going on. In the case of this boy, I felt he was taking charge of himself and fighting off the women in his life. He had entered treatment as a virtually mute, ten year-old, who was passive and disempowered. Not only was he now preparing to enter the man's world, he was feeling crowded and angry that he had to come to therapy every Wednesday afternoon. His sharp shooting soldier helped me be more aware of the importance of his desire to play basketball with his friends after school. His mother and I honored the progress he was making and moved his appointments to every other week. I was no longer used for target practice!

While it is true that clients place figures in the sand that may carry strong transference symbolism, it troubles me to hear therapists be overly focused on these issues. I feel discomfort when I hear therapists speak of the appearance of figures in the sandplay as representations of themselves. It is also disconcerting to hear therapists narrowly define particular figures, such as ambulances as representations of the therapist. These figures may carry transference, but we must exercise caution in limiting our conscious perceptions to so simple an idea. It is critical to remember that the ambulance may be concerned with the client's activation of healing and rescuing forces in his or her inner and or outer life. Symbolic process is never so narrow as to simply mean one thing. When we consider the broader issue of sandplay containment, there is transference in the entire process. Moreover, there is a mutual meeting of psyche of client and therapist in what we call the *co-transference*, after Bradway and McCoard (1997). We must be very careful about our identification of transference objects in sandplay. In any case, it must be done with humility and full awareness that this is the intrapsychic process of the client. It is not about the validation of the therapist.

Relationship to the Sandplay Space

In addition to the various spatial dimensions we have explored, there is profound significance in the relationship of client and therapist to the space of sandplay itself. As a therapeutic tool, sandplay creates a place specifically designed for the concretization of that which is beyond, for the grounding of the sacred in form. In sandplay the sacred manifests in material from. That is to say that what is beyond ordinary conscious awareness takes form in profane space. This coming together of the sacred and the profane produces a breakthrough in the perceived barriers between the planes of existence.

We recall that Eliade (1958/1996) spoke of the enduring quality of sacredness that develops when what is beyond ordinary conscious awareness breaks through in a particular place. He observed that the place becomes a seat of the sacred, and that all who partake of that space are affected by the power of the sacred that has manifested there. Seen in this way, the sand tray, as well as the entire sandplay environment, is a place that is set apart from the profane.

The sandplay room becomes a place where the sacred quality of the Self is repeatedly manifest by clients. The presence of the sandplay therapist reinforces the numinous nature of sandplay by serving as a container and witness to this process. Clients who have an experience of the numinous in sandplay become conscious of its capacity to hold the sacred. Importantly, sandplay also holds the potential to evoke the sacred for clients who are unaware of this possibility. From our discussion of Jungian personality theory, we recall Jung's central observation that human beings have an inherent need to move toward the archetype of wholeness. It is this hunger, this deep yearning for the Self that finds correspondence in the sandplay room as a seat of sacred possibility.

Examples of the relationship to sandplay in its broader context as an environment are children who work primarily with figures on the floor area around the sand tray. Because the sand tray is not used, we might conclude that there was no sandplay process taking place. It is evident to the therapist however, that these children are growing and strengthening within the broader context of this work in the sandplay environment. Perhaps they are undergoing the necessary inner preparation for later movement into the tray. Although not taking place in the sand tray, this activity can be considered as sandplay process, for the reason that it takes place in the watchful presence of the sandplay therapist and is *stimulated by the presence of the sand tray and the sandplay environment.* The psyche of the client is moving toward work in the tray. This comprises tremendous growth and development all occurring in the transformative field of sandplay. It is important to acknowledge even this as valid sandplay work.

Many years ago I worked with a twelve year-old girl, who was virtually mute during our weekly sessions. This girl's mother told me that her daughter had suffered several traumatic events that began when she was a toddler. At the time of treatment she was not doing well in school, kept to herself and had no apparent interests in life. During the course of our year together, she said next to nothing and responded only briefly to direct questions. She abruptly shook her head "No" in response to my many invitations to the sand tray. Although I was anxious and concerned that nothing was taking place, her mother assured me that she liked to come to sessions. Week after week we sat in silence at a small table, making earrings. One day, many months into our work together, she spontaneously wrote "Hi" in the tray on her way out of the door. Many weeks later, also on the way out the door, she quickly shaped the smiling face of a girl in the sand. With the simplest gestures, she re-connected to her authentic self in the sandplay. Something profound was taking place in our painfully long hours of silent jewelry construction on that tiny table beside the sand tray. When she wrote "Hi" she grounded her connection to me and to her deeper Self. From the perspective of psychic development perhaps this is the mother-child unity and the relationship to the mother. After this relational context was established she was able to manifest the Self, as a portrait of her own presence. This child never did talk with me, nor did she do much more sandplay. A ten-year follow up with her mother brought the wonderful news that she was socially well adjusted and enjoying an active college life. A great deal of healing and transformation occurred for this girl in the environment of the sandplay. Most of it was silent and unseen, yet the essence of the work was elegantly grounded and made manifest in the material body of the sand tray.

Ultimately there is no separation between the sacred and the profane. Its boundaries are illusory and are limited by our individual conscious awareness. When we consider Jung's definition of the archetype of the Self as the source from which all emanates and the goal toward which we strive, we see that ultimately, all of life is the Self. Sandplay provides us with a tangible, material environment, which functions to facilitate movement through the limits of our awareness and into the fullness of the Self.

~ Conclusion ~

Chapter 2
Spatial Themes in Sandplay

This concludes our discussion of the many facets of spatial themes in the sandplay process. To further develop our understanding of the healing and transformational dynamics of sandplay, we will now turn our attention to themes of motion and movement.

THE HANDBOOK OF SANDPLAY THERAPY
PART TWO: Process Concepts
SECTION II: Themes in Sandplay Therapy

Chapter 3

Motion Themes in Sandplay

Introduction

We have discussed the archetypal significance of a variety of figurative patterns, as well as movement along vertical and horizontal axes in some detail in our consideration of spatial themes. In this section we want to emphasize the importance of *motion* as a theme for understanding sandplay. Although the archetypal characteristics of the spatial directions continue to apply to our understanding of motion in sandplay, our concern here is to become more aware of the *direction and quality of energy flow* in the individual tray, as well as in the overall process. Paying attention to movement themes in sandplay can give the therapist a visual and almost kinesthetic insight into the activity of psychic energy in the sandplay process. The visibly physical characteristics of motion themes in combination with the more symbolic themes of content and spatial direction can contribute significantly to our understanding of the modification and development of psyche. We are better prepared to contain a process when we understand not only the implications of spatial dimensions in sandplay, but also how the psychic energy flows and where it is blocked.

Motion themes appear in sandplay in a variety of ways. Movement in sandplay can be indicated through figure choice, placement and sand configuration. For example, the appearance of any manner of vehicles, skateboards, running animals, birds, windmills and weaponry indicates various forms and qualities of movement. Roads, paths, waterways, bridges, ladders, and wells with buckets also imply motion, as they are channels for movement. Movement can occur as the actual physical movement of figures, often with the accompanying sound effects characteristically made by younger children during sandplay. Motion occurs in the active movement of sand, such as in sprinkling, pouring and dropping. Other activities with sand or figures also entail considerations of motion. These include the movement and repositioning of figures during the construction of a tray, as well as activities such as burying and digging up, or hiding and discovering.

Margaret Lowenfeld's *E*

In her work, Margaret Lowenfeld (1946, 1979/1993) talked extensively about a primary energy that she called *E*. I believe that it is valuable for us to review some of this foundational work, as it provides a conceptual map for understanding motion themes in sandplay. Lowenfeld postulated that E is the fundamental energy that vitalizes development and activity. She said that how it manifests depends on the quality of the channels through which it flows. Lowenfeld described three basic manifestations of E: that which vitalizes physical development, mental and intellectual functioning, and feeling and emotional functioning. Lowenfeld's concept of E is hydraulic in nature. She proposed that a blockage in any channel creates stagnation, pressure or flooding somewhere else in the overall system. Impaired conduits or lack of appropriate channels for E result in what Jungian theorists might refer to as unconscious conflict. Lowenfeld observed that this energetic obstruction manifests as symptoms across the gamut of physical, cognitive and emotional disorders.

Lowenfeld (1979/1993) made the very critical observation that the therapist needs to focus on how the child's work in the sandplay compares with his or her behavior outside of the therapy room. The differences in how the child uses the materials in the sandplay room and their behaviors at home or school may be key indicators of how their energy is blocked and how it needs to be released and channeled. This observation arose out of Lowenfeld's experience of children who were highly symptomatic at home and at school, but were able to create coherent worlds at the clinic. Lowenfeld surmised that these children lacked proper channels for E, which would build up in them and erupt in inappropriate and dangerous ways. Their work in the sand tray allowed them to access and develop proper channels for E.

I am reminded of a 12-year-old boy from my practice who suffered conditions of severe neglect, violence, and sexual abuse in his early years. Due to his propensity for violence and an apparent lack of conscience, his prospective adoptive parents feared what he might do to other children and were on the verge of removing him from the family. In marked contrast to his behavior and attitudes in his outer world, this boy's sandplay work was a breathtaking, highly coherent symbolic journey to find the center of the Self and to fashion channels for its expression and relationship in the outer world. Over time I am pleased to report that this young man has opened his heart. He is now honest, empathetic, and kind, and he is a happy, deeply caring member of his new family.

Paralleling observations from Lowenfeld's work, this boy had not had opportunities for proper development. Consequently, his energies had been improperly directed, arrested, and distorted. His work in the sand gave him the opportunity to rectify this wounding and to redirect his energies to more meaningful purpose.

Lowenfeld (1979/1993) used the client's progress in his or her capacity to manage E as an indicator of therapeutic improvement. She observed that as E begins to move from blockage and chaos toward order, the client develops the beginnings of purposeful relationship. Once the client's will and capacity to choose are properly ordered to E, they become able to develop healthy relationships and to develop their intellectual capacities. Lowenfeld noticed that as the client makes progress in his or her ability to manage E, he or she becomes able to confront the perceived enemy, or symbolic conflict. As the psyche moves to release and properly channel energy in sandplay, the client is able to address areas of inner conflict and simultaneously initiates the ability to enter authentic relationship to people and things in the outer world. Lowenfeld emphasized that the healthy ordering of E to the early childhood developmental accomplishments of trust and initiative are indispensable to the capacity for wholesome relationship. Lowenfeld's understanding correlates in fundamental ways with Kalff's (1980/2003) observations that healthy early parent-child interaction is foundational to the child's ability to form relationships, which is in turn, prerequisite to healthy ego formation and outer world adjustment.

Sandplay therapy provides a three-dimensional format for tapping and directing psychic energy. I find Lowenfeld's observations about E to be a helpful conceptual tool for coming into relationship with the movement of psyche in sandplay, particularly when working with early developmental wounding that is pre-verbal and non-rational. Because sandplay so fluidly accesses this level of psyche that cannot be spoken of in rational terms, the concept of an unseen energy that seeks to be tapped and properly channeled greatly supports the therapist's ability to hold this elusive, yet critical aspect of the work. Being able to envision the commerce of psychic energy along pathways that are new, blocked, clear and otherwise, can greatly assist the therapist's overall understanding of the psyche's travels in the conceptual field of ego, unconscious and Self.

Quality of Motion and Channel

When we examine motion in sandplay, we want to consider qualities of fluidity, strength, and direction. Throughout her work, Dora Kalff (1980/2003) emphasized consideration of the quality of the movement in the sand tray. In her studies, Kalff looked for places of constriction and blockage of energy with the intent to understand what it was that arrested the client's development. A wonderful example is her story of Daniela. In her first sandplay, a carriage pulled by two horses stands by a pasture of cows. The horses' legs are mired in the sand. Although all indications in the sandplay showed that the road to the outer world was clear, Kalff commented that the carriage was stuck near an area of motherly energy that somehow prevented its movement. In this example, Kalff was able to discern the nature of the energy that had been thwarted in its development by looking to the symbolism of the surrounding pasture and cows.

In another of her case studies, that of 12-year-old Kim, Kalff (1980/2003) worked with motion themes in a more abstract manner. Unlike the specific symbolic indication of the nature of the blockage she detected in Daniela's sandplay, Kalff was able to understand and contain Kim's work primarily by observing the general quality and changes of movement through the process. By tracking his initial movement through a series of diminishing barricades and armaments, Kalff held the process of change in this boy's psychic energy. His wounding, healing and transformation initially appeared in a skeletal, non-specific manner that did not become more identifiable until later in his work.

Without referring to them specifically as motion themes, it is interesting to note that most of Kalff's (1980/2003) case studies track movement patterns through the process as a means of understanding psychic transformation. Rather than attempt to repeat them here, the reader is referred to the beautiful accounts of this master sandplay therapist.

When we work with motion themes it is important to recognize that there are no generalities or patterns we can follow. Our task is to understand as well as we are able, each client's unique journey. We must remember that movement may occur within one sand tray, as well as from one tray to the next. We can say that weak movement needs strengthening, blocked movement seeks release, and directionless, chaotic movement requires channeling. Moreover, all psychic energy requires centering.

How, if and when all of this takes place is unique to each case.

Movement of Figures During Construction

A special type of movement occurs when the client moves or changes figures during the construction of the tray. What is moved or replaced, where it moves, and how the relocation is executed must all be taken into consideration to better understand the development of psyche that is taking place at that very moment.

Frequently the client will move or adjust a figure as the tray comes together. Perhaps, if we look carefully, we can discern the significance of these little snapshots of psychic change. The changed position of the object in the tray may help us understand the significance of the physical movement of a figure. Perhaps the new or changed relationships between the moved figure and those around it may indicate the nature or quality of energy movement.

Another type of movement during the construction of a tray occurs when the client moves, or replaces all or nearly all of the figures. In this circumstance a significant movement of psyche occurs. When this happens, the client in effect constructs two sand trays in rapid succession. As psychic change occurs rapidly in this form of movement, the therapist must track what happens as accurately as possible. This may be difficult to do and taxes our ability to keep good notes! I have found it helpful to reconstruct and photograph the first, or prior scenario after the session. Of course, its accuracy is limited by my recall. As limited as it might be, having a record of this part of the process can provide invaluable support for understanding and containing the client's work. Matters of time constraints and the practicalities of running a practice always figure in to our being able to reconstruct a tray. Whenever possible however, I strongly recommend doing so.

NORMAN Norman's Tray 1 is a good example of psychic movement occurring through figure replacement. In the completed tray, a formidable armored knight stands sentry in the far center. The knight was placed as the final figure to replace the more threatening skull and skeletons that originally manifested in the construction of the sandplay. In this tray, the movement of the objects underscores the level of threat and the need for strong defense. Being aware of the need for defense held in the movement of figures facilitates containment of the psychic fragility that necessitates it.

LENAE Interesting examples of movement occur in **Lenae's Trays 45 and 46**. In **Tray 45**, the mermaid on the far center edge of the tray is on the brink of diving into what is below her. In this case, the movement is held in the posture of the figure, as well as in its placement. As she began to work in the sand in **Tray 46**, **Lenae** spontaneously asked to see the picture of her first sandplay. After considering it in silence, she proceeded to pound on the sand saying, "It's neat to make a thousand handprints. It's like monkey prints."

She then constructed her tray, but in the reverse position of the end product. **Lenae** first assembled the arc of figures facing away from her. She positioned Glenda, the good witch, in the center area facing the semi circle of figures and herself. **Lenae** contemplated the sandplay silently, then with great intention turned Glenda toward the far edge of the tray saying, "She is going to face her."

Lenae rapidly put the dark witch on the far edge of the tray, facing Glenda. She walked around the tray, so she stood with the dark witch at her belly, identifying this side as the front of the tray and saying she was done.

The movement in this sandplay is remarkable. Once positioned facing the constituents of her domain, Glenda, the light feminine, recognizes that it is incomplete without the inclusion of the darker feminine qualities. She turns in the opposite direction to accept her dark side. In this example, the movement of the psyche is witnessed in the repositioning of the figure. **Lenae** moves toward even greater conscious integration of this formerly threatening aspect of her self when she physically moves to the side of the dark witch.

In **Tray 49**, **Lenae** establishes inner harmony with the archetypal parents of the sheltered seal family. She clearly affirms her identity as a girl child by placing her favorite doll in the sand in **Tray 50**. In her final **Tray 51,** the exasperated expressions of the caged cartoon figures indicate that **Lenae's** psyche also recognizes the reality of her captivity in her parents' continued discord.

Manner of Construction

The manner of the execution of the tray is an important consideration of motion. What we are referring to here is the client's movements and gestures while making the sand tray. The quality of construction may be graceful, crude, tentative, forced, and so on. It is important to consider the client's quality of motion against the background of what is normal for him or her. When for example, a client is customarily serene and gentle, it may be of no particular note when they execute their sandplays in this manner. If the client is ordinarily a clumsier, rougher sort, the motion of a serene and gentle tray construction may hold great significance. The therapist must be aware of the nature of the quality of movement in the execution of the sandplay and factor this in to the overall consideration of the symbolic process. We must also consider changes in the manner of execution over the course of the process.

Movement in Psychic Space

The direction of the flow of energy in psychic space is a feature of movement that merits close attention. The archetypal consideration of spatial direction is crucial to understanding where psychic energy is coming from and moving toward as healing and change take place. For this reason we have previously discussed the spatial features of sandplay in some detail. Our concern here is to become aware of how energy moves or is arrested as it travels along these spatial parameters. It is important to combine understanding of the *significance of the direction* of movement with an awareness of *the quality with which the energy moves.* Putting these two features of movement together lends deeper understanding to indications of arrest and motion in sandplay.

Being aware of slow or thwarted assents or descents for example, might indicate an uncertainty in the client's readiness for the psychic movement. The blocked movement could result from any number of factors ranging from the natural pace or style of the client's development, to a piece of unfinished work that must be undergone before the client is fully ready for the psychic movement at hand. Paying attention to such possibilities may facilitate the therapist's containment of the process by stimulating him or her to explore what may have been previously overlooked. On the other hand, a sudden ascent or descent in a sandplay process might alert the therapist to issues of readiness for the undergoing. Being alert to movement and direction can aid the therapist's ability to safely hold the work.

In some instances significant movement from left to right may indicate an influx of unconscious energies. Similarly, right to left may indicate movement toward the unconscious. Although it is essential to keep such factors in mind, we must be careful to not be formulaic about it. It is always best to consider possible implications of the sandplay and be patient while the story continues to unfold.

Another consideration of movement is whether psychic energy appears to be moving toward integration or disintegration. It is important to consider whether energies appear to be coalescing into some meaningful order or appear to be coming apart. As we have seen, psychic healing and transformation entail a cycle of death and rebirth. The therapist's awareness of movement toward integration or disintegration in the sandplay process strengthens containment and facilitates the client's safe and meaningful psychic development.

Lowenfeld (1979/1993) reminded us that time is measured by movement. Psychic identification with the movement of the figures in sandplay moves and channels energy in time and space. These are qualitative transformations of psyche, however they must be physically experienced and embodied. The movements in the sandplay process ground the qualitative changes of psyche in material form. Movement in sandplay embraces what is timeless in the field of time. The time measured by the movement in the sand tray is the psyche's time. In her studies, Lowenfeld observed that each coherent world focuses an aspect of E, which *activates* the making of an incoherent world. In Jungian terms we might say that, as the ego-Self axis is strengthened, the psyche is able to move deeper into the unconscious. The sandplay therapist can cultivate significant insight into the client's process by tracking the psyche's movements toward destruction or construction in relationship to the release and channeling of energy.

Sprinkling, Pouring, Dropping, and Burying Motion

Actions such as sprinkling, pouring, dropping, and burying are another form of movement in the sandplay process. Although we have examined some of these motions in our discussions of sand and water we will take another quick look at them here with a particular emphasis on the gestures of their execution.

Sprinkling

Sprinkling with sand or water in sandplay may derive from mythic acts of fertilization. In his studies of religion and anthropology, Eliade (1958/1996) detailed many agricultural rites across cultures that are concerned with the fertility of the earth. Regardless of location or culture, each entails rituals of sprinkling water or ashes as a means of ensuring continuity of the earth's fertility. Sprinkling in this sense is sacrificial. It is an act of reverence that sanctifies by giving back to the earth that which has been given. In sandplay, the act of sprinkling may reflect a participation in this deeply mythic act that acknowledges the sacredness of life. Sprinkling may be a gesture that demonstrates a profound awareness of the client's essential connection to all of being. Children frequently tenderly sprinkle sand over the figures in the tray. Many times I have heard children quietly utter, *...it's snowing.* This is a gentle, reverent motion that seems to carry a ritual significance. One little girl from a background of severe neglect and abuse said she was, *...salting.* Salting brings out the flavors. Salting food helps our bodies accept the nourishment. It was such a simple gesture from a young child, yet it had all the reverence of a sacred event. We quietly experienced it together.

Considered from an archetypal level, sprinkling is about the cycle of endings and beginnings. It reflects a deep awareness of participation in the round of being and is a profound acknowledgment of existing in and of nature. On the deepest level this is an acknowledgement of connection to others and to all of being. It is this awareness that initiates a way of being in the world that is quintessentially responsible, for the individual becomes aware that whatever he or she does or thinks has a very real, material impact on others, and ultimately on all of being. The gesture of sprinkling in sandplay is the initiation of this capacity. As the client sprinkles, he or she becomes aware of his or her capacity for impact on the world and on other people.

Just as sprinkling quickens a deep, inner connection, it is the beginning of the ability to respond and interact with the outside world and is the budding of relationship. To acknowledge one's inseparable connection to all of manifestation generates an ethic of caring and activates the heart center. Although it may not be conscious to the sandplay client at the time, becoming aware of one's connection in nature sets a profound psychic transformation in motion.

Dropping

Dropping sand may function as a less evolved gesture of sprinkling. It may be a rudimentary form of fertilizing and the beginnings of the awareness of connection and capacity. Crudely tossed, or *bombs* of sand may be angry or hostile gestures. To better understand the significance of this type of gesture, we must carefully attend to what is happening in that sandplay at that moment. Although we cannot generalize about their meanings, motions like this in sandplay are certainly significant components of the process.

Assuming we are talking about clients with adequately developed motor control, dropping figures into the tray may also be an exercise of anger. It may be an act of mastery in the sense of overcoming a wound or fear. In this way dropping is an action of capacity. When dropping occurs in sandplay, we must pay close attention to what is dropped and what it is dropped upon. The figures themselves may carry symbolic significance that helps understand what the movement concerns in the context of the overall process.

Pouring

Like sprinkling and dropping, pouring may also work as a form of fertilizing. What is being poured into the sand tray has a lot of bearing on its possible significance. If sand or water is poured into the tray, we want to consider the attributes of the element itself. Pouring water may have to do with creation by water and receiving the potential of the unconscious. Pouring of sand may be concerned with connecting with the element of the earth. It may be about the capacity to initiate, to take action in one's life. It may be about burying, or covering something up. Pouring jewels from a basket of marbles assumes a connotation of joy and abundance on the light side, and deprivation and desire on the dark.

Burying and Digging Up

Burying and exhuming are interesting gestures in sandplay, as they carry many possible implications. As we recall from our exploration of hidden and buried figures, when something is buried, the client may be hiding something precious, protecting something fragile or planting or nurturing something that is to grow like a seed. It may be a form of surrender or departure. It may be a laying to rest of a quality that is no longer needed for the process of transformation to take place. Burying something beneath the surface may indicate a quality that is not quite conscious, but is moving toward consciousness. Burying may also move to hide something that is intolerable, scary, or hideous. As we know, any quality that lurks in the shadows of the unconscious is frightening to the ego. Burying may have to do with being stuck, trapped, entombed or powerless.

Burial may be an attempt to control what has not yet been dealt with. To bury in this way is an attempt to put things out of sight. As a motion in sandplay, burial to hide something does exercise sufficient consciousness for the dreaded quality to be seen and acknowledged, at least in part, by conscious awareness. The conscious psyche engages in the act of dealing with the dark aspect by undertaking to bury it. Even though the shadowy psychic quality is temporarily put out of sight underground, the client's psyche is in charge of the action. The glimmer of conscious awareness that is involved in the act of burial is sufficient to set processes in motion that will gradually transform the shadowy quality. By intentionally engaging with the dark psychic aspect in this manner, the conscious psyche acknowledges its presence and initiates a relationship to it. This new relationship is prerequisite to the re-ordering of psyche.

In the gesture of burial, the psyche moves the quality downward with the intention of activating transformation. What happens subsequently is of great interest to the therapist. Observing where this energy moves, as well as how, when and where it changes can help the therapist contain the transformation process. The burying motion activates a new capacity to address the issues at hand. To bury something is a gesture that moves toward disintegration. Thereby, it initiates the process of rebirth and new growth. How this will manifest in time is unknown, but the movement itself plants the seed for something new.

Burying followed by digging up may indicate a new capacity to face things that were once overpowering. In burying and digging up the client may be exercising control over something that has heretofore been beyond his or her control. When the child exhumes a buried object from the sand tray he or she invites the therapist to see and hold a psychic quality, whether positive or negative. Even when the unearthed figure appears very dark, the process still points to rebirth and transformation. The process has simply not progressed beyond the death phase of the cycle.

Burying and exhuming may be about the client finding treasures in him or herself. It is not uncommon in work with younger children for the therapist to be asked to find and dig up the things the child buries in the sand. Frequently the child will say something like, *...okay, cover your eyes. Don't peek!* During this time the child buries objects in the sand for the therapist to seek and discover. I recall one little boy I worked with, who had me play this game with him over and over again. He was about six years old. He instructed me to cover my eyes while he buried jewel-like marbles in the sand. With playful elegance this little guy's psyche devised a game in which we could conjointly discover and hold the elements of the Self. Every time I found one, he would light up and giggle with delight. When I pretended to have difficulty, he would look a little worried and whisper, *..over there.* We always found them all!

Movement Between Two Sand Trays

Several types of movement are possible between two sand trays. Although we do not promote making two sand trays, there are a number of ways the client may make use of both trays during a session. In my experience this occurs far more frequently with children than it does with adult clients. I suspect that this may be accounted for by the child's level of cognitive development and less concern for the assumed boundaries of containment inherent in the adult world. Children discover and inhabit physical and psychic spaces that were closed long ago to the adult. They have private rooms behind sofas and caves under tablecloths. In this magical sphere I doubt that the boundaries of just one sand tray have much relevance to the inner necessity for exploration and expression. We are not talking about the *spilling over or flooding* that we might see in psychotic process. We have discussed this elsewhere. What we are examining here is a more integrated level of psychic functioning that moves between the trays in significant ways.

A client may make two trays in sequence during the session. Process is moving rapidly when this occurs. In order to understand what this phase of the work is about, it is important to consider similarities and differences between the two trays, just as if they were constructed in different sessions. The psychic process in the first tray may be moving so quickly that it is ready for expression in its changed form in the second tray.

The content of the two trays may represent the polar opposites of a psychic conflict. A look back through the process may illuminate how the conflict has emerged. The two trays may work as safe containers for oppositional qualities that are not ready to face each other in the same container. It is significant however, that the opposites have emerged and are clearly defined *within the overall container of the sandplay process*. Although still in two sand trays, they are regarded together by therapist and client.

A client may use both trays to extend the size of one sandplay configuration. Dora Kalff's (1980/2003) case study of Kim provides a wonderful example of putting the trays end to end to create a large race track. In Kim's work, a major objective was the release and free movement of energy. It is clear that this tray extension emphasized the therapeutic accomplishment of the boy's abundant and well-directed energy. A consideration to aid in understanding the meaning of two adjoining trays is the nature of the representations in the two trays. The situation where two trays are effectively used as one, as in Kim's case, is very different than when the two trays hold distinctly different material.

Clients may create two sandplays in the same sand tray during the session, disassembling the first before constructing the second.

A special kind of movement takes place when the client makes a complete tray, but disassembles it and returns the figures to the shelves prior to photographs. If I am able, I try to reconstruct the prior tray after the session. When a second sandplay is made, considering the changes that occur between the first and second constructions can help us better understand the process patterns that take place between the two trays. For example, it may be that the two trays are a rapid progression through the material or that they carry the need to hide what first emerged. There are many possibilities of which we must let the sandplays inform us.

Another form of movement in sandplay occurs when a client constructs two trays, alternating between them. I have seen this occur primarily in children. Children who are dealing with the divorce of their parents will frequently make two trays at the same time. The sand trays may even be nearly identical. In cases of divorce, I suspect that process in two trays is the child's attempt to make intrapsychic sense out of the division of a unified archetypal parent into two bodies. The psychic impact of divorce on children is not to be underestimated. This is clearly indicated in the children's sandplay work, where they struggle to mend the inner rupture that occurs when Mom and Dad are no longer together. In my experience, it is only in cases of separation from a highly abusive or substance addicted parent that the sandplay process of a child undergoing parental divorce does not appear to address this profound psychic rupture in some way.

Children may construct two sandplays to represent two sides of a conflict. As discussed above, the trays may hold the opposing poles of the conflict. Monsters may oppose super heroes. A team of *good* guys may stand against the *bad* guys with the battle transacted between the two trays.

Interactive Play

As we learned in our discussion of developmental issues in sandplay, interactive play is the client's activation of the sandplay figures in live, imaginative play. Young children for whom the curtain between what is imaginary and what is real has not been fully drawn almost exclusively do interactive play. Although it is difficult to set an age for the average age of interactive play, it generally occurs in children under the age of six. I have seen interactive play in older children, particularly in the battle scenes of boys in the eight- to nine-year-old range. Infrequently I have also experienced adult client's making interactive gestures with figures. These are typically more isolated movements that lack the extended dramatic context of interactive play in young children. Sometimes an adult will knock a figure over in a gesture of anger or disgust. The adult client may move a figure through a door, or into another significant position.

With regard to motion themes, the important thing to remember is that the psyche is moving through the client's active play gestures. I have found it helpful to pay attention to the general themes of the play. During interactive play I listen for the underlying mythic themes and make note of these. Perhaps bad things continue to happen, or children and animals are trapped and caged. I listen for indications of strength, rescue or safety. Perhaps one theme carries through the action, or it transforms into another. There may be several themes interwoven in the same story. I want to be as fully present as possible, which sometimes means that I am not able to make notes until after the work is done. I watch for the direction of the movement in the play and the characters involved. There may be a pattern of movement through the interactive play in one sand tray. On the other hand, the movement may not be discernable until we have some distance on a number of sandplays.

When an interactive sandplay comes to an end, or time is running short and the child needs to wind up the story for the day, I will frequently photograph the primary characters in the play. If time is running short, I may quietly say to the child, "I don't want to rush you, but we have just five minutes to finish today." When the play is done and the figures are simply abandoned by the child rather than intentionally positioned, I may suggest that we have all the characters line up and take a bow. This is much like a theatrical curtain call. I photograph them with the child present. My sense is that this helps the child make closure to the vigorous psychic activity he or she has undergone in the interactive play. The curtain call supports the containment and functions as a mutual acknowledgement of the importance of the work. I do not suggest a curtain call if the placement of the figures at the close of interactive play appears to be significant to the process.

~ Conclusion ~

Chapter 3
Motion Themes in Sandplay

Themes of movement and motion enhance and refine our relationship to sandplay. Movement occurs in sandplay in the client's physical gestures and it is implied by stationery figures and configurations in the sand tray. As movement occurs in the sand tray, psychic energy moves, channels for psychic energy are discovered and created, and new intrapsychic connections are formed. Patterns of psychic strengthening, disintegration and reintegration are unique to each person's work. By carefully watching the movements of energy we are able to develop greater attunement to the profound evolution of psyche in the sandplay process.

Chapter 4

Affect Themes in Sandplay

Introduction

In this section we explore the feeling and affective components of sandplay. As with the themes of content, spatial relations and motion we have discussed previously, affect themes may help the therapist better understand the course of the sandplay work by tracking changes in emotional content and experience. Following the affect through a sandplay process gives the therapist another means of maintaining relationship with the client's sandplay work.

The Affective Core of Symbols

As we are well aware by now, sandplay is a symbolic therapy that occurs in the context of a relationship. We know that the nature of the symbol is complex and always exceeds our capacity to fully comprehend it. Symbols are characterized by many different features, which we experience in a variety of ways. Our discussions about the various features of sandplay content testify to this fact. We see and touch symbols. They evoke memories and they move the unconscious toward individuation. Prominent among the features of symbols is the *feeling* they evoke.

An extraordinary aspect of the symbol is that it simultaneously carries all of its manifold features as an amalgamated whole. It is only our conscious awareness that reflects upon the symbol and describes it as this or that. The truth is that what the symbol holds occurs in advance of consciousness, so there truly is no way to describe it apart from little bits and pieces. Margaret Lowenfeld's theories provide helpful tools for understanding this type of pre-verbal, pre-conscious mental activity that occurs in sandplay. In her work, Lowenfeld (1979/1993) conceptualized an early, pre-verbal type of thinking, characteristic of the young child.

Lowenfeld postulated that the thought process of young children is a synthesis, consisting of fragments of experience, ideas and feeling into *clusters of mental functioning*. We have explored Lowenfeld's concept of clusters in our discussion of spatial relationships in sandplay. Our concern in this section turns to their affective components.

In what she referred to as early *proto system* thought, occurring prior to the development of cognitive functioning, Lowenfeld (1979/1993) observed that children categorize their experiences,

> By the quality of the personal experience the child has of the thing and event in question. (p. 21)

All things that the child experiences as pleasant go together and all things that are scary are grouped together. In addition, the child associates other elements of the environment to the highly charged emotional core of the cluster. Typical examples of this are the smells and sounds that are remembered with highly charged events.

Of great help in understanding symbols in the process of reordering psychic complexes to the Self is Lowenfeld's astute perception that everything the child experiences along with the particular event is also associated with the clustered experience. Because these experiences are new to the young child and he or she has no other way of understanding them, the clustered experiences combine into an indivisible whole.

Like complexes, clusters of experience carry varying degrees of psychic energy. Ideally, with further cognitive development and added maturity, the clustered experiences are later sorted out along the lines of more commonly accepted perceptions of reality. However, experiences of wounding and deprivation often interfere with continued development, leaving actively charged clusters to cloud experience and drain psychic energy.

A primary difference between the concept of a complex and a cluster is the relationship to the Self. In Jungian theory, the entire psyche is composed of complexes. We organize our psychic experience through complexes. Having the experience of the Self and ordering the complexes to the Self requires higher-order mental functioning, which is not the province of the very early cluster. Our point here is not to debate differences of theoretical definitions, but to create a way to relate to the richly fused qualities of the symbol in sandplay, understanding that a large part of the work that goes on in sandplay occurs on this early, affectively charged, preverbal level of awareness.

Dora Kalff (1980/2003) affirmed that all psychic change occurs on this very early level of awareness, which she called *matriarchal.* When we consider the significant affective component of pre-verbal experience emphasized by Lowenfeld together with Kalff's understanding that all psychic change and transformation takes place at this early level of development, the seminal role of affect in the symbolic process becomes apparent.

Dimensions of Affect in Sandplay

To meet the sandplay process in the realm of affect is to be with it quietly, making a still and open inner space in which to receive it energetically. To experience an affective relationship with sandplay, the therapist must operate silently, from inside the shapeless, pre-verbal energy. In this way, the therapist is directly informed by the affective content.

By attending to the felt quality of the symbol in sandplay we facilitate the differentiation process on a pre-verbal level. If we can shift to the notion of the symbolic process as a cluster and focus on its felt qualities, separating them temporarily from any notions of what it is that we see, we are better positioned to understand or contain the psychic glue that binds the symbolic experience together. Having a clearer sense of how the sand tray, or series of trays feels gives us a point of reference from the vantage point of pre-verbal experience and memory. By feeling the symbolic experience in this way we are better able to understand what it is that we see.

Several dimensions of feeling must be considered in sandplay. These include:

> How the client appears to feel, or says he or she feels while making the sand tray
> How the client feels or appears to feel after the completion of the sand tray
> How the therapist feels as the client makes the tray
> How the therapist feels after the completion of the tray

How the room appears to feel during and after the tray
How the sandplay feels as a completed tray
How areas of the sandplay feel
How feeling moves and changes through the course of the sandplay process

The therapist must take note of these varying dimensions of feeling. The therapist must also consider the possible significance of any coherence or incoherence among these many dimensions of affect. A coherent experience of feeling between the client, the tray and the therapist lends added significance to the overall sandplay experience. For example, if the client is visibly sad, the therapist feels the sadness and the sand tray itself feels sad, the affect is evident and is clearly contained.

Incoherent experiences of feeling between the client, the tray and the therapist pose more complex possibilities that may be more difficult to understand. Such inconsistencies in affect must be considered in the context of the sandplay process. For example, if the sand tray appears very frightening or ominous and the therapist feels an intense apprehension, but the client appears cavalier and not particularly moved by the experience, the therapist may want to pay attention to the client's attitude toward the unconscious, his or her sense of denial or lack of conscious preparation for deeper transformation.

Another possibility occurs when the client is deeply moved by the sandplay, but the therapist is untouched. In this circumstance, the therapist must examine what he or she is not seeing and holding. The therapist must also be mindful of his or her own issues of resistance to what is being evoked by the client's work. Consultation and personal therapy are always indicated when we suspect our own issues are inhibiting the proper containment of the sandplay work.

There are any number of possible experiences of affective coherence and incoherence between client, therapist and sand tray. Tracking affect over the course of a sandplay process can help the therapist remain in relationship to the process. The operative considerations are to watch and hold carefully. As we can never be completely certain that the feeling qualities we perceive as the therapist are precisely those of the client, we must remain open, compassionate and inquisitive.

Because the symbolic content moves us affectively the sand tray generates and carries its own feeling content. The therapist must be clear and inwardly still in order to allow the sandplay to resonate within him or herself. To become better attuned to the affective component of a sand tray, I will frequently consider it as a *landscape* or a *place*. I then consider the *quality of the place*. Imaginally, I enter this place or landscape to attempt to experience it from within its own context. Does it feel barren, rich, foreign, familiar, vast, constricted, remote, and so on? Is it ebullient, or chaotic? If the tray is empty I sit and experience its feeling. Does it feel depressed and bereft, or is it quietly serene? When there are significant empty or full areas in the tray, I check to see if this is consistent throughout the tray, or if there are distinct areas and regions. I let each area of the sand tray speak to me before inquiring about the possible relationship of these regions in the same sandplay. We explore this method of being with the process in more depth in our discussion regarding understanding sandplay.

~ Conclusion ~

Chapter 4
Affect Themes in Sandplay

Truly said, the whole of the symbolic process occurs in a formless dimension of affect. Before the creation of words, which define and describe things in life, the symbol moves the psyche along powerful waves of felt experience that evade our conscious abilities to describe them.

While the affective dimension of sandplay is likely its foremost thematic component, its pre-verbal nature leaves little to say about it. The important consideration in sandplay work is to not underestimate the significance of affect and moreover to cultivate a lived, working familiarity with its word-less domain.

~ Conclusion ~

Section II
Themes in Sandplay Therapy

This concludes our exploration of process themes in sandplay. We have examined elements of content, spatial relationship, motion and affect as means of attending to the progress of psychic change through symbolic process. Understanding and attending to these thematic features of sandplay gives the therapist a rich variety of ways to enter into relationship with the symbol's powerful, unseen movements of psyche.

Having familiarized ourselves with these tools and points of reference, we will next explore some approaches for their use in developing understanding of the overall sandplay process.

Section III

Understanding Sandplay Therapy

Introduction

At this point in our study we have explored sandplay therapy from a variety of dimensions. We have examined Jung's personality theory to develop a template for engaging with the phenomena of psyche and its changes. We have studied how symbols form and how they exert an effect on the human psyche to produce growth and change. We have taken a close look at the quiet, but formidable, role of the therapist in the process of sandplay. We have explored the dimensions of thematic content present in sand trays in order to facilitate a living relationship to the rich, comprehensive possibilities of sandplay. We have also explored the developmental dimension of the psyche's growth and healing functions through the diverse lenses of ancient mythology, neurobiological research and psychological theory.

In this section, we explore ways to put it all together and look at the issue of understanding the sandplay process. As you might well imagine after our many discussions, to even speak of *understanding sandplay* is somewhat misleading. In Jungian sandplay, understanding has little to do with the dimension of knowledge and is truly concerned with the matter of *holding*. *To understand* in sandplay is not to *know* rationally, but rather to be psychically positioned to provide an adequate container for what transpires. *To understand* sandplay is really about the therapist's preparation and readiness to *stand under and hold* the sandplay process. It is about containment.

This being the case, some people may wonder if it is necessary to undergo such an arduous study to work in sandplay. The answer is yes and no.

YES, it is imperative to undertake the continued study of the various subjects we have reviewed. In addition, it is crucial that the therapist undergo his or her own sandplay work with a well trained certified sandplay clinician. In fact, the therapist may find it essential to undergo several sandplay processes over the course of his or her career. Growth and development does not stop, rather it continues to press us to learn and deepen. Likewise, work in sandplay continually challenges the therapist to grow and evolve. Sandplay is never static.

The *NO* part of the answer has to do with the rational component of the learning in sandplay. While we must learn and continue to do so, we must also set it all aside when it comes to dealing with sandplay. When we sit with the client and the tray, we must be completely empty. We must be open to receiving whatever occurs in as present a way as possible. No amount of knowledge or rationalization can result in this serene, clear presence. When the therapist's relationship to sandplay is correct, the preparation or study he or she undergoes readies him or her to be present to the work of the clients.

In consideration of the above, we will continue our study in this section by exploring some of the documented methods used to decipher the meanings of sand trays in both the Lowenfeld and the Jungian traditions.

We will first look to the early *World Technique* research of Margaret Lowenfeld and Charlotte Buhler, after which we will examine Dora Kalff's approach to understanding Jungian sandplay therapy. Following this we will examine the contributions of some more contemporary research on the subject of comprehending work in the sand. We will briefly discuss two important aspects of understanding sandplay, first trays in a series, and the so-called quadrant theories. Finally, we will briefly explore the subjective immersion analysis tool I have developed to facilitate sandplay understanding.

Chapter 1
Understanding the World Technique—
Margaret Lowenfeld

Introduction

Margaret Lowenfeld (1979/1993) developed the *World Technique* as a means for the direct expression of children's inner thinking processes. She observed that the World Technique creations (worlds) seemed to express a state half way between what is conscious and what is not conscious. Preferring to allow any theory to evolve out of her experience of world making with the children, over the course of time Lowenfeld deduced that there were four processes of world making.

Appearing either individually or in combination, Lowenfeld distinguished:

The making of a coherent story or scene
The creation of a pattern through use of sand or objects or both
The creation of a *moment*, as a photographic scene
The lack of a coherent story or scene

Her experience with world making led Lowenfeld (1979/1993) to the analysis of the worlds through the consideration of five axes:

1. Time
2. Movement
3. Coherence/Incoherence
4. Symbol
5. Patterning/Design

We will consider each axis individually.

Time

Lowenfeld (1979/1993) examined the sequence of worlds to discern patterns in coherent and incoherent worlds, as well as the symbols used. Lowenfeld studied the structure of time within the worlds to determine:

> If present or historic time was represented
> If time was moving, or static
> If worlds unfolded along story lines
> If episodes or incidents of a story were portrayed, and
> If the movement in a story had just taken place or was about to.

Lowenfeld felt that the analysis of these parameters of time indicated how the client perceived the passage of time.

Movement

Lowenfeld (1960, 1979/1993) felt that the suggestion of movement through the placement of objects, or the direct manipulation of the objects in the world making process were significant, as they allow the client to identify with the movement itself. This facilitates the expression or fixing of what Lowenfeld came to refer to as *E*. As we recall from our discussion of motion themes in sandplay, E is the term Lowenfeld assigned to the energy that activates human personality. Not unlike the early Freudian concept of libido, Lowenfeld perceived E to be a neutral force in the psyche and soma and felt that it could manifest or express itself in a number of ways. Much of Lowenfeld's analysis of world making came to be concerned with blocks and freedom of movement of E, which she saw expressed in the worlds.

Lowenfeld observed a developmental progression from what she referred to as early *proto-system* children, characterized by circular movements in early worlds, to horizontal movements in mid-range worlds, and vertical movements in later work.

Coherence/Incoherence

Lowenfeld (1979/1993) analyzed the organization, or lack thereof, in the worlds to explore a number of factors, noting that worlds more expressive of outer reality were further developed than incoherent expressions. Lowenfeld regarded expressions in the world as aspects of both the client's outer and inner worlds. She examined what the client did in the world making and how this compared with what he or she did outside treatment as indicators of possible lines of therapeutic inquiry.

Lowenfeld also observed the manner of execution of the world and any changes in execution from world to world. She looked for themes in the worlds and any changes in theme through the series of worlds. Lowenfeld analyzed the coherence or incoherence of a world to determine the quality of E and any changes in E toward orderliness and relationship to others through the series as well.

Lowenfeld examined any changes in the rigidity of concepts and observed how elements moved toward greater awareness. She spoke of therapeutic improvement in terms of *self realization* and *control and direction of E* (Lowenfeld 1979/1993, p.149). Through the study of many worlds, Lowenfeld (1948) theorized the existence of a *proto-system* to describe the nature and structure of preverbal thought. As we have seen, Lowenfeld thought that it was through the processes of sensory and affective linking that young children form *clusters*, as early organizational groupings of their inner experience. In order to comprehend what transpired in the worlds, Lowenfeld looked for clusters and particularly for the movement of elements to more adaptive and developed forms over the series of worlds.

Lowenfeld (1979/1993) postulated that the client uses the symbols in the world as a step toward healing in his or her outer life. Through the projection of the client's inner condition onto the objects of the world, the development of new and different skills comes about through the symbolic interaction and experimenting in the world. Lowenfeld defined reparation or healing in a child by the child's:

> Development of will and decision in relationship to E
> Development of normal human contacts, and
> Use of mind and intellectual powers

It is interesting that, unlike Jungian sandplay practice, Lowenfeld frequently interpreted the worlds for the client. She felt this became a meaningful conversation between client and therapist.

Chapter 2

The World Test—Charlotte Buhler

In the early 1950's, Charlotte Bertha Buhler (1893-1974) noted child development researcher at the University of Vienna, adapted Margaret Lowenfeld's World Technique to her studies of children's cognitive and developmental processes. Formulated on the basis of Lowenfeld's (1939, 1979/1993) World Technique, Buhler fashioned a diagnostic instrument to detect pathological symptoms (Buhler, 1941, 1951a, 1951b; Lumry, 1951). While Buhler's work was intended as a diagnostic use of miniature worlds, her findings do have bearing on the therapeutic use of sandplay.

Calling her research instrument the *World Test*, also known as the *Toy World Test*, Buhler (1952) wanted to determine if specific groups of people, such as people with the same nationality, might evidence similar projective patterns in their worlds.

Taken with the ability of the World Technique to portray the workings of the child's mind, Buhler (1951) attempted to standardize the technique for use as a diagnostic test in the study of children's cognitive and developmental processes. With Lowenfeld's original support and encouragement, Buhler observed world making at the clinic in London. When Lowenfeld and Buhler later met in 1950 to discuss their work, Lowenfeld found Buhler's World Test to be at cross-purposes to her work with the World Technique (Bowyer, 1970; Lowenfeld, 1950a, 1950b).

The World Test (Buhler, 1951a, 1951b) is done on a tabletop or on the floor, without sand, and uses between 160 and 300 miniature figures. The client is instructed to, …*create whatever they wish.* Using a standardized rating scale, Buhler discerned what she called *signs* in her analysis of the worlds, noting that one sign was generally found in all worlds, but that the presence of two or more signs indicated emotional disturbance or mental retardation, particularly if one of the signs is what she called *closed, rigid* or *disorganized* (CRD).

A-Signs *Aggressive World Signs*, which might include scenes of accidents, fighting soldiers, threatening wild animals or violent storms.

E-Signs *Empty World Signs*, which include less than 50 elements or fewer than 5 types of elements. These Worlds often have no people in them.

CRD-Signs *Closed, Rigid or Disarranged Worlds*, which may be unnaturally cut off or enclosed, unnaturally schematic in arrangement, disconnected or chaotic.

Buhler (1951a, 1951b) scored the World Test on the basis of the type and number of figures used in the world, generally regarding an abundance and variety of figures used in a more coherent pattern or thematic scheme to be healthier indicators than the obvious scarcity or absence of certain figures in a world. Scoring was based on the administrator's sketch of the subject's world and was recorded on a scoring sheet (Buhler, Kelly [Lumry] & Carrol 1951).

Buhler noted that at least one CRD sign was present in the worlds of all emotionally disturbed subjects she tested. She observed that the CRD signs appeared to be used interchangeably by the disturbed population. That is to say that at one time they may create a closed world, and at another time a disarranged world. Buhler surmised that CRD signs might be indicators of insecurity.

Chapter 3

Understanding Sandplay Therapy—Dora Kalff

In her analysis of sandplay, Kalff (1966, 1980/2003) studied the series of sand trays as a *process*. Kalff recognized that the process of sandplay entails a descent into the psyche to a centering in the Self, which is followed by the development of a healthy, more adaptive ego.

What Dora Kalff meant by the term *process*, can be deceiving. Due to the limitations of language, we often use the word as a noun. Sandplay therapists frequently speak of *a process*, *my process*, and so on. Our tendency is to think of it as an artifact, a *thing*, when what we are actually describing is the active, alive phenomenon of the psyche in movement. Although the three-dimensional content of the sand tray is a representation of a part of the client's inner world, Kalff (1980/2003) considered sandplay to be a direct, immediate process of psychic change that takes place within the client as the client makes the sand tray. When we study a sandplay process, we actually enter that eternal dimension, which is removed from the limits of time and space. Thus, to study a series of sand trays is literally to *experience this active process* with the client.

Kalff's analysis of sandplay and her approach to teaching was the case study method. It was a marvelous experience being taught sandplay by Dora Kalff. Her classes followed a rather typical format. Class assembled at nine-thirty in the morning and consisted of a 2 ½ hour session. This was followed by a lengthy lunch and rest break at noon. Class then reconvened at three-thirty or four, running another 2-2 ½ hours.

Dora Kalff frequently began a class series with a short lecture, which she delivered from a podium. I would like to share my notes, taken from her lecture in Carmel, California March 31, 1989, to impart the tone and profound nature of Kalff's teachings.

> The depths in ourselves knows what we do not know consciously. We touch the collective unconscious with

> sandplay. This shows us the path where we need to go. Sandplay facilitates the individuation process, becoming conscious of unconscious contents and integrating them into our lives.
>
> Inner and outer happiness simultaneously is a synchronistic event. What is displayed with the symbols is a coming together of an inner and outer happening. This provides for the next step of development in the person.
>
> Thus, it is vital that we understand, not necessarily verbally, but with our intuition, what is going on.
>
> When we see repeated images in the sand, we must ask what is going on. As soon as I grasp the client's unconscious, the images will change.
>
> This inner understanding is known more in the Far East. Here we are trained to understand things consciously. No real transformation takes place just in the consciousness.

Following the lecture material, Kalff showed slides of a completed sandplay case. This was a slow, in-depth process. The sand tray slide frequently remained on the screen for an hour or more. Kalff asked the members of the class to discuss what they saw. Her training occurred through the dialog created by the responses from the class members. Kalff and her students joined in the active process of the sandplay, allowing it to inform them on deeper and deeper levels of awareness. It was arduous. Thus, the long rest break. The regular rest period Kalff adhered to reminds us that doing sandplay demands much of us and that we must take care of ourselves.

Through the examination of symbolic content and process, Kalff sought to allow the uniqueness of each individual sandplay case to reveal its meanings to her. As we have learned, Kalff drew upon Erich Neumann's (1971) theory of development to track the psyche's growth and change through the symbolic content of the sand trays. While Kalff honored the particular meaning a client might apply to a figure, her understanding of the symbolic content of the sand trays was grounded in an in-depth, case by case examination of the archetypal content of the symbols considered over the course of the entire process.

Chapter 4

Other Principles for Understanding Jungian Sandplay Therapy

Jungian sandplay therapists who have studied with and followed Dora Kalff's teachings tend to conform to the case study approach of analysis with minor variations in theme. Irrespective of the various approaches, central to all analyses is the core process of descent to Self and reintegration of the ego structure.

Some of Kalff's students have created tools and guidelines to facilitate the study of a sandplay case. We will examine some of the more significant and helpful of these below.

Understanding the Sandplay Process—Estelle L. Weinrib

Following Kalff's tradition, one of Dora Kalff's earliest American students, Jungian analyst, Estelle L. Weinrib (1983/2004) drew upon Jung's individuation process for analytic guidelines in the sandplay process. Weinrib observed that the sandplay process includes four primary stages.

Weinrib's Four Primary Stages of Sandplay Process

1. Partial resolution of the key complexes
2. Manifestation of central archetype of totality, or the constellation of the Self
3. Emergence of the differentiated contra sexual element (anima/animus)
4. New ego relativized to the Self

Weinrib (1983/2004), as did Kalff, used the case study method to illustrate examples of these stages of individuation. Weinrib focused her analytic guidelines on the transformative process of sandplay, rather than on the specifics of its construction.

Guidelines for Understanding Sandplay
Katherine Bradway and Barbara McCoard

Katherine Bradway, Jungian analyst and an early student of Dora Kalff, and her co-author, Jungian psychiatrist, Barbara McCoard, delineated guidelines for understanding drawn from many rich years of sandplay experience (Bradway & McCoard, 1997).

Bradway and McCoard (1997) looked for levels, stages, sequence and themes in their analysis of sandplay.

1. Levels

This refers to the level of consciousness at which the client is working.

Observing that these levels may interact, this may involve trauma, of which the client is conscious, as well as traumatic events that remain unconscious. Feelings and experiences about significant relationships and events may be evidenced or activated by the sandplay, as may indications of either negative or positive transference toward the therapist. Archetypal experiences may also be activated and evidenced in the sand tray.

2. Stages

This refers to the beginnings and endings of the sandplay process.

Bradway noted ten guidelines for the analysis of an initial sand tray:

1. Respect for and awareness of the client's feelings
2. Awareness of the therapist's own feelings
3. What is buried or hidden in the sand tray and may be discovered later on
4. The presence of chaos or order
5. Indications of transference

6. Signs of nurturing
7. Use of the water areas, or water or water-related figures
8. Indications of a mother-child unity
9. Indications of a problem and/or a solution
10. The need for consultation if the sand tray evokes anxiety in the therapist.

Many possibilities exist between the beginnings and endings of a sandplay process, including periods of deepening, nurturing and constellation of the Self.

3. Sequences

This refers to the order of placement of figures.

The therapist must observe the sequence in which the figures are placed in a particular sand tray. Also, it is important to be aware of the sequence of figures and their placement throughout the series of sand trays.

4. Themes

This refers to thematic tendencies in the sandplay case. Thematic considerations may include:

Places of incubation, such as enclosures that may protect or shelter something needed for growth and transformation.

Sources of energy or blocks to energy, indicated through choice or placement of figures, as well as verbalizations and use of the sand.

Indications of a journey or path and movement.

Indications of the client's sense of control, authority and anger.

The emergence and development of the masculine or feminine energies.

The appearance and union of opposites and attaining the treasure.

Bradway and McCoard's (1997) parameters for analysis are particularly comprehensive in their attention to transformative process and thematic concerns.

The Sandplay Categorical Checklist Geri Grubbs

Jungian analyst, Geri Grubbs (1991, 2005) developed the *Sandplay Categorical Checklist* for the analysis of sandplay in her study of the sand trays of abused and non-abused children. Composed of qualitative and descriptive categories of sand tray construction and modes of expression in the sand tray, the Checklist emphasizes patterns of change from one sand tray to the next. Grubbs's Checklist encompasses 19 categories of analysis which utilize three aspects of sand tray construction:

Thematic content and process in the creation of the sand tray
The client's story about the sand tray
Progressive or regressive changes from one sand tray to the next

Grubbs also considered the therapist's subjective impressions and their implied meanings. The 19 categories of the Checklist are:

Direct Observation and Objective Analysis

1. Story

   What the client says during or after the sand tray construction, if anything

2. Figures

   Number and description of figures used. Meanings of figures if verbalized by client

3. Setting

   The theme or environment of the sand tray, (disorganized, family, spiritual, symbolic, etc.) Movement or relationship between figures

4. Creation Process/Dramatic Play
    Changes that occur in the sand tray creation. Dramatic play

5. Use of Human and Animal Figures
    Which human and animal figures are used and how they are portrayed

6. Use of Sand
    The choice of wet or dry sand, shaping and burying

7. Use of Tray
    Full or empty quality of sand tray.
    The primary focal area of the tray, empty areas and centering

8. Creator's Response
    Client's feelings elicited by the creation of the sand tray

Subjective Impressions and Implied Meanings

9. Main Psychological Expression
    The primary psychological expression of the sand tray, such as destruction, aggression, self-protection, celebration, etc.

10. Cognitive Development and Scene Progress
    Developmental age level of sand tray creation and progression or regression within the context of the sandplay process

11. Coordination of Whole and Parts of the Scene
    The degree of organization within the sand tray

12. Structuring of Relationships
    Degree and quality of interpersonal organization and interactions of humans and animals portrayed in sand tray

13. Boundaries
    The use and quality of the boundaries of the sand tray itself and those created by the sand tray maker

14. Movement/Obstacles
    Movement or blockage of movement indicated in the sand tray

15. Relationship of Parts and Opposites
    The appearance and relationship of opposites

16. Therapist's Impression
    The therapist's feelings or impressions during and after the sand tray creation

17. Significant Symbolic Representations and Thematic Play
    The symbolic content of the sand tray

18. Significant Repetitive Theme and Figures Used
    Symbolically relevant figures and themes used repetitively

19. Questions Raised
    Therapist's questions that occur when viewing the sand tray

In her *Guidelines For Sandplay Analysis*, Grubbs (1997, pp. 11-13) draws from Bowyer's (1970) developmental norms, Kalff's (1980/2003) discussions of the manifestation of the Self, and her own research (Grubbs, 1991) to formulate indications of disturbance and signs of strength, progress, working through and integration through the course of a sandplay process.

The strength of Grubb's work lies in its integrative approach to the analysis of sand trays, drawing as it does from the best of the Lowenfeld literature, particularly Bowyer, while maintaining a therapeutic, process orientation to the work with active therapist involvement, particularly the use of therapist's feelings, questions, etc., as vital elements of analysis.

Twenty Points of Consideration for Understanding Sandplay Therapy—Martin Kalff

Martin Kalff (1993) approached the understanding of sandplay from a multi-dimensional stance. Kalff detailed twenty points to be considered in the analysis of a sandplay.

1. Client's History and External Situation

As similar sandplay scenes may have differing meanings depending upon the clinical history of the client, the sandplay must be considered in terms of both the outer and inner condition of the client. Kalff (1993) emphasized that it is important to remember that sandplay scenes are often anticipatory of actual life circumstances, so may not be realized in outer life until sometime subsequent to their appearance in the sand tray.

2. Session Contents

The interactions between client and therapist during the session, as well as verbal and non-verbal expressions from the client must be considered for their pertinence to the sand tray. Comments and emotional reactions to the sand tray by the client, or even dreams might provide important indications of the meanings of the sandplay.

3. Therapist's Feelings

It is important to consider the emotional response the therapist has to the entire sandplay, or to elements of it, and to compare how he or she was feeling prior to experiencing the sandplay in order to sort out any projections. It is also important to compare the therapist's feeling response with the client's emotional reaction to the sand tray.

4. Space

The use of space in the sand tray can provide important information in the analysis of sandplay. Overly full images may indicate overflowing unconscious activity, and empty scenes may point to depression or low energy. In other circumstances a relatively empty tray may be an indication of inner clarity and calm. Consistently empty halves or sections of the sand tray may indicate the inability to express threatening inner experience or a deep imbalance.

5. Choice and Use of Sand

The client's choice of dry or wet sand and the comments they make about it can provide important information about the meanings of the sandplay process. How contact is made or not made with the sand may be similarly important. Hesitance or reluctance about touching the sand may indicate unconscious fears or difficulties relating to the physical aspects of life. Flattening the sand may indicate a desire to control emotions or be an obsessive defense.

6. The Arrangement of Figures and Shape of the Sand

The therapist must observe the quality or dominance of shapes in the sculpting of the sand and in the arrangement of the figures. Principally round shapes may indicate a predominance of feminine energy or a feeling quality, whereas geometric shapes may indicate a dominant masculine energy and intellectual value. The manner in which the sand is shaped and the figures placed may also provide important indications of aspects of the client's process. More careful shaping and placement may carry great intent, while random scattering may indicate a lack of will or intention. The physical level that is affected by the sandplay process may be indicated by the configuration of the sand or objects into body parts or organs.

7. Color

The choice of dominant colors in a sandplay may be indicative of meaningful parts of the process. Intense red may represent a longing for life. In the sand play of a depressed person this may act in a compensatory manner. A dominant green may indicate a quieter, vegetative inner attitude.

8. Use of the Blue Bottom of the Sand Tray

The blue base of the sand tray may be used to indicate a clean surface for a design pattern or a clean area such as a hospital, but it is used generally to indicate water. How the client moves down to the water level is important to observe. If the client avoids opening the sand to the water, it may indicate a fear of going too deep within the psyche. If the client gains access to the water level early on, it may indicate his or her access to deep, nourishing resources within. It is significant to notice whether the blue water areas are clearly used as water, or if confusion exists about them. The placement of land objects in the water areas and watery animals and vehicles on the land nearby may be indicative of an underdeveloped capacity to discriminate.

9. Figures

The therapist must be aware of which figures are used, as well as how they are used. In addition, the exclusive use or avoidance of specific categories of figures may provide important information regarding the client's process. Avoidance of particular figures may indicate defensiveness. The presence or lack of vegetation may also provide important information about the client's experiences of growth, inhibition, hope or desolation.

10. Placement of Figures Within the Space

The placement of objects in opposite diagonal corners of the sand tray is the longest distance possible between any two figures and may indicate opposite qualities of the particular symbolic content represented.

11. Level of Differentiation

The level of ego development is discernible from the differentiation of the sandplay scene. This bridges the spectrum of possibilities from the dumping of figures into the tray at the undifferentiated end, to random placement, to battle scenes with unclear distinction of sides, and to well organized scenes with clear boundaries at the most differentiated side.

12. Relationship Between Figures and Elements of the Scene

It is valuable to notice if the figures are related to each other and how they interact. This can indicate how the client feels in relationship to other people or how aspects of his or her psyche are related. Changes in the quality of relationships among figures and elements over the course of the series are important indicators of the direction of healing. Unrelated and parallel scenes may indicate a severe disturbance. In this case it is crucial to observe changes from conditions of un-relatedness to greater relationship over the course of a process. The presence of bridges may indicate the connection of distinct aspects of the personality and access to greater levels of energy. Bridges connecting identical elements or placed randomly may indicate low energy or a lack of decision making ability.

13. Personal Expression

The need for uniquely personal expression may be observed in the client's shaping the sand into faces or bodies. Similarly, the client may make or bring his or her own figures from home for a particularly unique expression in the sand tray.

14. Dynamic or Static Quality

The presence or blockage of movement in the sand tray may provide significant information about the movement of the client's energy. It is essential to consider if the movement is contained, channeled, free or chaotic. In cases of blocked movement it is important to look for indications of any outlets for the obstructed energy. It is also valuable to explore the quality of a closed system, attempting to understand if it indicates a need for safety, concentration and demarcation, or if it prevents activity and indicates thwarted energy.

15. Two Dimensional Use of the Sand

The sand tray and figures may be used for the creation of a two-dimensional picture-like drawing. The significance of this use of the sand must be considered within the context of the entire sandplay process. It may indicate that the contents of the picture are not quite realizable in the fullness of a three-dimensional context.

16. Closeness to Consciousness

The level of consciousness or of unconsciousness of a sand tray may be indicated by the quality of everyday reality of the scene. Those sand trays with very far away, distant places and times, or even imaginary places are more remote from consciousness than are scenes of normal, daily life. Mixtures of varying levels of consciousness may also be observed.

17. Symbolic Content

Interpretation of symbolic content requires a thorough knowledge of myth, symbol, religion, fairy tale and dreams and must be considered in the context of the particular work of each client on a case-by-case basis. Although the client may use the collective meanings of symbols unconsciously, any associations or feelings the client has toward the particular symbol are to be given particular weight. By their nature all symbols have a wide variety of meanings ranging from the content at their negative poles to that of their positive poles. It is critical to demonstrate how a particular symbolic content is relevant to the specific case under consideration and it is insufficient to simply draw meanings from symbol dictionaries.

18. Interpretation in the Context of the Entire Process

The therapist must analyze each individual sand tray in relation to the sand trays that precede and follow it.

19. Interpretation Based on Inner Developmental Patterns

Careful analysis of the relationship between figures and elements of the scene may be indicative of the process of developmental patterns in the Jungian individuation process. The manifestation of the Self and the subsequent stages of ego development are particularly significant in the analysis of the sandplay process, as are the appearance of the shadow, the animus and the anima. Neumann's (1973) stages of development of consciousness may be discernible in the sandplay process, as may indications of development following patterns of development of other prominent theorists, such as Freud (Freud, 1966; Brill, 1966), Erikson (1963) and Grof (1976).

20. Relationship Between Client and Therapist

Sandplays and their elements may be indicators of the relationship between the therapist and the client and the quality of transference, counter-transference, or co-transference, as the complex interrelatedness of conscious and unconscious actions and reactions between client and therapist is often called in sandplay. The manifestation of the Self is the natural outcome of the relationship formed by the free and protected space of the therapist's containment of the process. The relationship between figures may be indicative of the ease or difficulty the client has in his or her relationship to the therapist. The client's choice of specific figures, whether consciously or unconsciously may express qualities of the therapist.

Martin Kalff's parameters provide a comprehensive inclusion of sandplay content and process. Kalff emphasized a firm grasp of the dynamics of symbolic process and the transcendent function. Kalff's guidelines for understanding sandplay therapy stress a thorough working knowledge of the individual client's history and experience. Importantly, many aspects of Kalff's guidelines focus on the quality and nature of the therapist's presence in the process of sandplay, a topic that we have emphasized throughout our explorations.

Martin Kalff's elements of sandplay analysis provide excellent guidelines for an approach to understanding sandplay. Used in conjunction with the various theoretical, thematic and developmental dimensions of sandplay we have explored, Kalff's guidelines of understanding provide the therapist with a comprehensive means for deepening his or her relationship with sandplay.

The Significance of the First Tray

Dora Kalff (1988) gave particular attention to the first sand tray in a series, noting that the first tray often contains indications of the issues to be addressed in the sandplay process, as well as indicators of the direction and resources for the client's healing.

As we recall from our discussion of spatial relationships, Kalff taught that figures positioned on diagonals running the greatest distance possible in the sand tray, frequently hold the opposing polar forces that define the conflict the client will address in the ensuing sandplay series. When such a polar opposition does occur in a first tray or early in the series, the symbolic content of the figures often identifies the nature of the work to be undertaken. If for example, the figures carry dark and light faces of mothering or fathering their diagonal opposition in a first tray or early in the series may indicate that the client's process is concerned with the healing and transformation of wounding of the archetypal constituents of mother or father. In addition, Kalff (1988) emphasized that a first sand tray can indicate the client's relationship to the unconscious and the client's feelings about therapy in general.

Weinrib (1983/2004) cautioned that the first tray in a series may be a more conscious, realistic scene, but nonetheless may indicate the direction of the client's problem and the possible solution. Friedman (Mitchell

& Friedman, 1994) suggested examining first sand trays to identify areas that are particularly energetic or troubled, to examine what types of groupings are present in the tray, and to notice indications of problems and strengths, as indications of the direction of the client's work.

My experience shows that the first tray is a vital and critical aspect of sandplay process containment. When the client does his or her first sandplay, a door is opened. The client extends an invitation to the therapist. The first tray is the threshold over which the client's psyche invites the therapist to join in one of the profoundest and most sacred possibilities of human relationship by traveling together into the unknown depths of his or her soul. The first tray is the initial meeting of these souls who will travel together. It establishes the tone of the journey and is the therapist's initial opportunity to join with the client in the intimacy of the non-verbal, symbolic interior regions in an appropriate, respectful and sound manner.

First trays are replete with the process that is ahead. Even as the sandplay progresses, it is very important to continue to refer back to the first tray. It may be a great help to the containment to consider the position of the client's current phase of the work in relationship to the overall process held in Tray 1. Perhaps even more importantly, a frequent reference to Tray 1 functions to attune the therapist's lesser conscious understanding of the client's process to the overall course of the work.

AARON We have examined **Aaron's Tray 1** in our discussion of diagonals. We will take another look at it here as a wonderful example of the rich capacity of a first tray to hold the course of the entire sandplay process.

Aaron's inner challenges are clearly evident in his first tray. The diagonal configurations in this tray carry the symbolic polarities of volatility and a deeply spiritual nature that appear at cross-purposes to **Aaron's** continued development. Also present are the perplexing issues he faces regarding his own developing masculinity and his frustrations with the irresponsible masculine role modeled by his father. The widely different qualities **Aaron** needs to integrate to achieve inner peace and psychic wholeness that are carried by the dramatic symbolic tension of the diagonals, literally cross in the center at the position of the defensive and imprisoned, armored knight.

In **Tray 1 Aaron's** psyche presents a symbolic road map of the journey, which pictures the inner and outer conflicts, the defenses, the isolation and the solutions to be found in his conscious integration of his spiritual nature. In his final sandplay, **Tray 15, Aaron's** psyche brings his work to a close in the triumphant loving cup. Cast from the heavy metal defenses in his first tray, even this final trophy of his victories was foreseen in the armor of the knight **Tray 1**. As a learning tool, I suggest reading through **Aaron's** sandplay case, examining each sand tray with reference to **Tray 1**. The psyche's presence in sandplay is elegant. It is our job as the therapists to be ready to accept its invitation.

Quadrant Theories of Sandplay Analysis

Some therapists have attempted sandplay analysis by assigning particular meanings to regions, or areas of the sand tray (Ammann, 1991; Ryce-Menuhin, 1992). These analytical tools are commonly referred to as *quadrant theories* for their tendency to divide the sand tray into four quadrants through the imagined vertical and horizontal division of the sand tray.

Ryce-Menuhin observed three levels of psyche - conscious, personal unconscious, and collective unconscious - projected into the sand tray alone and in varying combinations. Ryce-Menuhin observed that the more conscious psychic material tends to be toward the far and right side of the tray, while the unconscious, more archetypal material on the near and left sides of the tray. Ryce-Menuhin consigned the anima or animus, contra sexual elements to the far left corner of the sand tray and family constellations to the near right corner with Self constellations in the center of the sand tray.

Ammann (1991), who also employed alchemical themes for the analysis of sandplay process, ascribed matters of the inner world to the far half of the sand tray and instinctual, more conscious matters to the near half.

To the left half of the sand tray, Ammann relegated the more unconscious matters and the conscious outer world matters to the right. It is in the center of the tray that Ammann observed matters of the ego manifesting in the sand tray.

Bradway and McCoard (1997) observed that Dora Kalff experimented with the use of regions of the sand tray in analysis, but later abandoned the practice, noting that the entire sand tray is the unconscious. Bradway and McCoard noted that neither of these quadrant theories correlates to their experience with sandplay.

Martin Kalff (1993) admonished the use of quadrant theories, noting that it is questionable whether such a two dimensional grid is even applicable to a three-dimensional medium such as sandplay. I am in agreement with M. Kalff. To attempt to assign regions of the tray to regions or pieces of psychic process appears to me to be an attempt to rationalize and quantify something that is, by its very nature, non-rational and qualitative. While archetypal influences of direction and space do factor into symbolic process, it is unwise to attempt formulaic assignations of meaning. For example, a movement toward the unconscious may be indicated by figures moving toward the left side of the sand tray in a particular sandplay. But to apply a blanket meaning to an area of the tray, saying it *means* this in all or most cases is incorrect. We must move into relationship with each individual process and *allow it to inform us.*

Chapter 5

Subjective Immersion Analysis

Introduction

Subjective Immersion Analysis (SIA) is an analytic tool I developed for the understanding of sandplay process. It emerged out of a chance observation made in my office when I was preparing to disassemble a sand tray one evening. I noticed that if I imagined I was one of the small figures in the client's sand tray, I had a sudden *felt sense* of understanding what it was like to be in the context of the symbolic process. I recall a small spotted wild cat surrounded by massive architecture, with monsters and assorted threats looming nearby. Imagining I was the cat, I felt the sense of apprehension, of readied awareness, of the necessity to continue moving ahead and the sense of my (the cat's) own inner strength and balance, albeit in the midst of imposing danger.

This chance experience led me to wonder if *entering* the sand tray, imagining I was a central figure of a particular sand tray might be a way of more directly engaging in the energetic matrix of the symbol, in this way eliciting a deepened understanding of sandplay. I wondered if this might be a way of engaging in sandplay analysis that would honor the lack of specific definition, characteristic of the symbolic process.

Application of Subjective Immersion Analysis To the Sandplay Case

Following more casual experimenting with subjectively identifying with figures in sand trays, I formally applied this method to the analysis of a completed sandplay case. I set up my slide viewer next to my computer keyboard and studied the sand trays in sequence, one tray at a time. The particular case I used in this initial study was the work of nine-year-old **Aaron**.

In each sand tray I chose a central or prominent figure and subjectively identified myself with it, imaginatively immersing myself in the context of the sand tray. From the vantage point of the selected figure, which I refer to as the *focus figure* I described *myself* (as the figure) and my location. I made notes of my thoughts, feelings and reflections and made no attempt to censor what occurred to me. When I felt I had exhausted my awareness of the focus figure, I shifted awareness to the other elements in the sand tray, still speaking in the voice of the focus figure. That is to say, as the focus figure I described the other elements in the sand tray, their location, my, the focus figure's, observations about them, feelings, thoughts, memories, and so on. I continued this process, extending it to all areas and elements of the tray until it felt complete. This process was repeated with each of the sand trays in the fifteen tray series. The entire transcript of the SIA of this sandplay case is included in the Appendix.

The application of the SIA to this completed sandplay case was richly rewarding and beneficial to my deepened understanding of **Aaron's** process. Even though I had worked with this client and knew a great deal about him, I found the subjective immersion analysis of his sandplay work enlightening. I had the opportunity to review the entire case with **Aaron** and his mother six years after completing our work together. The insight gained by employing the SIA was borne out by **Aaron's** own understanding of his sandplay process and the course of his subsequent development.

During our review of his sandplay work **Aaron**, then fifteen, saw in his sand trays the great struggle he had had between his own deeply religious, sensitive nature, and his father's wild and angry ways of being in the world. This young man's more mature reflections on his work done in the sand tray as a little boy paralleled the analysis I had done of the case using SIA. In **Tray 2**, for example, he said that the odd looking pair in the upper left corner, "...was like the struggle he felt between Mom and Dad. They were so different and always fighting.." Later, in **Tray 5**, looking at the wide variety of men watching the baseball game, **Aaron** quietly commented, "These are all parts of my father."

A Study of the Subjective Immersion Analysis Method

This initial experimentation with SIA indicated that it had the potential to be an effective and potent aid in sandplay analysis. I subsequently conducted a study involving 17 sandplay therapists, using the SIA method (Turner, 1998). All but two of the test therapists found the SIA tool helpful and simple to learn. Most commented that they were startled by how aware they became of the relationships between the various elements in the sand tray. Most observed that the SIA tool greatly deepened their awareness of the symbolic dynamics present in the sandplay. Some commented that using SIA was emotionally intense and taxing and may be too demanding for the study of an entire case.

Two of the therapists in the study had difficulty with the SIA method. One was inexplicably resistant to experimenting with SIA to understand a sand tray. The other participant appeared to lapse into near delusional perceptions about the dynamics present in the sand tray.

Clearly, the SIA method is not right for everyone. Some therapists may find it helpful, while others may not. SIA is a very deep and intense engagement with the sandplay process. It is taxing to apply the SIA method to an entire case, albeit highly rewarding. SIA might best be used as needed to form a relationship with a puzzling or troubling sandplay case. Perhaps using the SIA method for the first tray in a series might benefit the therapist by cultivating a deepened awareness of the nature of the client's process.

My study confirmed however, like any work with sandplay, the stability and preparation of the therapist is of fundamental necessity. The SIA method has the capacity to thrust the therapist into the immediacy of the symbolic process in the sandplay. The therapist must be a sturdy, clear and ready vessel to hold what emerges.

Following are the instructions for the SIA method, as given in the formal study. Therapists may want to experiment with this method of engaging with the sandplay process to see if and how it facilitates their engagement with the symbolic process.

Directions for Subjective Immersion Analysis

You will be studying a sand tray by entering in to its reality in your imagination.

Select a prominent figure in the sand tray, which we call the focus figure. Using your imagination, you will become the focus figure, assuming its identity.

Begin by describing yourself, making notes on paper or on the computer. Please include everything that occurs to you: your thoughts, feelings, reflections, associations, etc.

When you have completed your description and reflections as the focus figure, proceed by following the same process with the other elements in the sand tray.

Remain identified with the focus figure and describe all other elements in the sand tray in the voice of the focus figure. As before, record all of your thoughts, feelings, associations, reflections, interpretations of meaning, etc.

For example, if a sand tray has a large red apple in one part, you might select it as the focus figure. Your transcript might read something like this:

I am a large, red, juicy apple. I'm so heavy and plump, full of juice. My skin is very shiny and reflects what is going on around me. I have two fleshy green leaves that shade and protect me. I feel so content and full.

Perhaps there is a squirrel in the tray, as well. The focus figure might say,

Behind me, to my left, comes a tiny squirrel. He is so little and frail. Perhaps he will take a bite out of me and fill up and get stronger.

The advantage of the Subjective Immersion Analysis method is that it facilitates a lessening of conscious viewing of the sandplay and can assist the therapist in entering the symbolic work more immediately. This requires that the therapist be centered and well anchored in the Self. Un-tethered, the imagination may be given to random flight, as we saw happen with one of the SIA study participants. As with all aspects of sandplay work, the SIA method should be used only if it feels appropriate to the individual therapist.

~ Conclusion ~

Section III
Understanding Sandplay Therapy

The various approaches to understanding the sandplay process we have reviewed provide a wealth of tools that are of great value some of the time, and are irrelevant at other times. As a part of our preparation to work as sandplay therapists, it is essential that we be familiar with all of these well-documented approaches to understanding sandplay. Then, as with all other aspects of sandplay we have studied, we must set them aside gently and allow the sandplay itself to guide us. We must listen to each tray with intense stillness in order to hear its unique directives.

~ Conclusion ~

PART TWO
Process Concepts:
Healing and Transformation
In Sandplay Therapy

This concludes our discussion of Process Concepts in Sandplay Therapy in which we have explored the growth and development of the psyche in sandplay, the themes through which this healing and change manifests in the tray and a variety of means of coming to understand this process in sandplay therapy.

Now we turn to the practical matters of using sandplay in our discussion of the Procedures of Sandplay Therapy. Having examined the process of sandplay therapy from many different angles, we are ready to look at putting sandplay into practice. In the next section we will explore the activities of both the therapist and the client before, during, and after the sandplay session.

PART THREE

Procedural Concepts:
Implementing Sandplay Therapy in Practice

THE HANDBOOK OF SANDPLAY THERAPY
PART THREE: Procedural Concepts
SECTION I: Before the Sandplay Session

Section I
Before the Sandplay Session

Chapter 1
The Therapist

Training

The responsible practice of sandplay therapy entails extensive inner and outer training. As we have seen, the apparent simplicity of sandplay is highly deceptive. Sandplay therapy is likely one of the most complex psychotherapeutic modalities that exists. Because sandplay symbolically penetrates to the core of being itself, there really is no end point to training and study. The training and preparation we discuss here is for purposes of embarking on the journey.

Sandplay training begins with the inner experience of a meaningful sandplay therapy process of one's own. This is best undertaken with a skilled, experienced, highly trained sandplay therapist. This phase of sandplay training is essential. It is the only way we can personally engage in the medium of sandplay, and experience it from the inside out. If we attempt to do sandplay without having completed a sandplay process ourselves, there is no way we can be properly prepared to adequately hold and contain this depth of work for our clients.

The *International Society for Sandplay Therapy (ISST)*, founded by Dora Kalff, has established rigorous training guidelines to become certified as a sandplay therapist. These guidelines are available through the Society's regional branches. In the United States this organization is the *Sandplay Therapists of America (STA)*. While it is currently not legally necessary to be certified to practice sandplay therapy, the training guidelines provide a sound, structured approach to sandplay. In addition to professional licensure and clinical training, these training guidelines currently include a personal sandplay process, a comprehensive coursework program of well over one hundred hours and a minimum of seventy-five hours of clinical case consultation. The certification process includes the submission and approval of a number of written materials, including a fully documented completed sandplay case from the therapist's own practice.

A course of training that adheres to these guidelines and that entails the subject matter we have explored in this book sets the stage for the practice of sandplay therapy. It is imperative that the therapist, after undergoing all of this work, feels ready to begin sandplay practice. This degree of self-awareness and self-respect is an essential quality of preparation to practice sandplay therapy.

Equipment and Supplies

Shelves

To bring sandplay therapy into your practice you need an area for shelves, which people can easily access. The shelves can be tall, so it is important to have a stool, or small ladder available. In this way, children and smaller adults will have no trouble reaching the higher shelves. Some people use bookcases for shelving. Others build narrow shelves along the walls. I have always used the deeper bookshelves, but think the narrower shelving makes the figures more accessible. On the narrow shelves, the figures are easier to see than they are deep in the recesses of a twelve inch shelf. Another difficulty with book shelves is that figures frequently tumble over when clients reach to the back for a particular figure.

Sand Trays

Two sand trays are suggested. Dora Kalff recommended having both dry and wet sand available. The sand trays are rectangular in shape, 28.5 X 19.5 X 3 inches deep. The trays are colored blue on the inner floor and walls. Choose a blue that is sky-colored, cerulean. This is a medium yet bright blue that works in a more neutral way in the sand tray than does a darker shade that might tend to psychically *pull* in darker directions.

People use all sorts of containers for sand trays, including dresser drawers and plastic buckets. There are some beautiful trays professionally made for the trade. It is also possible to have your sand trays custom made. I did this many years ago. I went to a cabinet shop, chose the wood and beautiful light blue kitchen counter material for the inner lining. I love these trays and still use them.

Perhaps a word about the quality of materials we use for sandplay is appropriate at this point. Because sandplay is so profound and meaningful, my feeling is that we need to honor it and our clients by having good quality equipment. The idea of telling an adult client that sandplay is a profoundly effective therapy, then asking him or her to sit on the floor in front of a plastic wash tray, strikes me as absurd, if not embarrassing. Remember that our environment *is the container*, also. Our equipment need not be extravagant, but it must be respectful to the work we are undertaking.

Sand Tray Carts or Tables

You will need tables or carts for the sand trays. It is important, if possible, that the client be able to move freely around the sand tray. The height of the table depends on the therapist's preference. Some therapists have them at a comfortable height for adults and children to stand. Some have their trays at a level comfortable for adults to sit in a chair. Dora Kalff had hers positioned this way. Kalff sat on one side, the longer side, of the tray, the client on the other. It can be helpful to have the carts or tables on casters, so they can be moved easily.

The size of your space will dictate some of the choices you make. I formerly worked in a luxurious space, where I had ample room for two trays in the central floor space, surrounded by shelves along the walls. My current office space is quite small. It all works out just fine. Our preparation and presence as therapists can compensate for many deficits in available space.

Water

We need to have water available for the client to add to the sand. This can be in an attractive container or a water jug.

Finger Bowl

I like to have a bowl of clean water available near the sand tray for rinsing sandy fingers. I have seen some beautiful glass bowls, with shells or beautiful rocks in the water, used for rinsing hands after sandplay.

Sand cannot go down the plumbing, as it collects in the curved trap at the bottom of the drainpipes, leading to some serious plumbing repairs. I empty the sand and water from the bowl outside in the garden.

Towels

I keep a supply of clean, folded cotton tea towels for clients to dry their hands. It is so interesting how just offering a child his or her own fresh towel can support the loving, safe, respectful container of the work. These little things make a difference.

Tools for Sand

A few simple tools for sculpting, digging and moving sand need to be available. I keep mine directly under the sand tray on the bottom shelf of the cart. Helpful tools include small shovels, rakes and spoons. Something with a straight edge for smoothing the sand, like a narrow piece of wood, can be useful. Small, medium and large flat-headed paint brushes are good for sweeping and tiding up edges where sand and water come together in the tray. Large-holed and fine sieves can be useful for sprinkling, or sorting sand. They can be helpful to the therapist later, during the disassembly process, as well.

The Collection

The collection is a vital extension of the therapist, as a result of the deep symbolic connection the therapist has with the figures. In a very literal sense, the collection is a living aspect of the container. The therapist's active, unseen psychic participation in the choice of figures activates an archetypal connection to each object. The collective presence of the figures as a whole body thus holds profound archetypal energy, as well as, the unique qualities of the individual therapist, who has assembled them.

There is no formula for the sandplay collection. The objective of the collection is to have a representation of all parts of life and fantasy. Remember however, that what is needed to carry symbolic process is not necessarily elaborate. The psyche can express and move itself with proper containment and a very small collection. Additionally, if a client needs to make a figure that is not in the collection, it is a good idea to have building and craft materials available.

Although the sandplay collection can be extensive and grand, it need not be. I feel that it is important to issue a health warning at this juncture, as it seems that every sandplay therapist I have ever known is quickly overtaken by a passion for collecting figures that can only be likened unto a disease! Of course, I am kidding. The fact is however, that the work of sandplay demands the fullness of who we are, body, mind and spirit. Sandplay therapists are fascinated by symbols and their sandplay figure collections. Our passionate pursuit of figures to augment our collections is driven by something deep within us.

Figures for the Sandplay Collection

A basic sandplay collection might include the following items. The basic collection may include multiples of some of these items, such as soldiers, people and animals. In some cases, it is apparent that a single figure in a category will be adequate. For example, one unicorn or one king may be all that the collection requires. I offer the following list as a guideline.

People
- Babies, Children, Adults
- Different Ethnicities
- Familiar & Foreign
- Young & Old
- People in action, doing various tasks
- Police, Fire & Rescue Workers

Household Furnishings
- Furniture
- Common Household Items
- Food

Architecture
- Houses, Towers, Churches
- Temples, Shops
- Domestic and Foreign
- Old and New

Vehicles
- Land, Air, Water
- Old & New
- Rescue & Helper
- Military

- Military
  - Contemporary Soldiers & Weapons
  - Historical Soldiers & Armaments
- Animals
  - Land, Sea, Air
  - Wild & Domestic
- Magical Creatures
  - Unicorn, Pegasus, Dragon
  - Archetypal Horses (pure white, blue)
- Magical People
  - Magicians, Fairies, Wizards
  - Fairy Tale, Cartoon Characters
  - Super Heroes and Villains
- Ancient Creatures
  - Dinosaurs
- Archetypal Figures
  - **Mythic Figures**
  - **People** – King, Queen, Prince, Princess
  - **Shapes** – Cube, Sphere, Circle, Square
    Triangle, Pyramid, Sun, Moon, Stars
  - **Jewels** – Glass Marbles, Beads
    Gold Chains, Treasure Chest, Gifts
- Shadow and Death Figures
  - Skeletons, Gravestones, Coffins,
  - Bones, Monsters, Dark & Scary Figures
- Religious and Spiritual Figures
  - People and Artifacts from Different
  - Traditions, Eastern and Western
- Elements
  - Fire, Ice, Windmill, Waterwheel, Well
  - Balloon, Flag, Shovel
- Items from Nature
  - Rocks, Shells, Wood
  - Trees, Shrubs, Flowers, Greenery,
  - Fruits & Vegetables
- Connectors and Dividers
  - Fencing, Bridges, Road &Traffic Signs
  - Telephone
- Building and Craft Materials
  - Tiles, Sticks, Clay, Paper, String, Glue

Acquiring the Collection

There are several companies that sell sandplay starter kits. A kit can be an excellent way to begin a collection, but is not necessary. There are so many places to find small figures. Toy stores, flea markets, dollhouse shops, toy train suppliers, craft stores and souvenir shops are but a few. How and where we acquire the figures is a personal reflection of who we are. These are only suggestions.

It is also rewarding to make some of the figures for our collections. For example, sturdy trees can be difficult to locate, but are easily made by mounting artificial greenery in a plaster base. Plasticine modeling clay can be shaped, baked and painted to make some of the more difficult to find items, such as fires. I recommend spraying hand-painted figures with a finishing coat of liquid plastic in order to prevent water damage in the sand tray. Found objects, such as stones and driftwood, bring meaning to the collection by being discovered and gathered in nature and places we love. Each piece carries memories and feelings.

The size of sandplay figures is also a matter of taste. Some therapists prefer that all figures be in proportion to one another. Others find the imposing size of disproportionate figures to be an important part of the symbolic process. I lean toward maintaining a level range of size in my collection, but do have a couple of large monster figures and some very small items, as well.

Arranging the Collection

Arranging the collection is a matter of the therapist's personal taste. Therapists approach this issue in very different ways, which reflect aspects of their personalities. The arrangement and maintenance of the collection becomes a significant aspect of the individual therapist's unique way of holding and containing the overall sandplay process. After all, a great deal of the therapist's personal energy, personality and style is invested in the selection and arrangement of the collection.

I have seen collections that vary widely in arrangement from precise, neat and orderly on one side of the spectrum, to completely random and messy on the other. Personally, I am most comfortable with a general pattern of organization that groups items in a meaningful way. This accomplishes two things. First, when a client asks for a particular figure, finding it in its general category on the shelves is not too difficult. Second, I simply feel more comfortable presenting the collection to the clients in a way that is not jarring or chaotic to the psyche. In other words, I suspect that the client is more at peace scanning for a particular type of person among groupings of human figures, rather than having to look about randomly to locate what they need. I group the figures in the general categories listed above under *Figures Needed for the Sandplay Collection.*

If you opt to arrange the figures in groupings, then the issue arises as to how to place the groups. My preference in is to follow a combination of developmental and archetypal guidelines. The developmental aspect of the placement considers the general size and height of the client and the easy access to figures that children of that general range of development might typically want to use. What this means is that categories such as animals, people, common household furnishings, cartoon and fairy tale figures are placed on lower shelves. I place the soldiers, military vehicles and horses in a middle-range area for easy access by the elementary school aged children. The archetypal dimension of my placement preference includes putting the earthly, natural items, such as rocks, trees and shells on the lowest shelves, or the floor, while putting the more spiritual, religious figures on the higher shelves. I further divide these by putting Eastern religious items and people toward the upper left side of the collection, and their Western counterparts on the upper right side. I also place the death figures up on higher shelves. Developmentally, children do not typically need these figures for their work, so they are generally out of view. However, when and if a child does require a more archetypal figure, they will find it. The psyche compels them to look higher and they ask to climb up on the ladder, "To see what's up there." It takes some doing to find our own comfortable way of being with the collection. This is all a part of sandplay containment.

Room Preparation

The sandplay room must always be in a state of receptive readiness, when a client is present in the room. This creates the *temenos*, the sacred place that is apart from ordinary time and space. In this way, the sandplay is always available, inviting the client to move into his or her depths in a safe and respectful way.

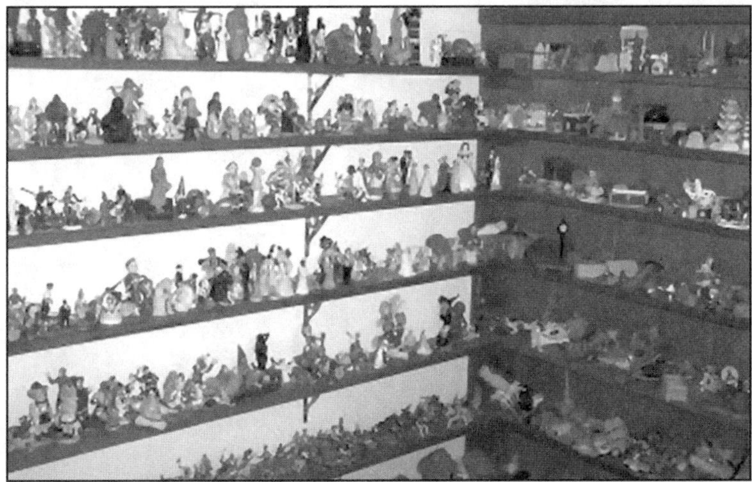

Photographs B. Turner, 2003

Views of two sandplay collections. A colleague's, using narrow shelving (above) and the author's, with deeper shelves (below).

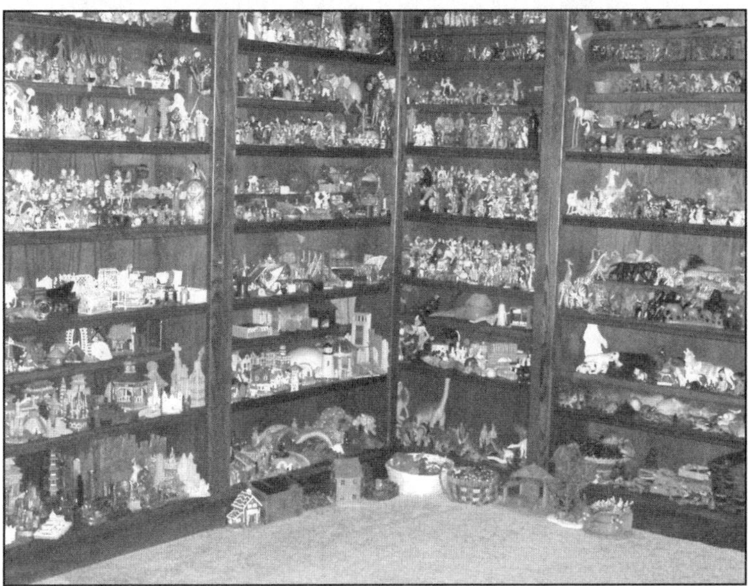

This means that figures are returned to the shelves, the sand cleared and smoothed. The water, tools and towels are all available. It is an important part of containment that the client always finds the sandplay in this state of readiness.

Chapter 2

The Client—Introducing the Client to Sandplay

Before a client works in the sand tray, he or she will want to know something about it. How the therapist introduces sandplay therapy has a great deal of bearing on whether or not most adults will work in the sand. In the case of child clients, the children tend to dive right into the work, but their parents need to understand why sandplay is important and how it differs from playing at home. How we as therapists *carry, or hold* sandplay therapy in our initial contact with new clients is an important aspect of containment that may powerfully influence the entire course of therapy. Our first impressions of anyone or anything new are significant. This applies to our work in sandplay in profound ways.

Explaining Sandplay to Adult Clients

When an adult client enters the office for the first time, he or she sees the sand tray and the collection. The client may say something like, *…Oh, I see you work with children.* Or, they may simply glance at the collection. This is the opportunity to introduce sandplay. Given the nature of the trepidations of any first session, this is a gentle, brief introduction. While greeting the new client and showing them through the office, I say something like this,

> This is the sandplay therapy. We use it for children and adults, as well. It is a powerful therapy, like a dream, that allows us to work through deep issues in a safe, non-verbal way. I do not know if this will be right for us or not. We will see.

I then invite the client to sit down, so we can get started.

Later in the therapy, the client may indicate interest in sandplay. At this time we can show them how it is done. When this occurs, I invite the client to come over by the sand tray and say something like this,

> Let me show you how we do sandplay.
> This is called the sand tray. The method is known as sandplay.
>
> (While I move the sand around to demonstrate) The tray is blue on the bottom, if you want to make a river, a lake or a design.
>
> What you do is move the sand around for a while. You can shape it. The wet sand holds more firmly than the dry, which feels softer. (I demonstrate with the two trays.)
>
> (Demonstrating, choosing two or three figures randomly from the shelves) Then you go to the shelves and pick out whatever grabs your attention and put it in the tray.
>
> As you do that, a scene or a world may develop, or not. You can have an idea about what you want to make, or not. It absolutely does not matter and it is not an art contest. It is simply a way of allowing what is inside of us, the stuff that doesn't have words, to come up and out in symbols.
>
> While you do that, I sit quietly over there (indicating my chair) and make a little map of what you do. Don't be concerned about changing things around, because I can keep up with it just fine.
>
> You will know when you are finished. Then I'll come around and look at the sandplay with you. I may ask if you had any associations while you were doing it. (Pointing to what I have done in the tray) You may say something like, "Well, that one is chasing that one. This one is sick. And I have no idea about the rest of it." I just write that down, then take photos for your file. Some time after our work together is complete, we can go through your pictures together to understand what the work was about. By then, you will be able to tell me.

That is it. You never take your tray apart, but just let it live inside of you.

Perhaps you would like to do a tray now, or later?

In the event an adult client does not mention sandplay, after a therapeutic trust is established and I feel sandplay is appropriate, I will say that I really think that sandplay would be very helpful and that we might seriously consider beginning a series of sand trays. I then invite the client to the tray and introduce the method, as above.

Explaining Sandplay to Parents and Children

Introducing Sandplay to Parents

My practice is to meet with the parents of child clients without the children, before seeing the children. This accomplishes several important tasks, which benefit the child's therapy. By doing this, I am able to take a thorough history that will help my assessment. This meeting establishes a good working rapport with the parents, gives them a sense of confidence in the therapist, who will be working with their child and it informs them of what to expect from therapy. I tell the parents I will see the child two or three times, then have another session with them to review my assessment of their child and any treatment recommendations.

The confidence of the parents in the therapist is a critical aspect of the containment of the work, as they feel included in the treatment. This can circumvent any apprehensions they may develop when the child bonds closely to the therapist, or when the child begins to change and they do not exactly understand how this is taking place. When working with children we depend upon the therapeutic alliance of the parents to hold and sustain the work. This is never so important as in the sandplay process, when the child's psyche demands the time necessary to undergo the fullness of a completed piece of work. Any early termination is a rupture in the sandplay process. In therapy with children, the alliance of the parents is essential to the continuation of the work.

During this first session with the parents, I introduce sandplay therapy, using much the same language, as we discussed above. I tell the parents that we also draw, play games, and so on.

Additionally, I say to the parents,

> Because of their age and level of brain development, children aren't able to stand apart from what they experience, to analyze it the same way we adults might. The language of children's minds IS imagery and symbols. They talk to me with their sandplays.
>
> So, even though it appears that they are JUST PLAYING, they are deeply engaged in their inner work. Play IS how they do their work. On some level, they know this. They want to come here and work.
>
> It's so funny though, if we ask them what they did in their session, they will say, "…I colored. I played checkers. I made a sand picture."

When I meet with the parents again for the assessment interview, I share my general clinical impressions of the child's needs. I draw most of this information from the first two or three sandplays the child has done, as these trays are filled with indications of the child's wounding, assets, strengths and therapeutic direction. This meeting underscores the parents' confidence in the therapist, because the therapist demonstrates that he or she understands what is going on with their child and is clear about the therapeutic possibilities.

In cases where the parents are resistant to having their child in therapy or are in denial about the child's needs, it is critical to both secure the parents' confidence and to communicate the child's real needs to them. This can occur when the child is referred for treatment by the school or a community agency. In the early phases of the treatment process the therapist must have the parents' cooperation to work with the child, yet must sensitively and respectfully deal with their resistance. In some cases, I will show the photos of the child's early sandplay work to the parents. This is a way of communicating what I attempt to say in words directly with their deeper selves, through the symbols. Seeing their child's sandplay pictures visually impacts them far more than my words. I do not always show the parents the first two or three sandplay pictures during the assessment interview, but when I do, I comment,

> We don't usually share the sandplays with the parents, because the kids need a place of their own to work through their troubles. But sometimes pictures say a lot more than words.

This tells the parents that seeing the child's sandplay is not a usual practice. In some cases however, it can secure the parent's confidence and cooperation.

Certainly, being with the child and understanding the family's circumstances and history have a lot of bearing on an assessment. It is fascinating however, that the inner work a child may undergo in sandplay is often of a different nature than what appears on the surface. An example of this is the case of **Ivy**, who was brought into therapy for fighting with her brother and not doing well in school. As we have illustrated in several prior discussions, her sandplay work concerned her identity roles and authenticity as a female. Of course, she did better in school and got along better with her brother after the sandplay work, but the relationship between the inner and the outer circumstances was not immediately apparent and was certainly unknown to her mother and father.

Abrupt Termination of Child Clients

Perhaps a word about abrupt terminations is necessary at this point. A great peril in work with child clients is the parents' unwillingness or inability to see the child's work through to completion. As all child therapists are painfully aware, early or abrupt termination is a fact of life.

Although we do our best to engage the parents' trust and cooperation, it is a sad fact that children's treatment can come to abrupt and premature ends. When this happens, the child and the therapist can be left feeling raw and hurt. For the child a sudden termination is abandonment and the loss of a safe, trusting relationship where he or she was seen and honored for perhaps the first time. For the therapist, an inappropriate termination can feel as if he or she has caused a child hurt, rather than the hoped for healing.

When we are properly ordered to the work of sandplay and we believe we have done our work well, such painful endings become a living component of doing child therapy. These losses are a living reality of holding and containing the pain and powerlessness suffered by many children. I know however, from the deepest part of myself, that being with a safe, respectful adult in a free and protected environment for even a brief time ignites something profound and powerful in a child. Even if the child's life is unpredictable, dangerous and ugly, the experience of being recognized in his or her truth, Self to Self, by the therapist, awakens this possibility in him or her. Hell may exist around them, but children that have been honored in the free and protected space of sandplay know that what goes on around them is not right and that something else is possible. The child that has been held in the sandplay temenos NEVER forgets it.

As therapists we must question ourselves to be certain that we have done all we can for the parents and children in our care. When we do err, we must make amends and learn from our failings. When we have done all we can and therapy comes to an abrupt and inappropriate end, we must have faith in the power of the safe, loving relationship in Self, where the child has been allowed, albeit briefly, to be real and free to heal and grow.

The therapist's loving connection to the child in the energetic field of symbolic process does not end simply because the child is taken away. The affective resonance with the child, which is gained at the very profound level, defies the boundaries of time and space, as long as the therapist is able to hold it. When a child is taken from therapy abruptly, I turn my attention to this eternal aspect of containment and continue to hold with love.

Introducing Sandplay to Children

Introducing sandplay to children is rarely difficult. Frequently children are playing in the sand before the therapist has said anything to them about it. The readiness of children to dive into sandplay continually reminds me of Jung's observation that the psyche has a natural tendency to heal and be whole. Play and images are natural to children, so they take to it like fish to water.

Even when the child is already scooping and moving sand, I tell them a few things about sandplay. This establishes a mutual understanding about sandplay. I tell the child,

> This is sandplay. We call this the tray. We've got wet and dry sand. They feel different.
>
> The trays are blue on the bottom, to make lakes and designs.
>
> You can use any of the toys in here to make a picture in the sand. …Just like making your own world.
>
> Sometimes when you come in, I'll have things for us to do, drawing, games, and such. Sometimes you'll get to choose what we'll do. But you can always do a sandplay.
>
> I've got only one rule with sandplay… Don't throw sand at Dr. Barb.

Saying this is part of the containment. It is permission-giving and at the same time, establishes some boundaries. I believe it is important to have this communication with children, although one little girl, who was already busy in the sand, did look up at me and comment, "Boy! You sure do talk a lot!"

Introducing Sandplay to Adolescents

When I introduce sandplay to adolescents, my primary concern is to overcome any suspicions they might have about it being infantile, or child's play. I generally say something like this,

> This is the sandplay therapy. We use it for adults, as well as children. Anytime you are here, please feel free to do a tray. Let me show you how it's done.
>
> (I explain the procedure as I do with adults)
>
> Sandplay is a very deep therapy, but of course, kids just think they are playing!
>
> It's a good way to do our work without talking, or having to understand what is going on.

Some therapists comment that adolescents are hesitant to do sandplay. This is my experience. The mix of the psychic depth that is tapped in sandplay and the developmental upheavals of adolescence may explain their reluctance to work in the sand. However, there are therapists who do work well with adolescents in sandplay. Swiss Jungian analyst, Kaspar Kiepenheuer (1990) worked very successfully with this population and has written valuable material on the subject.

Client Readiness for Sandplay

Whether sandplay is an appropriate treatment for a client is largely a matter of containment. Whereas we once said that sandplay was inappropriate for treatment in schizophrenia and psychotic disorders, there are highly trained, capable sandplay therapists, who are well-versed with this population and are using sandplay effectively. With this population, sandplay has significant therapeutic qualities as an external container for their inner torments (Baum, 2002). This is more of an expressive use of the sand tray and is different from the classic sandplay process of the non-psychotic client. It is nonetheless, highly effective in the watchful containment of clinicians who are at home with these clients.

The same advice regarding sandplay therapists working with psychotic clients extends to all therapeutic populations. Sandplay is appropriate *when the therapist can properly contain* it. Whether a client will want to do sandplay, or not, is another matter, which brings us to the topic of resistance.

Client Resistance to Sandplay

Adult Resistance to Sandplay

Resistance to sandplay may occur at any phase of the process. Resistance to beginning a sandplay series may arise from a variety of psychic processes. One cause of resistance is fear. The level of the trepidation can range all the way from mild apprehension to full-fledge terror. The source of the client's fear can vary widely. For example, it may stem from a deep terror of loss of control over reality and portend a deep psychic instability. It may stem from fears of having to perform, of judgment or criticism.

When the adult is fearful of doing sandplay the therapist must make an appropriate assessment of what is transpiring with the client in relationship to the sandplay, and whether or not it is even appropriate or timely to facilitate the conscious holding of that fear in the therapy. Sometimes it is appropriate to gently ask the client if the sandplay feels a little scary. This can be a sensitive way of beginning to carry the fear together in a more conscious, open way. Sometimes it is not at all appropriate to inquire about the fear of sandplay. The therapeutic container is a living organism that changes from moment to moment. Only the sufficiently prepared sandplay therapist is able to discern what is right at the time.

The client's *resistance* to sandplay differs from *reluctance* to doing a tray, once having started the process. When a client, child or adult, has done three or four sandplays without displaying any hesitance, subsequent reluctance likely concerns a need for more processing time for the work they have already done in the sand. In this instance, the reluctance may indicate growing self-awareness and the need to honor their own pace with psychic change. If the therapist feels that it is therapeutically appropriate, he or she may confirm this with the client, using the reluctance to do a sandplay as a means of acknowledging the client's consciousness of his or her inner life.

When a client appears resistant to begin sandplay or to move forward in the process we must be mindful of the tendency of the ego to hold on for dear life in the presence of the unknown. As we recall from our discussions of sacred time and space, resistance to the sacred is a characteristic of all deeply transformative experience (Eliade, 1958/1996). In the terms of Jungian psychology this might be regarded as the ego's resistance to releasing its hold on identity. It is important to remember that the psychic processes undergone in sandplay can be fearsome.

Many adults will resist doing sandplay, as they think it is silly. This is a common occurrence, as Western culture tends to direct our energies outwardly and does not honor the inner life. For this reason many adults grow painfully dissatisfied with their lives and enter therapy, overly rational and disconnected from their depths. During the client's first session I introduce sandplay therapy as we discussed above and after a strong therapeutic alliance is established, I initiate a new discussion about sandplay in terms of trust and distrust of their own inner resources.

Developmental considerations may impact a client's apparent resistance to sandplay. Adults who have suffered wounds to the development of their own initiative at a very early age will not go to the sand by themselves. If the adult was raised by highly fearful or controlling parents, this adult's internal sense of control and empowerment may be so thwarted that he or she always waits for external direction. In these cases, the client's apparent resistance to sandplay has more to do with their inability to initiate. In some cases, it may be appropriate to direct them to the sandplay.

Resistance to sandplay may also result from inadequate containment on the part of the therapist. The therapist must frankly ask him or herself if there are important elements of the sandplay process of which he or she is unaware. The therapist must also carefully examine his or her psychic relationship to the client and the sandplay process. Perhaps there is something being constellated in the therapist that is impeding the client's process. In either case it is crucial to seek consultation to assist the therapist in his or her work with the case.

HAROLD **Harold's** sandplay work is a good example of wounded initiative. Although **Harold** was well into his sixties at the time of treatment, he still took direction from his elderly mother, who issued opinions and criticism about every aspect of his life. **Harold** entered therapy, because his wife told him to. He began sandplay because I told him to. Once engaged in sandplay he began to tap his own authentic inner resources.

In the process of constructing **Tray 6**, **Harold** mused out loud, "I need something to use for an ice rink." Thinking nothing about it, I said, "There are some things over..." Suddenly, with fire in his eyes, he looked directly at me, shouting, "I'll do it myself! " I was never so happy to have been put in my place!

Harold chose a plastic tablemat that was used to keep paint off of the craft table. Significantly, **Harold's** ice skating rink is messy and covered with smudges. It contrasts dramatically with his otherwise obsessive need for perfection. With this choice, **Harold** lays a foundation for himself. His psyche configures a new ground upon which he can glide with freedom and joy. In the symbolic context of the sandplay **Harold** overcomes an early developmental arrest, tapping his own ability to initiate action with authentic intent.

SHANNON **Shannon** overcame her resistance to sandplay through her trust in the therapeutic container. A strong, highly rational thinking type, **Shannon** made it clear in her first session that she just wanted some pointers and would be out of treatment in less than a year. Eventually she began sandplay, because she trusted me. She frequently would adamantly posture, "This is stupid! I only do it for you." Many years later, she lovingly shared, "You know, I still don't get this. I only do it because you want me to!" Even so, **Shannon's** sandplay took her to the depths of her soul, grounding her in a profound source of loving power that transformed her and sustained her through inordinate losses. In her final sandplay, **Tray 39 Shannon's** psyche settles in a bucolic marketplace just beyond the rainbow. In the center, a baby frog sits peacefully with its mother. Beside them stands a small conical spiral shell, indicative of the tremendous inner and outer transformation **Shannon** has undergone. Nursing piglets foretell an abundant future by a small clear, crystal ball.

Child Resistance to Sandplay

When a child client shows fear of doing sandplay, my concerns are about interruptions in development that have impaired the ability to play freely. Knowing the child's history is helpful in most cases, but even with this knowledge, we can be surprised. Whether or not the child has ever been able to engage in play behavior is a critical factor in determining if he or she has developed sufficiently to do sandplay therapy. The youngest age by which a normally developing child can begin to use the sand tray meaningfully is three. My experience shows that some three-year-olds are ready for the sand, while others are not. The less developed three year-olds will use the sand for pouring, mixing and cooking. While these are certainly important forms of age-appropriate play they are developmentally prior to the symbolic use of the tray. My experience indicates that the therapist can expect to see a meaningful use of sandplay in four year-olds that have suffered no impairments to their ability to play.

In the normal course of development, babies begin to play simple peek-a-boo games with their parents at just a few weeks of age. Children that are unable to play have experienced such early trauma and deprivation that the normal development of play has been lost. These children are not going to dive into the sand as other healthier, children will. They are not ready to do sandplay and have earlier developmental requirements. Therapeutic interventions that address early attachment and sensory needs may be necessary before they are ready to move into the sand.
Children that have developed the ability to play but are now fearful of doing so present a different clinical picture. Although this scenario is not common, when it does occur the therapist must understand what it is that has robbed the child of the natural ability to play. Being mindful of the child's fears and understanding their origins becomes a central containment issue. The child may suffer from an endogenous anxiety disorder. He or she may have endured severe trauma, historical or current. There may be something looming in the family unconscious so terrifying as to nearly paralyze the child. These are but a few of many possibilities that would give rise a child's resistance to sandplay. With trust building we would hope that such children would slowly move to the sand and figures, gradually becoming able to express themselves in the sand tray.

I have seen elegant sandplay work where the therapists have gently handled figures, sharing them with a terrified child. Over the course of many sessions, the therapists gradually place a figure or two in the sand, as if to remind the child that it is safe to play again. Such patient and loving containment by the therapist can restore the child's vitality and capacity to play and allow them to move more fully into their sandplay work.

Frequency of Sandplays

There are no rules about how often a client ought to or will do sandplay. Each circumstance is unique. The proper containment of the process is unique to each therapeutic relationship. There are adult clients who will do a sandplay each session. There are others who will do sandplay infrequently, with months or even years lapsing between trays. Even so these processes can be deeply transformative. **Shannon's** sandplays were sometimes years apart, yet the process was coherent and transformative. A total of eleven years transpires between **Shannon's Tray 1** and her final **Tray 39**.

Children will frequently want to do two trays per session. Some children will complete two trays with no hesitation and without asking about it. Some children will ask if they can make two sandplays. When they do ask, I reply, "Well, we try to keep it in one, but if we just can't, two are just fine."

My use of the phrase ...*keep IT in one* is purposeful. When saying this to the child, I am speaking to the deepest part of him or her. Rather than responding in a restrictive or disciplinary manner, as might be implied in ...*we try to do only one,* I convey the message that *IT* is meaningful work and process.

The watchful presence of the therapist's containment must be sufficiently flexible to meet each unique client in each moment with what *is* transpir-*ing* at that time. The primary concern is for the therapist to be mindful of the client's inner process and needs and to facilitate the client's growing awareness of same.

Integrating Sandplay with Other Therapeutic Modalities

Adults

Sandplay therapists agree that sandplay combines well with other modalities such as dream work, verbal analysis and active imagination (Donelan, 2000). There are however, distinct differences in the modalities. Whereas the therapist may actively interpret and offer insight in dreams, verbal analysis and active imagination, no interpretation is made in Jungian sandplay. The reason for this is that the content of verbal therapy is closer to conscious awareness than the material that is accessed in sandplay. More time is required for the content and process of the sandplay work to become conscious.

When sandplay is integrated with other modalities in adult therapy, it is almost as if there are parallel treatments happening simultaneously. While more conscious issues are addressed in the verbal therapies, what is moving in the sandplay is likely completely unknown to the client at the time. What results are content and process differences between the conscious and the unconscious aspects of the therapy. The therapist must contain both levels of the client's process.

Children

In my work with children I have always integrated sandplay with other play therapy modalities. As we saw above in the introduction of sandplay to the child, I make it clear that sandplay is the central activity we do. Some sandplay therapists have no other materials available and restrict their work with children to sandplay alone. My experience is that children will not always be ready to do sandplay and need other means of expression and release.

If a child does not feel like doing sandplay and says something such as, *...I really want to paint!* My heart and intuition tell me to follow that child's needs. Jung's observation that the psyche has a natural tendency to heal and grow toward wholeness applies to the child's realm of play. I firmly believe that everything in the vicinity of the sand tray concerns sandplay. Sandplay is the heart of the child's work. The child will return his or her work to the tray when the time is right.

The child has far less separation between the conscious and unconscious aspects of therapy than does the adult. Younger children especially, are directly engaged in the lived reality of symbol and myth. Therefore, there is less separation between what they do in the sand tray and what they do around it. It is important to watch their play, study their paintings, carefully note what play appeals to them, then consider its relevance to what is transpiring in their sandplay process.

AARON Aaron's work is a good example of the integration of other modalities with his sandplay process. Throughout the course of his sandplay series, Aaron was fascinated with volcanoes. Although he never used a volcano in his sandplays, between trays, he sculpted volcanoes out of plasticine. He later painted a series of volcanoes in progressive states of eruption.

The rage that had built up as a result of Aaron's disappointment and embarrassment over his father's irresponsible behavior and the resulting confusion about what it meant for him to grow into manhood was worked through in the sandplay. The rage was expressed and vented through his artistry.

Section II
During the Sandplay Session

Chapter 1
The Therapist

Introduction

The activities of the therapist during the sandplay session are much the same with adult and child clients. There are some special considerations with children, which we will discuss below. We have examined the therapist's role as container at great length throughout our study. What concerns us in this section is what the therapist needs to do as the client works in the sand tray.

Stance and Stillness

The stance of the therapist during the sandplay session is critical yet it is so subtle as to be nearly impossible to describe. To be present as the client does sandplay is an honor. The shared experience of the sandplay session is a sacred engagement where the client entrusts the therapist with the deepest, unknown regions of him or herself.

It is not enough to say that the therapist must remain quiet during the sandplay session. Being outwardly silent but inwardly noisy will not work. Also, there are times when a quiet verbalization or exchange with the client is completely appropriate. It is probably better to say that the therapist must remain *still.* All of the sandplay therapist's training and preparation is about the ability to sit in this stillness in the presence of the unfolding process of the client. The therapist must be acutely present and, at the same time, remain completely out of the way.

Record Keeping

Maintaining comprehensive records of sandplay is a critical aspect of holding the work. We depend on written and photographic records to reflect on and maintain an abiding relationship with the sandplay process. It is not possible to properly hold sandplay by memory alone or without good records. The reason for this is that much of what transpires in the client's sandplay is unconscious to us. It is important that we have ways of sitting with the work in order to allow it to continue to inform us. When we look at a sand tray, we do not see the greater part of it. Only by creating time and space to quietly witness sandplay, are we able to enter into its symbolic matrix in a vital, meaningful way.

The client's psyche *moves* as he or she engages in the symbolic dimension. While doing sandplay, the client is changing his or her psychic structure through the manipulation of concrete images of his or her inner world in the tray. Having this physical participation in the symbolic dimension, the three-dimensional manifestation of each sandplay is like a sculptural mold, which casts the configuration of a new psychic form in the client. With the sandplay the intrapsychic die is cast and is working on the client's psyche to re-order consciousness into the new configuration shaped in the sand tray. Said another way, once the client has completed the tray, it is working on him or her to transform the psyche, to the direction and condition held in the symbolic context of the sandplay.

The sandplay does work on the therapist, as well. However, the sandplay is primarily the psychic movement of the client, not the therapist. Thus, to contain what transpires in the symbolic constructs in the client's sandplay, the therapist needs images and records. In order to maintain a vital relationship to the client's symbolic process, the therapist must have ways of engaging with what is working on the client.

As the client makes the sandplay, the therapist sits quietly and makes notes and sketches of what the client does. My preference is to sit across the tray from the client, a few feet away from the tray. This allows enough room for the client to move freely around the sand tray and it provides me a clear view of what the client does. The only problem with sitting across from the client is that the therapist views the tray upside down, or opposite of the view from the client's position. Some therapists prefer to sit off to the side or slightly behind the client. I have done both, given the available space in various office settings. The important considerations in deciding where to sit are to be close enough to the tray and the client to be involved in the process but distant enough to give the client the physical and psychic room necessary to work.

The Sandplay Record Form

Through the generosity and shared experiences with colleagues in consultation over the years, I have developed a *Sandplay Record Form*, which works well for me during the note-taking portion of sandplay. I have included a copy of this form as an illustration. Please feel free to copy it and alter it to suit your needs.

I keep a stack of these forms on a clipboard near my chair in the sandplay area. When the client begins to work in the tray, I record the client's name, the date and the number of this sandplay in the client's sequence. For example,

Name: Mary Brown **Date:** October 15, 2003 **Tray No.** 14.

I then check whether the tray is **dry** or **wet**, and note if the client adds water to the tray.

Any comments the client makes while beginning the tray, I note verbatim in quotation marks in the top section, marked *Comments.* I also use this area to make my own comments about what might be transpiring in the client's life that may have significant emotional and psychic impact. If there is a significant amount of such information, I write, …*See session notes.* If the client were to hum a song, begin to weep, have trembling hands, behave aggressively or defiantly, or do anything of note that is related to the sandplay process, I write it in the *Comment* area of the form. If the client touches and works the sand, or does not touch it at all, I note this as well.

As the client begins to place figures, I chart them in sequence according to their position, in the little rectangular sand tray map on the upper right corner of the *Sandplay Record Form.* As I sit across the tray from the client, my map will end up being upside down. Nonetheless, it provides an accurate record of what went in, where it went and in what order. Figure 1 is marked first as a number 1 on the map. I then note what the item is in the numbered column on the left edge of the form. In this way we are able to track the sequence of the changes. It may be quite significant that the hen no longer belongs in the tray, either after the snake arrives, or before what follows. I make similar notes of process between the numbered sequence, about moving the sand, making a pond, extending the river, and so on.

SANDPLAY RECORD FORM Client ______________ Date ______________ Tray No. ___________ Wet ___ Dry ___	**(Map of figure placement)**

Initial Observations/Remarks—(Therapist) or "Client"

Placement Sequence

1	**14**	**27**
2	**15**	**30**
3	**16**	**31**
4	**17**	**32**
5	**18**	**33**
6	**19**	**34**
7	**20**	**35**
8	**21**	**36**
9	**22**	**37**
10	**23**	**38**
11	**24**	**39**
12	**25**	**40**
13	**26**	

Client's Closing Remarks

Using the Sandplay Record Form, let's follow the beginning of a hypothetical sandplay construction. First, I make a note of the client's position at the tray, and I also indicate where I am sitting.

If the client places a large red barn in the center of the tray, I write a number 1 in the corresponding location on my map, and I note the word "barn" as item 1 in the Placement Sequence section of the record form.

Map of Figure Placement

Placement Sequence
1. Barn
2.
3.

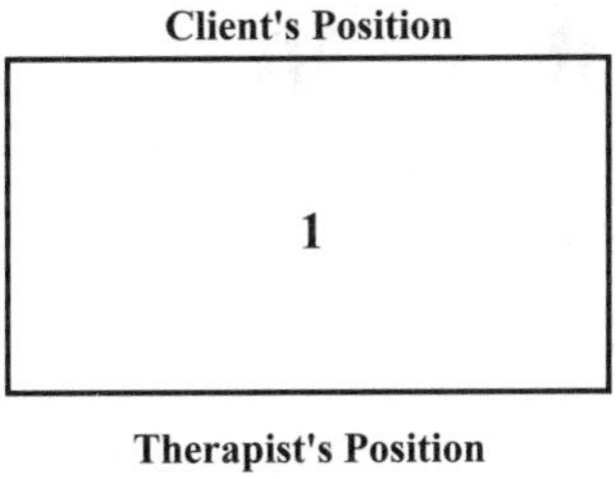

Client's Position

1

Therapist's Position

If the client then places a hen in front of the barn, I note a 2 where the hen is, from my vantage point, and write,

Placement Sequence
1. Barn
2. Hen
3.

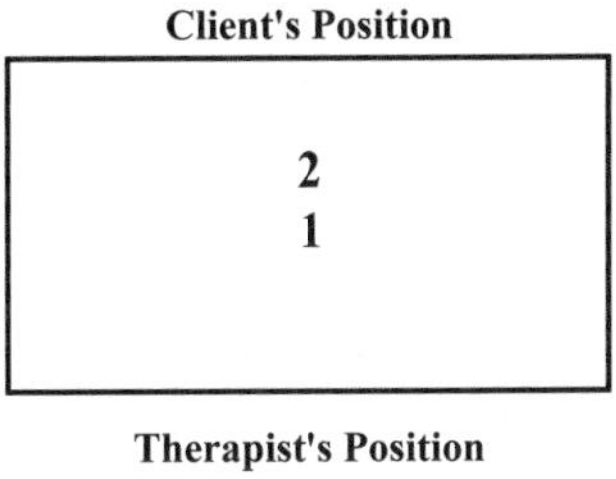

Client's Position

2
1

Therapist's Position

Sometimes the placement of the figures is so rapid that it is only possible to map the numbers. I can later, either during the session, or from photographs, note what the objects are that I missed during the session. Sometimes a client will put several figures in simultaneously. Just note what happens. Do the best you can. It can be rather challenging!

When a client removes a figure, I cross it off on the map and on the numbered list. I also make a note at the point in the sequence that the item was removed. For example, our sample tray has progressed to item 5, then the client removes item 2, I do the following,

Placement Sequence
1. Barn
2.x Hen
3. Farmer
4. Squirrel
5. Snake
   (Removes 2)

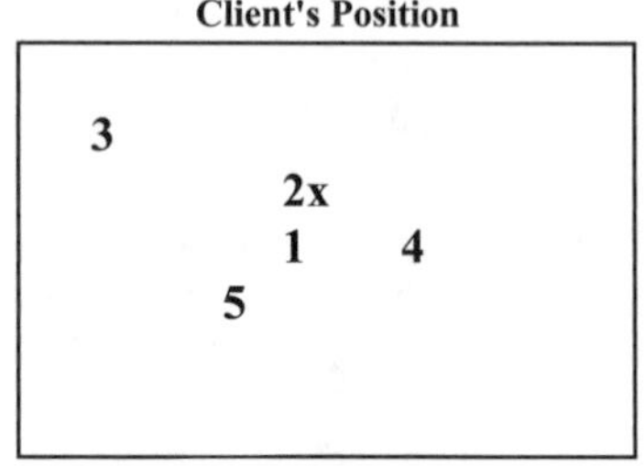

ADRIENNE Let us take an example from **Adrienne's** work. By following the sequence of placement on the sandplay record form of **Adrienne's Tray 1**, we see that she first places a man in the center and calls him *Father*. That she refers to him as "Father" is indicated by the quotation marks around what she said. **1. "Father".** **Adrienne's** second figure is the baby, which she places on the Father's lap. I indicate what she does within the parentheses, **2. Baby (on father's lap).** During **Adrienne's** reflections on her tray, she moves the baby, knocks over the motorcycle and the cup. These gestures are recorded in parentheses as they occur during the course of her verbal reflections.

The movements of the baby, motorcycle and the cup carry important aspects of **Adrienne's** process. By being able to review the sequence of the figure placement, her affect and her gestures, it is clear that a significant aspect of **Adrienne's** process concerns a proper "seating" in the masculine (father's lap) the "freedom" (motorcycle) and the nurturing (the cup) that this central issue holds. The movement of the three figures underscores the intimate psychic connection between these wounds to **Adrienne's** development and allows her to begin grieving their loss.

While the therapist keeps these notes, he or she must also note the client's affect, anything they might say while picking up a figure, etc. When the tray is completed, we will take photographs for a visual record. What we attempt to do with the note taking is to keep track of the *process of doing the sandplay*. The Sandplay Record Forms for a complete sandplay case are included in **The Case of Aaron** in Part Four. Following the sample trays sequentially through their construction process deepens our relationship to the client's work and aids the capacity to hold the psyche's movements. Studying the Record Forms in **Aaron's** work will also familiarize the newer therapist with the use of the form and the necessary record keeping in sandplay.

Example Sandplay Record Form

Client: Adrienne
Tray: 1
Date: 8 months into therapy
Wet Tray X
Dry Tray

Client's Position

2/1
5 5
3
5 4

Therapist's Position

Initial Observations/Remarks
(Works tray from left side)

Placement Sequence

1 "Father"
2 Baby (on Father's lap)
3 Motorcycle
4 Cup
5 Balloons

Clients Closing Remarks
(sadness)
When I first met my husband he had a motorcycle. It was exhilarating. Freedom, letting go of the restraints.

I don't want to take this anymore. It's obvious what this means. I never realized what I really missed out on... what a father-daughter relationship is about. It's hard for me to related to men. I always feel that I am being judged. If there had just been a time for him to be together with me, so I could feel special to him. But it was Mother that was important to him.

(Moves baby away from father. Knocks over motorcycle and cup)

Recently I'm having the urge again to have a baby.

Interaction With the Adult Client

The sandplay session is largely silent, however there are some appropriate verbal exchanges. If a verbalization becomes necessary during the session, it is critical that the therapist maintains the quietude of the setting, speaking in a soft and slow manner. For example, if a client asks, *Do you have a fire?* The therapist may be able to show the client where it is without even saying a word. If the client asks, *Do you have a poodle with fire coming out of its head?* The therapist may quietly and slowly respond, *No...but perhaps you can make one with clay,* indicating to the client where the clay is kept.

Although I use humor in this example, it does remind us that shocking things can occur in the sandplay session. The client is highly vulnerable while making his or her unconscious contents three-dimensional and sharing them with the therapist. The stance of the therapist must remain steady and not reactive. The therapist must openly and safely receive the client's process. The therapist must soundly hold the process in a silent collaboration of the deepest nature with the client.

If the therapist does have a strong reaction to what emerges in a client's work, it is imperative that he or she seeks consultation immediately. It is likely that the client's work has touched some wounded aspects of the therapist that need attention and healing. In such circumstances, it may be critical for the therapist to return to analysis or therapy to work through the issues.

Although the sandplay session generally occurs in silence, there are moments when the depth of the shared sandplay experience elicits a verbal exchange with the client. For example, I recall a sandplay session where, upon completion of the tray, the client touched a prominent figure in the tray and tearfully remarked,

> "She is beautiful, isn't she?" (looking directly into my eyes) I quietly responded, "Yes. She is very beautiful."

As this new aspect of herself emerged from her depths, this client reverently and joyfully invited me to acknowledge it with her. It was the right thing to do at that moment.

We know by now that there are no fixed rules to sandplay therapy. This is why the therapist's preparation is so essential. In order to be able to join with the client in the moment, the therapist must enter a state of emptiness. In this way, whatever is necessitated by the sandplay session will emerge out of that stillness.

The Talkative Adult Client

Sometimes the therapist encounters a client who talks excessively during the sandplay session. When this happens it is important to determine what all of the chatter is really about. Does this just occur during the sandplay session or is it the client's way of coping and defending against anxieties? The uniqueness of each situation must be assessed and addressed individually by the therapist.

When I sit with an overly talkative client during sandplay and feel that it will be important for him or her to move more inwardly, I generally wait to see if the sandplay process itself will gradually facilitate this end. Frequently the client will settle into the process after a few trays, no longer feeling the original apprehension as he or she becomes more at home in the depths. If the client persists in chattering and I feel a well-developed sense of trust in our relationship, I may touch the client gently on the hand and say something like,

> "Let's see what your soul wants to say. Sometimes we can't hear it with our ordinary words."

The therapist must be very careful making an intervention like this, because it can easily be taken as shameful criticism.

Chapter 2

During the Sandplay Session—The Client

The Client's Approach to Sandplay

The client may work in the sand in any number of ways. The client might follow the procedures we demonstrated to them, moving and shaping the sand then going to the shelves to select figures. My experience is that each client appears to have his or her own approach to work in the sand tray. Some gather a number of figures, setting them aside or in a corner of the sand tray, while they shape the sand. Some alternate between shaping the sand and placing figures.

The client's procedure can take many turns. Sometimes a client will do a complete, or nearly complete tray, take a deep look at it, then suddenly remove everything and do something else. I recall doing this myself when working with Dora Kalff. I did my tray with Frau Kalff sitting opposite me. Observing it, I suddenly knew it was not right and immediately took it apart. Dora Kalff remained silently present. I did something else and was finished.

For record keeping purposes, when this occurs I draw a diagonal line through the sand tray map on the *Sandplay Record Form*, and score a line between the numbers on the left side of the form, indicating the point in the process it took place. For example, if the client puts seven items in the tray, then disassembles it, I draw a line between 7 and 8. I make a notation, such as,

> (Suddenly disassembles tray)
> (Slowly disassembles tray) and so on.

I then label the diagram of the first configuration as *Tray A*. I draw another rectangle for the second configuration and label it *Tray B*. I continue numbering the figures with the next number available on the left-hand list. In our example, this would be number 8. Although this procedure sounds somewhat involved, the advantage is that it records the process undergone in the construction of the sand tray. With good records we are able to meaningfully review and join with that process, even years after its completion.

The Client's Demeanor During the Sandplay Session

As the client goes about doing a sandplay, his or her demeanor will most likely undergo some changes. The client's mood can shift dramatically. Mood can also fluctuate throughout the sandplay session. The therapist must remain aware of these shifts and hold them appropriately. The therapist might experience a shift in his or her mood during the sandplay session. He or she might suddenly experience an image, thought or bodily feeling, which is related to the sandplay session. As with any counter transference, the therapist must discern whether this is his or her material or that of the client. All of these fluctuations in mood and feeling, regardless of origin, need to be recorded and held.

During the sandplay session, the client may display a reaction to the sand or the collection. Sometimes these are verbalized. Many times they are silent gestures or expressions. Frequently these expressions and reactions are rich with information. I recall one client in her late thirties, who had been told to seek therapy by the members of a Board of Directors of the organization for which she worked. The Board had advised her that her job depended upon her doing something about her anger problem. When she approached the sizable sandplay collection, she commented loudly,

> "You just don't have what I need!"

Evidently, I did not have what she needed. Sadly, at the same time I became painfully aware that she had never received what she really needed.

Sometimes a client will make a comment about a figure or aspect of the work that is similarly telling. The client may pick up a female figure and say, "Boy, he's a mean one!" Another example is referring to a building clearly marked "Fire Station" across the front, as *Home.* The therapist needs to listen carefully to the client's perceptions.

Children's Interactive Play

Depending upon their age and phase of development, children may play actively in the sand. As we saw in our discussion of sandplay behavior and development, children are able to make more representative sandplay scenes at about age six or seven. Around this age the child's growing cognitive skills allow him or her to place figures in the sand tray, making a scene that *holds its own action and relationships* without the child having to physically animate it.

Interactive play is normal and appropriate for younger children. Four year-old children are particularly adept at interactive play, given their growing verbal skills and their highly imaginative inner world. Capturing all that transpires in interactive play is not possible. Not only do figures move, they frequently transform into new personae and assume new roles. Figures are put in the tray, or trays and then removed. Important symbolic components are repeatedly buried, unburied, killed, resuscitated, lost and rediscovered.

MARK Four year-old **Mark's Tray 5** is a good example of interactive play. Upon completion, **Mark's** tray had no figures remaining. He finished his work by impressing his handprints into the sand. Here is what transpired during the session. My notes are in parentheses. **Mark's** verbalizations are in quotation marks.

(Lines up four Ninja Turtles facing two construction plows. One plow pushes through the sand.)

"I think I don't want to play with these guys."

(Puts turtles away. Adds tow truck and forklift.)
(Puts tow truck and forklift away.)
(Removes the two plows.)

"This is the Daddy."

(Adds two alligators, a snake.)
(The Daddy alligator bites and fights the snake.)

(Adds lizard.)
(Daddy bites and fights the lizard.)

"The lizard wanted to kill his baby."

(Daddy fights with lizard and throws lizard across the room.)
(Adds cat and a moose)

"Meow. Meow!"

(Daddy fights with the cat.)

"He (cat) isn't doing anything to the babies. Now the babies are running after their daddy and they are going to eat this guy." (the moose)

"They saved their dad! " (outside of tray)

(Adds weapons)
(Moves to dry tray)

"They are cutting the sand." (with saw and swords)

(Buries weapons in the dry tray. Pats sand down)
(Puts Daddy in the dry tray, uncovers a spear and kills him.)

"Killed other baby one, too!"

(Removes buried saws and swords, replacing them in their container.)
(Puts alligators away. Puts weapons away. Puts the top cover on the dry tray. Picks up the animals from around the room, putting them back on the shelves.)
(Makes hand prints in the sand.)

As we can see, a great deal transpired during the course of **Mark's** sand-play. Undoubtedly I missed important features of the play in my note taking. However, there is enough recorded to be able to discern the themes and progression of **Mark's** work and to contain the process adequately. **Mark's Tray 5** is a clear example of the insufficiency of having only a final photograph in this mode of sandplay work. With interactive play we rely upon our process notes to contain the work.

Interaction with the Child Client

Additional considerations in the interactive play of younger children involve the therapist's verbalizations and engagement in the play with the child. As with all features of sandplay, the need for the therapist's more active participation can only be determined in the moment. Whether or not to engage in the play with the child is a much clearer distinction than whether or not to make a verbal reflection.

Young children, chronologically or developmentally, will use the sand tray for cooking, mixing and pouring, which I refer to as *cooking behavior.* I feel it is completely appropriate to cook and eat with the child when invited to do so. Such play fulfills many early nurturing, sharing and capability tasks for the child. Done in the sand tray with the therapist, it also acknowledges the special nature of the sand tray and facilitates a deep connection between the child and the therapist. When the child is finished with this phase of play, he or she will move on. At this point in development the child may not invite the therapist to play, or may say or do something to indicate the work is taking a new direction.

Children who are able to play in a more representational manner in the sand may also invite the therapist to play. When this happens my concern is to hold a place in which the child is free to do as he or she pleases. Generally speaking I do not feel it is appropriate to join the child in interactive play with figures in the tray. There will no doubt be exceptions, but for the most part it is of great importance to stay out of the child's way. The therapist is likely to influence the direction of the child's play with even a minor participation. In my experience, some children who invite the therapist to play are accustomed to paying too much attention to the needs of the adults in their lives. Of course, the child may simply be highly social by nature. In any case, we must remember the essential nature of the *free and protected space* and allow the child's psyche the place and safety to open to healing and transformation *in its own way.* Depending upon the situation, I may say something such as,

> ...You know, lots of times kids just need a place where

> they can do whatever they need to all by themselves.
> ...Oh, thanks. I want you to have a place to do whatever you need to by yourself.
> ...Thanks, but this is all for you.

During a child's interactive play, I sometimes feel it is appropriate to verbally reflect upon a component of the child's play. My tendency in determining whether it feels appropriate to engage in the process in this way is to err on the side of restraint. I do it at the moment it feels right and this is not often. I also make mistakes.

MARK **Mark's Tray 4** is an example of a verbal reflection by the therapist.
Mark: One at a time! (Running tractors through the sand)
Therapist: (quietly) One at a time...
Mark: He's clearing the path.
Therapist: He's making a way...
Mark: He's trying to get to his home.

In this example, I based my decision to respond primarily on the fact that it *felt right* to do so. Reflecting back on it, I see that it was a way of acknowledging the break-through **Mark** was making in his work. On another occasion, I was off track. This example is from **Mark's Tray 20.**

Mark: (Scoring shapes and lines in the sand with a sword that look like a head, eyes and mouth)
Therapist: Are you making a face? (quietly)
Mark: No! (sharply)

I felt terrible and deeply regretted intruding into his work in this way, but the damage was done. I was considerably quieter after that, and consoled myself by reflecting on D.W. Winnicott's concept of the adequacy of a *good enough environment* (Winnicott, 1958/1975, p. 214). Fortunately our therapeutic relationship was sturdy enough to tolerate the error.

Section III
After the Sandplay Session

Chapter 1
Client and Therapist

Completion of the Sand Tray

When the client says, "I'm done," the therapist walks around to the position from which the client primarily worked. This is the front, or the *near side* of the sand tray. This is a vulnerable moment when the client and the therapist share the sandplay together. By moving to the front of the tray the therapist is invited into the client's very sacred space. We must honor it as such. It is important to quietly and to reverently take in what the client has brought into the therapeutic container. We must not hurry and take care to maintain the quietude that surrounds the sandplay, only gently beginning to ask,

> **(To Adults)** Were there any associations that came up for you while you were doing this tray?
>
> **(To Children)** Is there a story or a title for this one?

The therapist then records, verbatim, what the client says. This can range from a silent tilt of the head to a lengthy, detailed story. It can be difficult to record a child's long, involved story. I take some shorthand and still have difficulty at times! Do the best you can. Capture the themes, the flavor and the main points. Try to record its essence just as we do with interactive play. In this way we can continue to carry the client's process in a living, vital way.

The therapist must also be careful to not attribute his or her own perceptions to the client's work. This can be tricky, as the genders and identities of figures may appear so obvious to us that we take them for granted. When reviewing the completed sandplay with the client it is wise for the therapist to be especially mindful to avoid using names, or attributions of gender when referring to the figures. Using the terms *this, here, that one* are fairly safe. For example, if a client's comments about the completed tray are,

If the client says, "They are all going to see the god," and it is apparent that the god figure is male, the therapist must still be very careful. The therapist might say, "They are all on their way over here. It can be highly disruptive to the client's process if the therapist refers to the deity as *Him,* and the client says, "She's a goddess!"

The continuity of the container and the joint experience of the sandplay by client and therapist can be jarred by something like this. The therapist will make mistakes. The crucial matter is for the therapist to get back in harmony with the client as smoothly and as soon as possible. In the above example, the therapist might say, "Oh, of course! Forgive me."

The Client's Desire to Interpret the Sandplay

Upon completion of the sandplay, highly rational adults may turn to the therapist and say, "Well! What does it mean?"

An imperative like this from an intelligent adult client can be very challenging to the therapist. The client's insistence on having answers and information confronts the therapist with the strength of his or her own confidence in the depths of the unseen inner life to guide and direct us. In a sense, a demand such as this confronts the sandplay therapist with the entire value system of Western culture, which prizes what is tangible and quantifiable far more than anything that is unseen and qualitative in nature. It is not at all easy to sit alone in your little office with a box of sand and hundreds of little figures in total certainty that the ordinary values and perceptions of our world are upside down.

On occasion, I admit I have sat in my sandplay room wondering to myself if I am crazy to tell clients to make sandplays. Yet, even with my own conscious doubts about the value of our inner, unconscious driving forces toward wholeness, something keeps me deeply engaged in sandplay. I witness miracles of transformation in some people and I continue to grow and evolve as well.

As products of Western culture, we will inevitably have doubts about the value and validity of sandplay. Sandplay challenges everything we *know* to be right and stands our values on their heads. As Westerners, we ask questions and we want proof. Of course sandplay clients and therapists will challenge sandplay. We cannot help ourselves! What we must do as therapists is to continue to turn our awareness inward to listen to the callings of the silence and to encourage our clients to do the same. Thus, when the client challenges, *Well! What does it mean?* We might say,

> Let's just let it live inside of us. We don't want to rush to analyze sandplay. Let's allow it to tell us what it's about. It will tell us, in time.

Upon completion of a sandplay, some adults will begin analyzing it themselves. When this happens, I say something like the statement, above. I may add something such as,

> Sandplay works in a way that is quite different for us. Instead of facts, figures, words and causes, it works in deeper parts of ourselves with images. It heals parts of ourselves that sit underneath all of our words and reasons. Let's just give it time.

Photographs of the Sandplay

Maintaining comprehensive photographic records of sandplay is also essential for the proper containment of the process. Because the symbols are alive, the images continue to work on the client and the therapist once they become manifest in the sand tray.

Necessary Photographs

Two forms of photographic records are necessary for the therapist to maintain adequate records. A printed photo of the tray is needed for the file. A quick printout of a digital photo works well. A series of slide or digital photographs showing the entire sandplay with detail shots and different views is required for study and containment.

The digital prints allow the therapist to easily and quickly scan through the client's sandplays. By doing this, the therapist's psyche is reminded of the course of the client's process, as well as at what phase of the work he or she is currently. On a deep level of the psyche, just looking through the prints attunes the therapist's psyche to the client's inner process. Looking quickly through the photos in the file before a session can be an asset to containment by positioning the therapist's psyche to be better able to energetically meet the client in the session. When using slide photography, having the print in the file can help the therapist sort slides when they return from the photo lab. Additionally, should the detailed images or slides of the sandplay be lost or destroyed, the file photo is still available. My procedure is to attach a print of the side of the tray from which the client worked to the Sandplay Record Form and put it in the client's file immediately after the session.

The slides or digital photos allow the therapist to study and reflect on the sandplay in great detail.

Photographic Equipment

Changes in photo technology continue to offer us more choices for recording sandplay. I used a Polaroid camera for my instant photos and a 35 millimeter camera with a micro-macro lens for many years. Now I am using a digital camera, which permits me to print out a picture for the file and save digital image records on the computer and on discs. Sandplay therapists have traditionally used color slide film in order to be able to project the pictures onto a screen for in-depth study. With the newer digital option we can use a digital projector or have color slides made from the digital images. Of course the technology will continue to change, offering sandplay therapists more options for these important records.

Which equipment to choose is a matter of taste and budget. It is not at all necessary to have a highly expensive camera to adequately record sandplay work. When consulting with the camera sales people it is important to remember that this is indoor, close up photography. This information will help the sales person direct you to the equipment that will work best. Many camera stores offer classes in specialty photography such as close up, landscape, and so on.

Taking Photographs

The photo record of a sandplay begins with a picture of the tray from the front. This is the main position from which the client worked, and how he or she primarily viewed the tray. My procedure is to take a photo of each of the remaining three sides. When the tray is very simple, these four views may not even be necessary. Depending on the nature of the sand tray and its elements, I may take an overview photo, looking directly down on it from above. I may also take close up pictures of significant details that do not show up in the more distant shots. When objects are hidden or buried, I uncover them in the course of dismantling the tray and photograph them. Thus, for any one sandplay, in addition to the instant photo I will have anywhere from one to ten photographs.

Some sandplay therapists like to write the client's initials and a date on a card, placing it in the sand tray for ease of identifying the slide later on. This can work well when it comes to filing the slides. However, this *identifier slide* is for the therapist's purposes only. For purposes of containment and of confidentiality, the identification card is not a part of the sandplay process. An additional photo of the front of the tray must be taken without the identification card. Later in consultation, the therapist is thus able to clearly contain the client's process without risk of a breach of confidentiality or the interference of an additional element in the sand tray.

Digital cameras allow the therapist to store the images in a client file on the computer and/or burn them to a disc immediately after the session. This greatly facilitates record keeping by eliminating the time delays that are necessary in sending slide film to the lab for processing and later filing the slides. As with all important electronic files, be sure to back them up (save in two or more locations) to avoid loss.

Photographs In Presence Of Client

Some sandplay therapists take their photos after the client has left. Others do it in the presence of the client. The choice is a matter of containment and what feels appropriate to the therapist. My preference is to take photos while the client is present. As a part of containing the process, my sense is that this affirms the importance of the sandplay to the client and therapist. In the case of child clients, photographing their work is a powerful acknowledgment of their individual significance and their growth. It is a way of joining with the children to value the very real importance of their non-verbal play. Children feel that their sandplay is significant, even urgent. Having the therapist photograph it affirms that he or she knows this as well.

For the therapist to whom it feels important to do the photography after the client has left, it is important to let the client know that you do take photos. The therapist may remind the client that one day, long after therapy is completed, they may want to review the sandplay pictures together.

Children Who Request A Picture

When we take instant pictures in the presence of a child client, they frequently ask to take a picture home with them. Although some sandplay therapists do give the client a photo, my preference is to say,

> Let's just let it live inside of you and do its work from the inside out.

However, with photos, as with all other aspects of sandplay, there are no rigid rules. I will give a client a photo to take home when I strongly feel that it is the right thing to do.

Child clients may use the photo issue as a means of testing the therapist's limits just as they would demanding three pieces of gum, rather than just one. In this case the issue is about safety, accountability and containment, not photographs of sandplay.

Leaving Sandplay Intact

Upon completion of the sandplay session, the sand tray is left intact. This may be one of the few real rules of Jungian sandplay therapy. The therapist *never disassembles the tray in the presence of the client.* The symbolic content of the client's heretofore, unseen and unknown inner world has manifested in a three-dimensional form within the boundaries of the tray. Witnessed by the client and the therapist in its material form, the symbols move the client's psyche at depths that exceed the vision of the client's conscious awareness. To disassemble the client's budding transformation in his or her presence is unthinkable.

Most adult clients do not question leaving their sandplay intact. For some children however, this may be a new concept. I say to them,

> Sandplay is the one place where we don't have to clean up after ourselves!

Saying this may delight the child. The concept of leaving something of theirs behind, particularly something that is so significant and personal to them may also have a subtle but powerful impact on their work.

The therapist's receptivity to the child's or the adult's presence is profoundly honored by allowing this unique piece of themselves to remain in the office. On a very deep level, the unique quality and inherent worthiness of the client is fully accepted in the therapist's gesture to hold the completed sandplay.

Showing Sandplay to Parents

Children will frequently want to show their parents the wonderful work they have done in the sand tray. This can be a challenging issue to handle. The motivation to show the sandplay to the parent may stem from a variety of sources. The child may simply be delighted and enthused about sharing his or her wonderful creation with Mom or Dad. The child's enthusiasm is completely understandable. He or she has expressed something uniquely his or her own. Of course, they want their parents to witness it. In other cases the child has little or no autonomy, resulting from the parents' own wounding. A child such as this lives with the imperative to give every aspect of him or herself to the parent. This child knows no other form of existence apart from being in service to the parents' deficits. Other children may feel compelled to give the parents an urgent communication through the symbols of the sandplay.

When the child asks to show the sandplay to the parents, after the first tray, or very early in the process, I say,

> We don't generally show the sandplays to the parents. It's not that it's a secret, but everyone needs a place where they can do what they need to do, without worry about what someone else might think about it.

This is a profound, permission-giving statement about the nature of our work. It tells the child that the therapist recognizes his or her need to do some important work. Moreover, it establishes the therapist's support and alliance with the child in doing that work.

This being communicated to the child, we then need to address the other therapeutic dynamics that might play into the child's insistence on showing the tray to the parent. How we respond is a decision made in the moment, based on therapeutic necessity and appropriate containment. When it is the child's first session and he or she is about to burst with excitement, I may say, ...*Well, just this one time.* Subsequent to the initial adjustment to the procedures with the child, the issue of showing the sandplay to the parent is unique to each situation. I have said everything from,

> You know, Johnny, I really think you need someplace in your life where you can just be yourself. Let's not show it to Mommy, and
> Hmmm… You really think Mommy and Daddy need to see this one, don't you? Okay, to
> No. I don't think we need to, and
> Nope! We don't do that with sandplay!

The Parent's Response to the Sandplay

When the parent does see the child's sandplay, their response can be enlightening about the nature of the relationship to the child. The parent with more appropriate boundaries may say nothing, but may appear interested and appreciative. He or she might say something like, ...*Oh, that's wonderful!* The less appropriate parent may do any number of things, ranging from attempting to explain and define what is happening in the tray, to curtly criticizing, "Why did you do that?"

Discussing the Child's Sandplay with Parents

When working with a child, my practice is to schedule parent interviews frequently enough to keep abreast of what is happening at home and how the child's behavior might be changing. I usually begin the parent meeting by asking how things are going at home. This makes the parent a valued part of the child's work and gives them an active way to participate. This is a good way to address issues of parenting, as well.

I also want to keep the parent informed about the child's progress in therapy. I generally discuss this with the parents in terms of themes and trends in the child's work. I may say things such as,

> Her sandplays show me that she is beginning to be able to face the trauma more directly and that she is getting in touch with her anger about what happened. This may explain some of the obstinacy you are seeing at home.

The parents are an active part of the overall treatment picture. Children need their parents and their treatment needs their parents. Appropriate collateral parent meetings in no way compromise the child's sandplay work.

Chapter 2
After the Sandplay Session

The Therapist

Disassembling the Sandplay

Sandplay procedures do not end when the client leaves the office. The therapist must first be certain that all necessary photos have been taken and that any remaining process notations are recorded on the Sandplay Record Form. Following this the sandplay must be disassembled, the figures cleaned and returned to their places on the shelves. The sand must be smoothed and the sandplay room returned to a neutral position in readiness for the next client. Frequently, the demands of client scheduling require that all of this be done in the ten or fifteen minute break between clients. This can be challenging, so I will share some helpful procedures that I have learned from colleagues or have developed out of necessity on my own.

Cleaning sand off of figures before returning them to the shelves helps avoid accumulating sand on the shelves. In spite of my sometimes overly ambitious efforts, I have resigned myself to the fact that there will be sand on the shelves. When a client uses a number of figures from one area, I use the opportunity to wipe off the shelf with a damp cloth.

A dry, two-inch flat paintbrush is good for dusting sand from the crevices of figures when cleaning up. When figures are buried, or are especially covered with sand, I put them in a large-mesh sieve and dip them in a bucket of water. The sand falls right off and gathers at the bottom of the bucket for disposal in the garden, or return to the tray. I dump the wet figures on a cotton towel and blot them up quickly. The sieve is also a good tool for collecting large numbers of buried items from the tray, which are easily cleaned by dipping in the water bucket.

There are times when it may not be possible to clear the tray between sessions. This can occur when the tray is so full of tiny, buried figures that finding them all will require more time. This can happen when hundreds of small plastic ants are buried in wet sand, or when many small objects have been mixed together in the sandplay and require sorting out to return to the collection. When the tray cannot be cleared and prepared for the next session, it must be removed from the room and be stored where no one can see it. When this happens I keep a small, dark-colored table cloth on hand to cover the tray and move it to a closet. In offices that have no closets, be sure to make arrangements for this contingency in advance. Sometimes the unprepared tray can be tucked behind a potted plant in a corner, hidden by furniture, or hidden under the sofa. The dark color of the covering cloth will help mask it from view. Another firm rule of sandplay is to *never allow a client's work to be seen by another client or anyone outside of the holding container.*

When the tray is flooded and too wet to return to the neutral condition, we have to remove it from the room or replace the sand. I like to keep an empty bucket for overly wet sand and two extra buckets of dry sand for these purposes. It is also wise to have extra sand for the times when a client wants more sand to build a higher structure in the tray.

Disassembly of the sandplay and all it entails is actually a ritual behavior the sandplay therapist undergoes in order to clear the container and return both the physical and energetic space to a neutral condition. Being a primary component of the sandplay container, the therapist simultaneously clears, cleanses and re-orders him or herself to a centered stance. In this way the therapist and the setting are ready and welcoming for the work of the next client.

Organizing and Managing Sandplay Records

We have explored the records we need to keep in some depth. How the therapist will organize and maintain those records is an important consideration. Each case has many Sandplay Record Forms and frequently hundreds of photographic records. Over the course of a sandplay career the therapist will accumulate thousands of records and photos, all of which must be safely stored and easily accessed. Considering an organization plan early in the sandplay career will go a long way toward avoiding problems in the future.

There are many ways to organize sandplay records. Some sandplay therapists have a separate folder or binder for the photo records of each client. Some keep their written notes with the photos. Others hold them in a separate file. I have always kept my written session notes, the Sandplay Record Form and the instant photo together in an individual file for each client. When I used slide photography, I kept the slides in the files, as well. With the digital photos, I now keep a compact disc that holds the digital images in the file.

It is important to store slides in archival quality clear plastic sheets in a dark place. A filing cabinet, or container of some sort works well. The slides fade over time, so taking good care of them will extend the life of the color and detail.

It is of critical importance to keep up to date with photo records. If slide photography is used, filing the slides when they are returned from the lab can avoid serious problems. Allowing the photos to accumulate and attempting to file them accurately many months after the sandplays are done is a terrific challenge.

Filing and saving the digital pictures as soon as possible is somewhat easier than dealing with the slides. It is easy to upload the digital images directly into the computer and to save them in the individual clients' files. From there they can be burned onto compact discs for back up. This can all be done on the same day the sandplays are completed, avoiding future filing and storage tasks.

The best advice regarding sandplay records is to develop a system and use it. Make it work for you, while amply considering all features of containment.

Carrying the Sandplay

After the sandplays are completed, annotated, photographed, stored and organized, the sandplay continues to live in the therapist. The therapist carries the sandplay process of each client in body, mind and spirit. In order to sustain the viability of the transformative energies of the symbols, the sandplay therapist must continually engage in cultivating understanding of all aspects of the process. This involves deep study of all features of theory and psychic process. It also entails the relentless exploration of the therapist's own inner depths and the tireless quest of Self in all aspects of life.

The materials we explore in this book provide a good guideline for the direction and subjects of sandplay study. In addition to these features of sandplay, it is critical that the therapist listen to his or her inner directives. With meaningful reflection, meditation and attention to dreams, the therapist will receive inner guidance for the direction of study that is necessary for his or her growth and understanding.

Studying sandplay work from his or her practice is deeply informative. Simply contemplating the pictures with *soft eyes*, loosening the hold on conscious rationality, activates the necessary directions for learning and growth in the therapist. This may evoke dream images, bodily sensations, ideas or awareness that leads to the investigation of a particular theory, mythology or symbol image. The sandplay therapist carries the process by listening to the inner stillness.

When taking formal classes on sandplay therapy, it is important that the therapist choose his or her teachers well. Knowing something about the teacher's background and their approach to sandplay can help the therapist decide if he or she would like to study with this person. It is important that sandplay teachers carry the spirit of the work. It is also a good idea to study with several different teachers in order to acquire a breadth of approaches to sandplay from a variety of voices. The *International Society for Sandplay Therapy* certifies master teachers of Jungian sandplay therapy. The ISST American affiliate, *Sandplay Therapists of America*, is a good source of information regarding sandplay classes and study. (www.sandplay.org)

Sandplay Consultation

Sandplay consultation involves the therapist taking his or her sandplay cases to a sandplay consultation group or to an individual consultant for review and study. We have discussed consultation in an earlier chapter regarding the role of the therapist in sandplay therapy. Following a brief review of the importance of professional consultation, we will turn our attention to the details and procedures involved.

Consultation is a vital aspect of the sandplay process. In fact, it is essential. There is far too much happening in sandplay for the therapist to contain it individually. To work in sandplay therapy without on-going consultation is dangerous and irresponsible. This brings us to our third firm sandplay rule. *The sandplay therapist must always participate in consultation.*

Individual sandplay consultants are frequently certified sandplay teachers and have many years of experience in sandplay therapy. The individual consultant becomes a part of the sandplay container, respectfully holding the client's work. The sandplay consultation group is led by a certified sandplay therapist and has up to six members. Consultation groups schedule regular meetings, wherein group members take turns presenting sandplay work from their practices. Just as with the individual consultant, the group becomes an extension of the sandplay container. The purpose of consultation is to create a free and protected space for the sandplay therapist. The consultation group needs to be a safe, respectful environment in which the individual therapist's sandplay work is informally reviewed and studied.

Finding and joining a good consultation group is a vital asset to sandplay therapy work. Sandplay groups often evolve into deeply meaningful gatherings with rich and profound exchanges of insight and support. Many sandplay consultation groups continue for years. Sometimes the therapists have to travel quite a distance to join a group or to seek individual consultation. Until there are more groups and qualified consultants available, this is simply part of what it takes to work in sandplay therapy. The Sandplay Therapists of America have information regarding available consultation groups.

The Structure of Sandplay Consultation

There are some variations in the approach to consultation, but it tends to follow a consistent pattern. In individual consultation the consultant and therapist share and review slides of the therapist's sandplay case material. Without attempting to impose or affix a meaning to the sandplay process, the therapist and consultant review slides of the sandplays in sequence. Together they come to an understanding of the nature and process of the client's work.

Many dimensions of the client's sandplay work become more conscious to the therapist as a result of the conjoint sharing of the sandplay in individual or group consultation. Among many possibilities, a better understanding of the issues with which the client is grappling develops. The nature of the symbolic and archetypal constituents that are activated to move the client's psyche begins to emerge. The course of the process to date and the phase of the process at which the client is working becomes clearer. Elements of the process that were previously unknown appear. And importantly, the less conscious or unconscious elements of the therapist's psyche that are necessary to contain the process are activated.

Consultation gives the therapist the rich gift of learning from others and a support system to help contain the challenging work of sandplay. As a group member the therapist is enjoined to respectfully hold the group's work and assumes the responsibility for carrying the work of colleagues.

Preparing to Present a Case

Preparing to present a case in consultation differs from the formal presentation of case material in a teaching setting. In the more formal teaching setting the teacher has already studied and reviewed the sandplay material in great depth. This requires that the teacher do extensive study and planning in order that he or she is fully prepared to make a formal presentation of the material. Preparing for case presentation in consultation involves reviewing and organizing the case records, so the therapist is prepared to show the slides in order and is able to easily refer to his or her notes.

If I were scheduled to present a case using slides at my group consultation, I would put all of my slides in a carousel in advance of the meeting. This way I could quickly check them at home, using my own slide projector, to be certain I have them right side up and not reversed and in the proper order. The slides go into the typical slide carousel upside down, with the emulsion side of the film, (the duller side) toward the screen.

Loading the Slide Projector

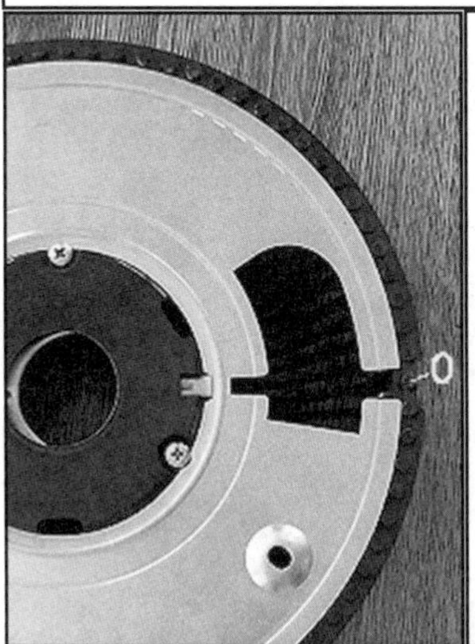

Prior to loading the slides, turn the carousel upside down and be certain that the loading slot (the open space) is aligned at "0."

A good way to load the slides correctly is to set the carousel on a table directly in front of you, slot number one in the 3:00 o'clock position. Progressively higher numbers, two, three, four, should be moving toward your tummy.

Holding the slide, just as if you were looking at the tray, the top being at 12:00 o'clock, rotate the top to the 6:00 o'clock position. In other words, continuing to look at the slide from the correct view just as the tray appeared when photographed (not with picture of sand tray backwards) turn it upside down. I have included a diagram for reference. Notice that the "up" arrow points down, as the slide is loaded.

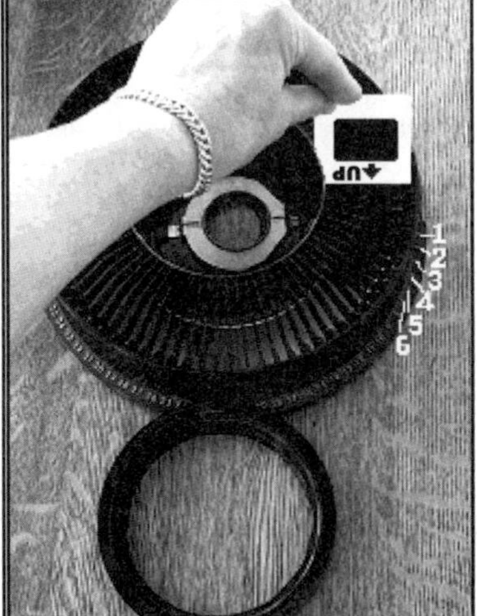

For example, if I were loading **Aaron's Tray 1**, I hold the slide up in front of me, seeing the tall knight in the center, the Asian wise men on the left and the cartoon figures on the right. This is the *front* of the tray, and is how it looked to **Aaron**. I rotate it so the knight is now upside down, the wise men are upside down on the right and the cartoon people are upside down on the left and then put it in the carousel slot in this position.

Another way to load the slide is to hold the slide in the position you want to see it on the screen. Lay it on the table in front of you, top of slide away from you and bottom toward your tummy. Rotate it two times to the right. Put it in the carousel slot in this position. As simple as this sounds, it is easy to reverse the slides!

For each sand tray in the series, I will first load the front view of the tray. If I have side views or close up shots that show details and figures that are not readily apparent in the front view, I load these in a meaningful sequence. I leave an empty slot in the carousel between each sand tray. If there are two views or slides of Tray 1, I load these slides into slots 1 and 2. Slot 3 I leave empty. The slides of Tray 2 go in slot 4 and following. When showing the slides in consultation the empty slot prevents me from running over into the next sand tray prematurely.

Digital Images in Consultation

Presentation of digital images in small consultation settings can be done by viewing the images on the screen of a laptop computer or projecting with a digital projector. Just as with slide presentations, proper preparation involves making sure the images are in the right order on the disc.

Presenting a Case in Consultation

My preference for consultation is to have the therapist present a brief client biography. It need not be greatly detailed as the sandplays tell us nearly everything we will need to know to review the case effectively. The introductory biography for sandplay consultation will include:

Age and gender of client
Nationality and religious background
Family composition
Presenting issues

> Significant developmental events, such as trauma and illness

For example, if consulting on the case of **Aaron**, we might say,

> This is the work of a nine year-old boy whose parents have recently divorced. Mother is Jewish by faith. Father is Catholic. Father is drug and alcohol addicted and is verbally and physically violent. This child lives with his mother, younger brother and older, teenage sister. Mom's parents play an active role in the boy's life. He is healthy, does very well in school, but has developed an explosive temper. His mother brought him in for therapy to deal with his anger. I have been seeing him for four months and he has done six sandplays.

This is plenty of information.

We then begin looking at the sandplay slides. In this example, if I were presenting the case in a group, I would probably have about an hour and twenty minutes to go through the six sandplays. That allows between ten and fifteen minutes to review each tray in the series. As the presenter, I want to pace the consultation accordingly.

The presenting therapist projects the first sandplay slide or digital image showing the front view of the sand tray. The therapist names and indicates the location of the figures in order of their placement, shows the side and detail views of the tray, then returns to the front view. It is helpful to have a pointer during consultation in order to be able to indicate the figures and images in the tray.

The group sits with the sandplay and under the guidance of the consultant, discusses the features of the sandplay that *come alive for them in that moment.* This may include any of the numerous aspects of sandplay content and process. Group members may share strong feelings and intuitions about the sandplay. It is important to remember that we can experience the same sandplay work many different times and be in relationship to it in as many different ways. Group members and the consultant need to be able to speak freely without fear of judgment, or feel comfortable remaining silent, as the moment dictates. The sandplays frequently generate questions about sandplay resulting in lively and stimulating learning. If there are several images to review, this process is repeated for each sand tray.

The consultation container must be safe for free discussion. It must be devoid of worries about needing to be right or of saying something wrong. Witnessing sandplay in consultation is a deeply evocative experience. The container must be secure enough to allow the deeper, less conscious aspects of the therapists to emerge and develop safely.

We never tell the client that we have taken his or her work to consultation. It is unnecessary to do so, as it is simply a part of our holding process. Advising the client that you are consulting about his or her work would disrupt the container and is inappropriate. Sharing a case in consultation is however, a powerful experience for both therapist and client. The added holding and enhanced containment of consultation have a material impact on the symbolic process, which is frequently reflected in the client's work. It is not uncommon to see dramatic changes and movement in the client's process after reviewing the case in consultation, although the client has no knowledge of it at all.

~ Conclusion ~
PART THREE

PROCEDURAL CONCEPTS

Implementing Sandplay Therapy In Practice

This concludes our discussion of the procedures of sandplay therapy, wherein we have explored the practicalities of practice prior to, during and following the sandplay session.

Although many people might open a book on sandplay with the practical procedures, this is by far the least involved aspect of sandplay. The vast complexities of the mystery of being underlie the simple procedures of doing sandplay. In order for sandplay therapy to have value and meaning, the therapist must first cultivate a deep understanding of the theory and process that supports these simple procedures.

This brings our examination of sandplay to a close. Book Four follows with our Case Illustrations and Appendices.

~ Postscript ~

PARTS ONE THROUGH THREE

As we are by now abundantly aware, sandplay therapy is a deceptively simple therapeutic modality, which when properly contained is a powerful vehicle to plumb the depths of being. Sandplay can transform the most subtle constellations of psychic energy. Sandplay has the potential to heal wounds, to re-order psychic contents to the center of the Self and to access untapped resources and latent capacities, freeing them to develop. Sandplay therapy can unlock a profound capacity for loving and open us to the realm of wisdom that is seated in the central quietude of the Self.

To undertake the practice of Jungian sandplay therapy is a serious decision, as it will affect every aspect of the rest of the therapist's life. Sandplay must be undertaken with sincerity and an open heart.

As bright as the potentials of sandplay shine, they can cast a grave shadow. Sandplay is very powerful and power is seductive. When the therapist mistakes the power tapped by sandplay for his or her own power, there is corruption. To mistake the vehicle for the wholeness and to fall into an ownership of it results in a dangerous inflation with a greedy, possessive face. When working with sandplay therapy we must remain mindful of our relationship to the medium as a vehicle for the discovery of wholeness in ourselves and our clients.

An adult male client once presented me with a precious gift of insight, which continues to remind me of the nature of sandplay and the proper relationship to it. With his kind permission, I share it with you.

> The sand trays seem to stay with me for so long, both in semi-conscious and more conscious ways.
>
> Sandplay is about opening a door for our depth to come out. It isn't that we have to delve into our stuff. We just have to get out of the way and let it open up.

> Sandplay becomes a living thing. It is like the dream state being brought into the moment. In the sandplay, I am looking at parts of myself and recognizing parts of myself.
>
> I used to feel that all of the figures on the shelves were just busy-ness in the room. Now I see them as friends.

As sandplay therapists, let us get out of the way and allow sandplay to open the door to the depths.

Learn and study all we have discussed and more. Continue to learn and engage in relentless self-examination. Then, when you come to the sandplay room, gently set it all aside. Be empty and listen...

PART FOUR

Client Case Examples

Case Examples

Case examples are arranged alphabetically by name of client used in the text, in this order. Approximately half of the case examples include all of the sandplay work done by the client. In those cases that are not shown in their entirety, the first and last sandplays are always included to show the beginnings and endings of their work.

*AARON	IVY	MARK
ADRIENNE	JASON	MARTINA
ANNIE	KAILEIGH	NORMAN
ARTHUR	LARRY	RACHEL
BILLY	LEELA	REGINA
CARY	LENAE	ROSA
CHARLIE	LEO	SANDER
ELIZABETH	LILLY	SHANNON
HAROLD	MAIZIE	TARA
ISAAC	MALCOLM	

***Aaron's Sandplay Case** is fully documented, including:

1. Sandplay Record Forms: The Sandplay Record Forms completed during Aaron's sandplay sessions. These contain complete records of the sandplay construction, the order of figure placement, maps of the sand configurations and figure locations, as well as client comments and therapist observations.

2. Written Case Analysis : A written analysis of Aaron's sandplay work follows the Case Examples as a sample one of many possible ways of understanding the symbolic process undergone in this case.

3. Subjective Immersion Analysis : The complete text of the Subjective Immersion Analysis (SIA) of Aaron's case is included in Appendix A to provide an example of the use of this method for a depth understanding of sandplay work.

Sandplay Record Form Coding

Words in (parentheses) = Therapist's notes and observations

Words in "quotation marks" = Client's words

Wave marks = Blue bottom of tray exposed

Dots = Sand area

"x" Beside figure number, for example "3x" = the original placement of figure 3, later moved or removed

"/" Between figure numbers, for example "7/6" = figures placed on top of others, in this case figure 7 is placed on top of figure 6

Client Profile

AARON

Boy, age 9

Second of three children, older sister, younger brother

Chronic parental conflict

Mother and Father divorced

Father drug and alcohol addicted, violent

Father Catholic, Mother Jewish

Brought to treatment by Mother, who is concerned about Aaron's volatile temper and angry outbursts

Sandplay	Discussed on Page Number
Tray 1	18, 67, 253-4, 269, 286-7, 342-3, 345-6, 376-7
Tray 2	67, 346
Tray 3	67, 160
Tray 4	67, 160, 287-8
Tray 5	346
Tray 6	81, 254
Tray 7	81, 157
Tray 8	
Tray 9	159
Tray 10	159
Tray 11	
Tray 12	245
Tray 13	
Tray 14	161, 165-6
Tray 15	85, 157, 343

Sandplay Record Form
AARON

Tray 1 ~ Session 1
Dry Tray
Wet Tray X

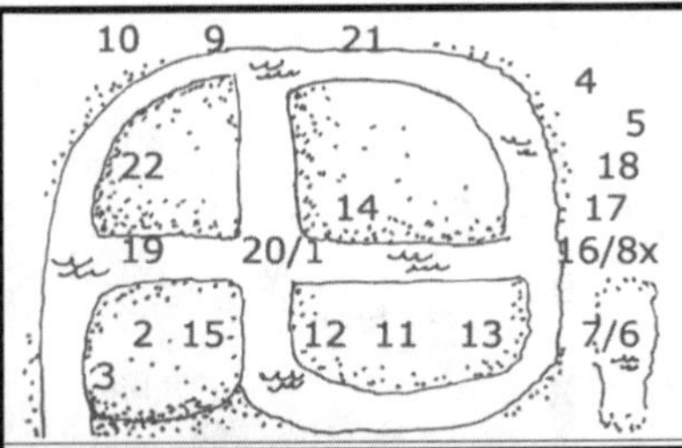

Initial Observations/Remarks—(Therapist) or "Client"
None

Placement Sequence

1) Bridge (Runs several cars and motorcycles over the bridge non-aggressively)
2) Crystal ball
3) Asian man with monkey
4 – 5) Skiers
6) Raft
7) Penguin (In raft)
8) Superman "He is looking for lions"
9) Tiger
10) Lion tamer
11 – 13) Ninja warriors
14) Large knight (On hill)
15) Asian man (Removes #8)
16) Batman
17) Joker (Lays down)
18) Robin
19) Police car
20) Car (On bridge)
21) Oak tree
22) Small tree

Client's Closing Remarks

"Batman caught the Joker. The police car is chasing the other car. The Chinese guy is doing magic. This (#14) is a statue of a guy who fought. This (#10) is a lion tamer. These (#4,5) are skiers."

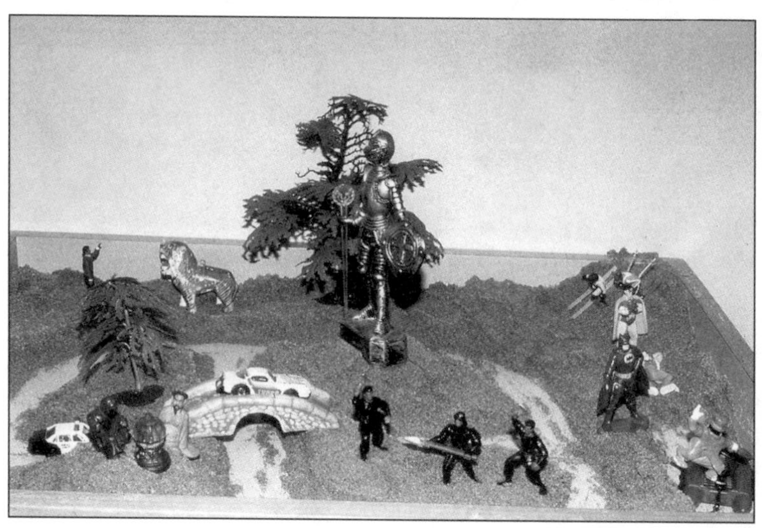

Aaron
Tray 1

Sandplay Record Form

AARON

Tray 2 ~ 2 Weeks Later
Dry Tray
Wet Tray X

Initial Observations/Remarks ~ (Therapist) or "Client"

"…I was thinking of making a cartoon land today!"
(Shapes a square in far left corner)

Placement Sequence

1) Small boxer hitting big boxer
2) Mickey with camera
3) Minnie Mouse
4) Mickey Mouse
5) Pluto dog
6) Duck with telescope
7) Duck
8) Smurf
9) Smurf with mallet
10) Girl
11) Wolf
12) Oak tree
13) Small tree
14) Rutabaga man
15) Banana woman
16) Witch
17) Dorothy
18) Cowardly Lion
19) Scarecrow
20) Tin Man
21) Small tree
22) Minnie Mouse cheerleader
23) Glenda Good Witch
24) Small boxer

(Note: Order of placement unknown)

Client's Closing Remarks

"This girl (#15) has fallen for the carrot man. (#13) This girl is watching this guy (#7) find gold. This guy (#8) is laughing so much that the other guy is going to hit him on the head. He is the guy that doesn't like anything. The witch is getting mad at them because they are eating the apples from the tree. The witch is hiding behind the tree and comes out. This princess (#23) is watching. He (#11) is trying to eat her."

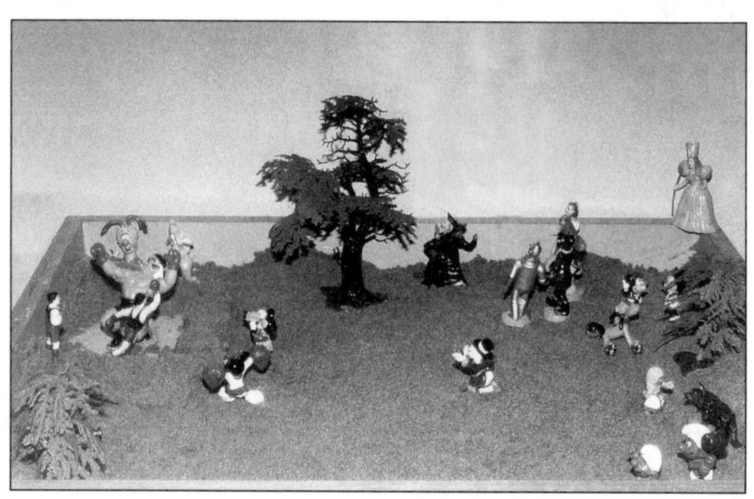

Aaron
Tray 2a

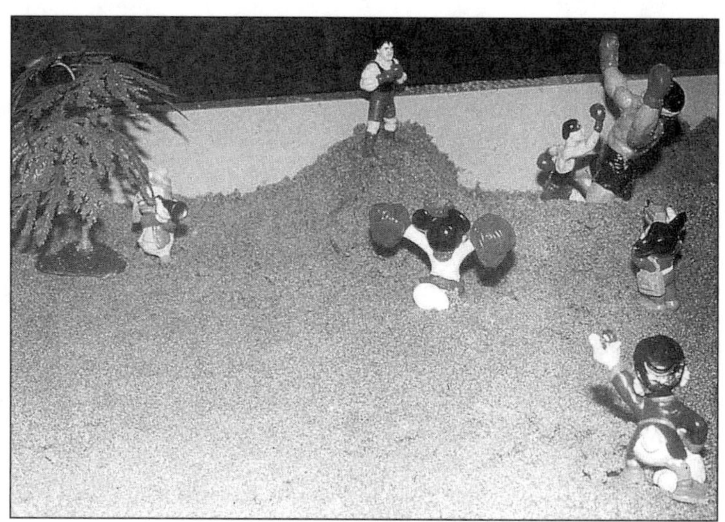

Aaron
Tray 2b ~ Detail

Sandplay Record Form

AARON

Tray 3 ~ 3 Weeks Later

Dry Tray

Wet Tray X

		12				
1			9		6	17
				14		
				7		13
2						
						4
		16				
	18		15	11		5
3						
	8		10			

Initial Observations/Remarks ~ (Therapist) or "Client"

"This is going to be a wonder land."

Placement Sequence

1) Cathedral
2) Coach
3) Space ship
4 – 5) Astronauts
6) Two headed dragon
7) Superman
8) Skeleton on grave
9) Cow skull
10) Hanging man
11) Pegasus
12) Unicorn
13) Three headed dragon
14) Two headed dragon
15) Alien
16) Warrior
17) Palm
18) Oak

Client's Closing Remarks

"It is a wonder land. The space ship has just come down. These guys in the suits will not be hurt when the aliens come out. This thing (#2) is going to a ball. Superman is fighting the lizards. These (#15,16) are the death people and their death animal."

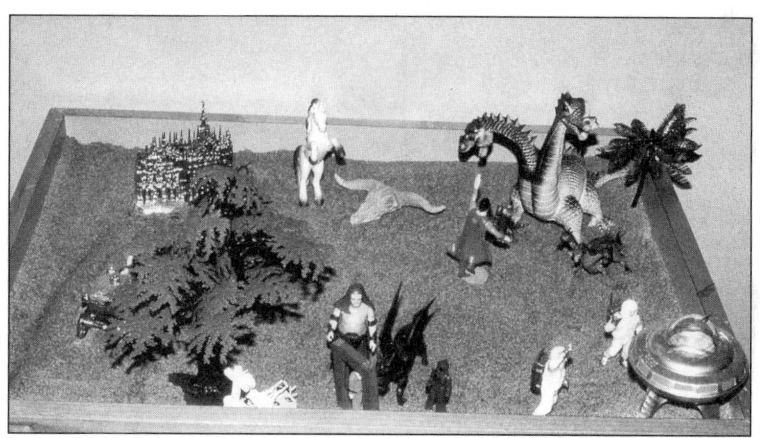

Aaron
Tray 3

Sandplay Record Form **AARON** Tray 4 ~ 1 Week Later Dry Tray Wet Tray X	15 20 23 22 18 14 24 6 5 10 9 2 8 17 19 1 4 11 3 7 21 13 12 16

Initial Observations/Remarks ~ (Therapist) or "Client"
None

Placement Sequence

1) Fire ring
2 - 5) Indians
6) Kachina
7) Mask
8- 11) Indian women
12) Davy Crocket
13 - 14) Ramayana masks
15) Indian child (On edge)
"I want this girl to be a spirit hanging above the fire."
16 - 19) Trees
20) Moon
21) Boa constrictor
22 - 24) Teepees

Client's Closing Remarks

"They are having an Indian ceremony. This one is watching (#12). This guy (#5) wants to kill him because he is invading their territory. They (masks) are the gods they pray to. This (#15) is the first Indian. Now she is dead, but she is a spirit. These (#22-24) are the tents that they sleep in. Here is a snake, who wants to get the warmth of the fire."

Therapist: Is he dangerous? "Yes"

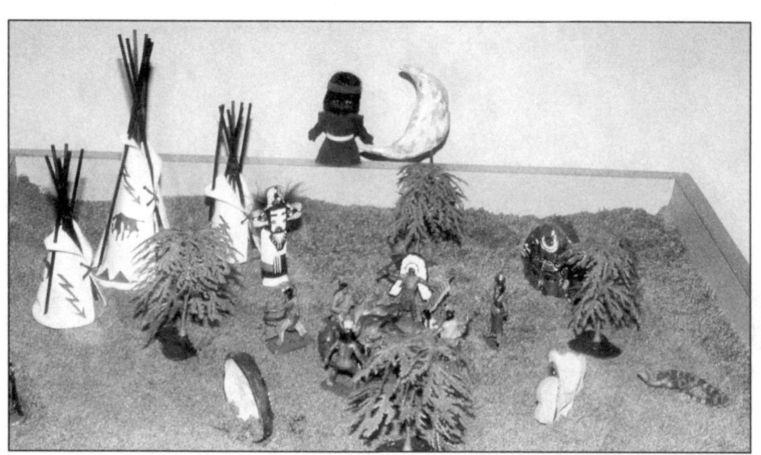

Aaron
Tray 4

Sandplay Record Form
AARON

Tray 5 ~ 2 Weeks Later
Dry Tray
Wet Tray X

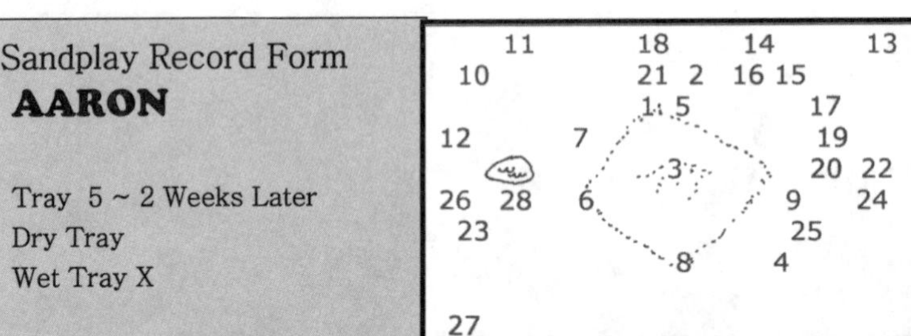

Initial Observations/Remarks ~ (Therapist) or "Client"
(Scores a diamond shape in sand with finger)

Placement Sequence

1) Catcher
2) Umpire
3) Pitcher
4) Baseman
5) Batter
6) Baseman
7) Camera man
8) Baseman
9) Fielder
10) Man in chair with beer
11) Man with sore thumb
12) Farmer
13) Drunk man with headache
14) Man with boy on shoulders
15 – 22) Men in tuxedos
23 – 24) Trees
25) Sun (Suspends on hook. Makes lake)
26) No Fishing sign
27) Pick up truck
28) Shrubs

Client's Closing Remarks

"They are having a baseball game. These guys (on left) live on a farm over here (left). They brought their chairs to watch. This guy (#13) got hit on the head with a bat. The pick up truck lost his way, be he finally found his way to the game. This guy (7) is watching the pitcher get all of his motion in. These guys (tuxedoes) are the ones who sang at the beginning. This guy is fishing (#12) and is breaking the law."

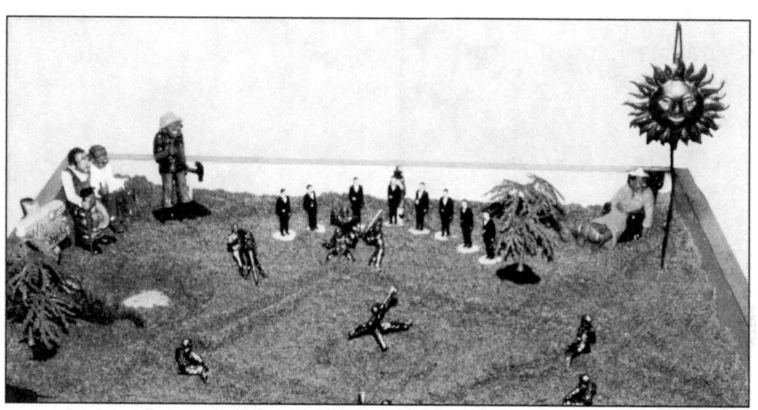

Aaron
Tray 5

Sandplay Record Form
AARON

Tray 6 ~ 2 Weeks Later
Dry Tray
Wet Tray X

28
23 10 9
18 1
16 11
15 24 2
4 25 19 26 12
5 20 13
8 3 17
6 14 21
7 27 29 22

Initial Observations/Remarks ~ (Therapist) or "Client"
(Somberly) "I am going to make a war going on."

Placement Sequence

1 – 8) Soldiers
9 –12) Mounted soldiers
13) Soldier
14) Civil war soldier
15) Contemporary soldier
16 –22) Civil war soldiers
23) Contemporary soldier
24) Adolph Hitler
25) Bugler
26) Sand bag bunker
27) Medics with stretcher
"That is it! Now the details…"

28 – 29) Oak trees

Client's Closing Remarks

"They are getting ready to start the war. When he (#25) blows the horn, it will start. This guy (behind the bunker) will be disqualified, because he already shot a guy. He is the bad guy. The good guys are here (left side) the bad guys are on the right. This (Hitler) is the commissioner of the bad team. This guy (#25) is the commissioner of the good team."

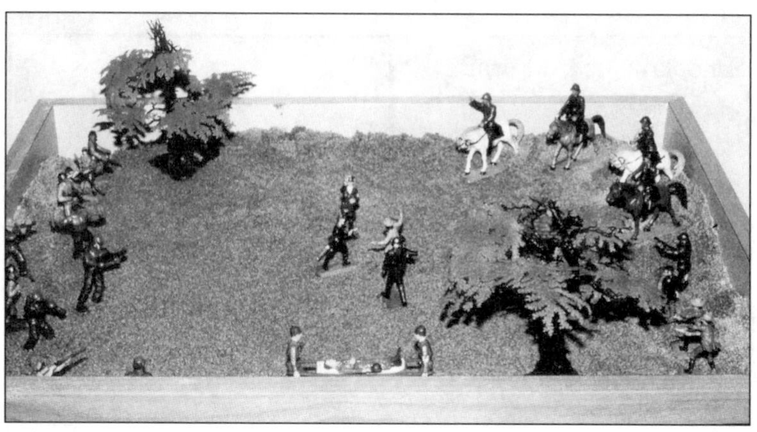

Aaron
Tray 6

Sandplay Record Form **AARON** Tray 7 ~ 1 Month Later Dry Tray Wet Tray X	15 13 2 14 3x 8 7/6 3 18/5 17x/1 16 12 11 17 10/4 19/9

Initial Observations/Remarks ~ (Therapist) or "Client"
None

Placement Sequence

1) Ping pong table
2) Bird in cage
3) Bed
4) Television
5) Dresser
6) Table
7) Computer (On table)
8) Chair
9) Trunk/box
10) Trophy (On TV)
11) Umbrella (Folded up)
12) Ladder (Adjusts positions of bed and table, shifting to right)
13) Bath tub
14) Toilet
15) Sink
16) Mirror (Positions behind dresser)
17) Foot ball (On table, then moves by ladder)
18) Small army jeeps (Lines up on dresser top)
19) Sail boat (On chest)

Client's Closing Remarks

"It's a little kid's room. His parents are rich so he has all of this stuff. This (#10) is a trophy he won in foot ball. I have a computer my father gave me, left over from his office. This bird cannot get out. This is a ladder to put things away. This is his umbrella by the winter box, where he puts his winter clothes away. This is his bird, named "Fred." He has his own mirror. "

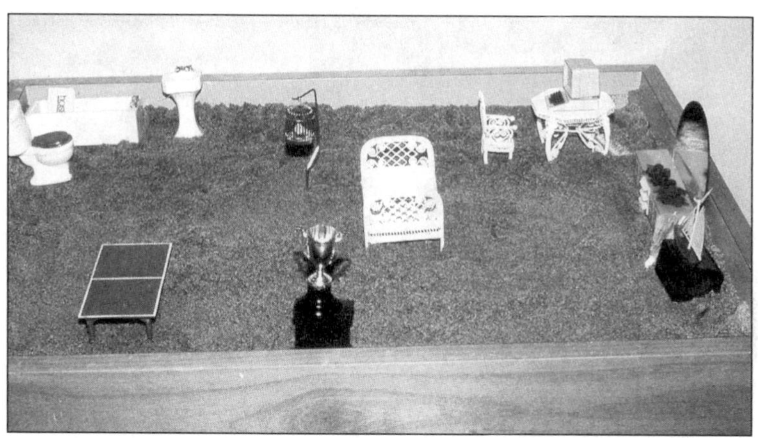

Aaron
Tray 7

Sandplay Record Form
AARON

Tray 8 ~ 11 Weeks Later
Dry Tray
Wet Tray X

Initial Remarks/Observations ~ (Therapist) or "Client"
(Firmly pats sand down)

Placement Sequence

1) Bridge
(Digs river out underneath it)
2) Gondola
3) Umbrella
(On gondola)
4) Oak
5) House
6) Fish - 3
7) Bench
8) Sea gull
9) Geese
10) Oak
11) Car
12) Dove
(Suspends on a string from hook above tray)
13) Dog (On bench)
14) Raft
15) Fisherman
16) Oak

Client's Closing Remarks

This is in the country by a stream. A guy is catching fish. This is someone's house.

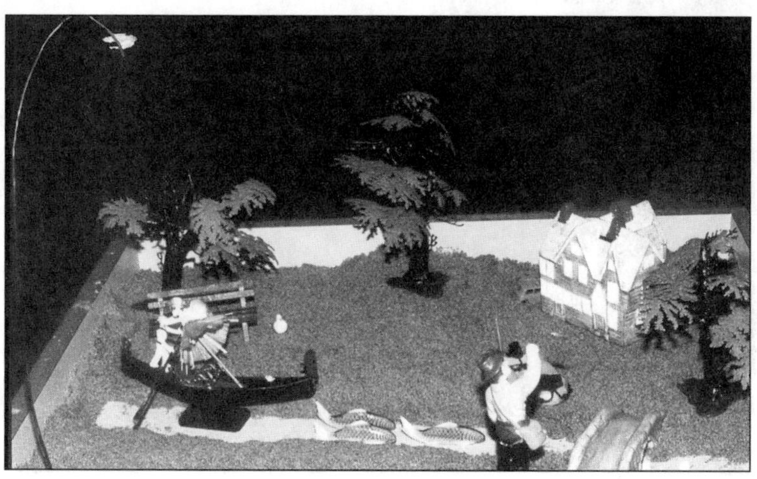

Aaron
Tray 8

Sandplay Record Form
AARON

Tray 9 ~ 1 Week Later
Dry Tray
Wet Tray X

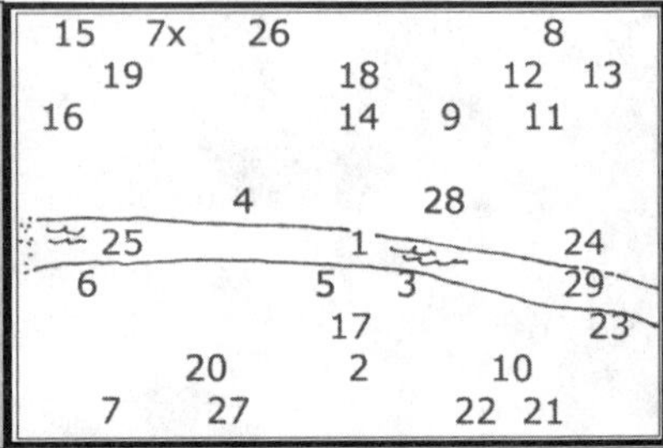

Initial Observations/Remarks ~ (Therapist) or "Client"
"I'm going to make a picture of San Francisco, because I am going there to spend the night at my great aunt's. I'll make China town!"

Placement Sequence

1) Large Chinese bridge (Makes river)
2) Temple
3 – 5) Pagodas
6) Gazebo
7) Pagoda
11 – 13) Bridges
14) Portal (Moves #7)
15 – 23) Chinese buildings
24) Tree (Widens river)
25) Boat
26 – 27) Trees
28) Silver pine tree
29) Large fish

Client's Closing Remarks

"This is China. Everyone is in their house. This boat is leaving. It's early in the morning, because it just dropped off food and stuff. This is a dolphin. It is swimming to the ocean. The fishers (men) tried to catch it, but it got away."

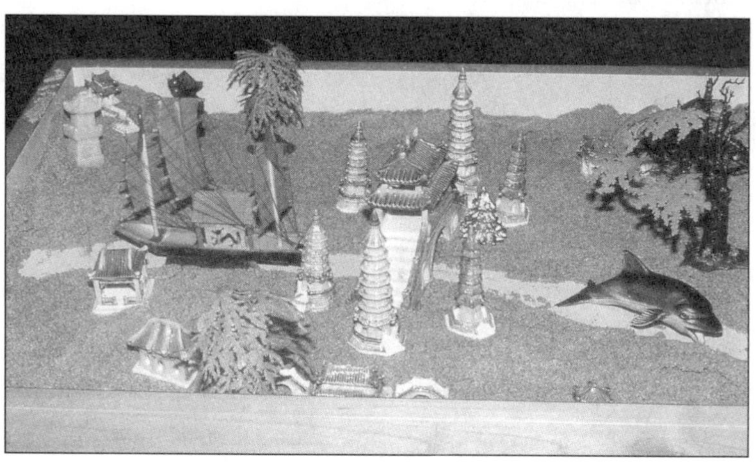

Aaron
Tray 9

Sandplay Record Form
AARON

Tray 10 ~ 2 Weeks Later
Dry Tray
Wet Tray X

Initial Observations/Remarks ~ (Therapist) or "Client"
None

Placement Sequence

1) Black board
2) Desk and 2 chairs
3) People (In the chairs)
4) Desk "Teacher's desk"
5) Chair
6) Brief case
7) Teacher
8) Desk and 2 chairs
9) People (In the chairs)
10) Swing set with people
11) Slide
12) Chart
13) Merry-go-round with kids
14) Bench with person on it
15) Stroller with toddler
16) Purse
17) Bench
18) Table (Moved teacher)
19) Television (On table)
20) Radio (On teacher's desk)
21) Waste basket
22) Chair with child (In corner)

Client's Closing Remarks

"These people (children at desks) are in class and these (on play-ground) are trying to be quiet at recess. The teacher wants them to be quiet, but they are not. They (in classroom) are showing a film about dinosaurs."
Therapist: What about this one here? (Child in corner)
"He is a dunce. He was playing with his pencil. This (#14) is a Mom with her baby. The teacher is going to get mad at this guy (on the swings) because he is standing up."

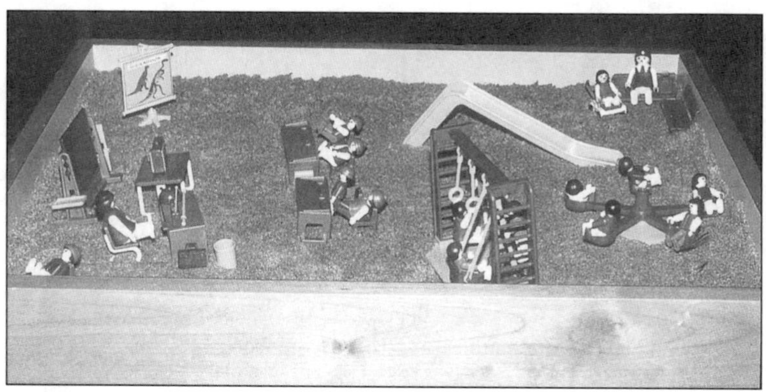

Aaron
Tray 10

Sandplay Record Form

AARON

Tray 11 ~ 3 Months Later
Dry Tray
Wet Tray X

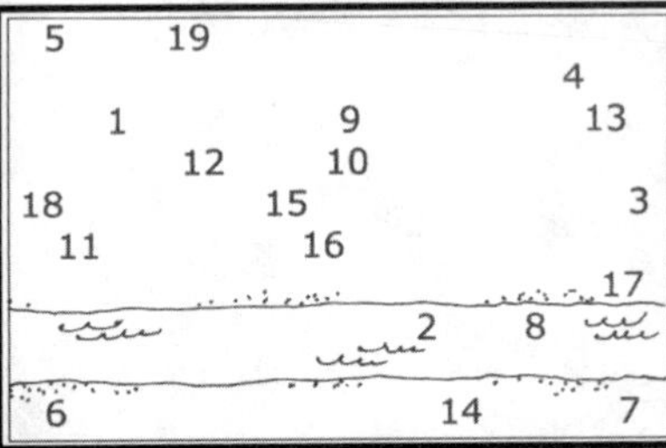

Initial Observations/Remarks ~ (Therapist) or "Client"
(Adds water from left end of tray, works from front)

Placement Sequence

1) Train
2) Bridge
3 – 4) Houses
5) Sun (Suspends from hook. Secures base of hook with large stone)
6) Rock walls (Along rear border of tray)
7) Bench
8) Fish – 4
9) Gazebo
10) Table and chairs
11) Well
12) Rock
13 – 15) Snow trees (Adjusts position of gazebo, moving slightly farther back)
16) Pine tree
17) Silver tree
18 – 19) Pines

Client's Closing Remarks

"It's Christmas time. It is a place where there is no snow, just sand. Everybody decorated everything and wants to see their families. That is where the train is going – to the families. That is why no one is around."

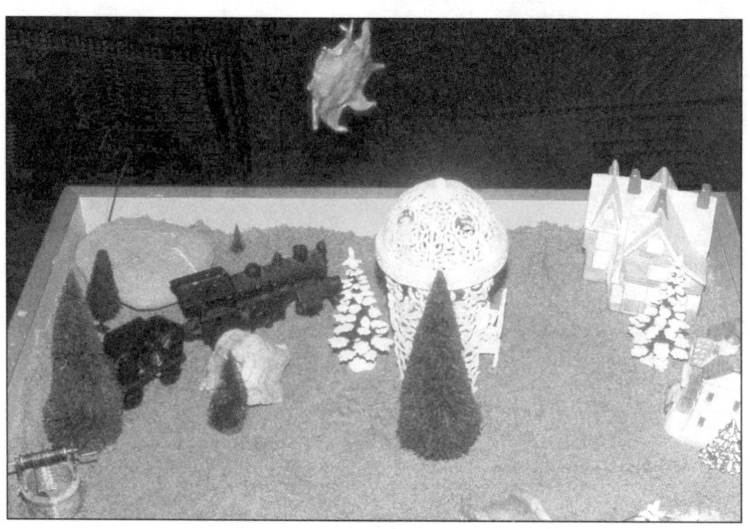

Aaron
Tray 11

Sandplay Record Form
AARON

Tray 12 ~ 1 Month Later
Dry Tray
Wet Tray X

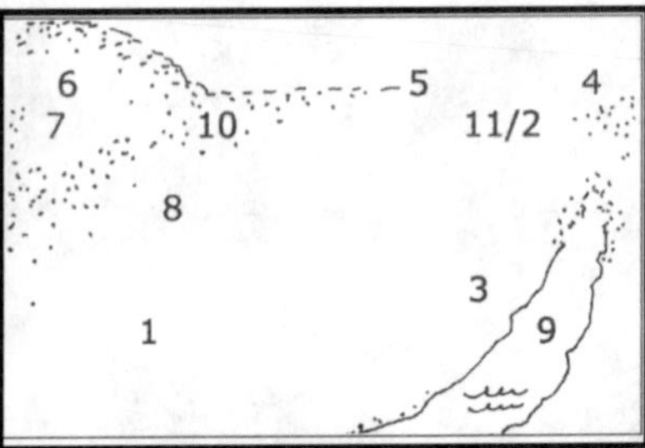

Initial Observations/Remarks ~ (Therapist) or "Client"
None

Placement Sequence

1) Galloping horses
2) Igloo
(Makes river)
3) Polar bear
"What are horses doing in ice land?"
4 – 5) Snow trees
6 – 7) Skiers
8) Snow flakes
(Sprinkles around)
9) Ice cubes
(In river)
10) Large crystal star (Suspends from ceiling above tray)
11) Crystal ring
(Top of igloo)

Client's Closing Remarks

"This is a Winter Land."

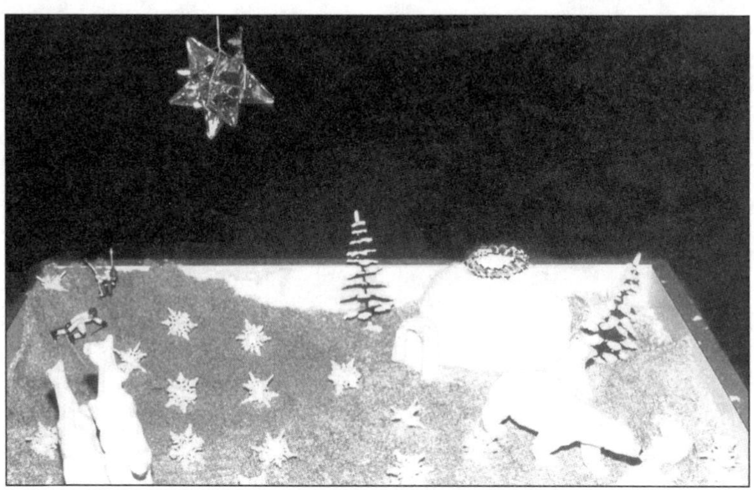

Aaron
Tray 12

Sandplay Record Form
AARON

Tray 13 ~ 5 Mo. 3 Wk. Later
Dry Tray
Wet Tray X

```
   2   21    28   16 17
  1     4  3    8   7         26
  12                 24     20
 14                    25
 29                        30
  22
 11                              23
                  9
   5  18      6    15  10  13
     27      19
```

Initial Observations/Remarks ~ (Therapist) or "Client"
(Circles around tray during construction)

Placement Sequence

1) Bunker
2 – 10) Soldiers (Arranges darks vs. lights)
11) Canon
12 – 15) Tanks
16 – 19) Jeeps
20) Tank
21) Canon
22 – 24) Military jets
25) Soldier
26) Medics and man on stretcher
27 – 28) Soldiers
29) Military jet (Suspends on hook above tray)
30) Walls (Forms a bunker)
31) Jet (On rock at base of hook)

Client's Closing Remarks
"This is the war in the Persian Gulf." (Persian Gulf War started today)
Therapist: How do you feel about it?
(Disgusted) "It stinks and they are acting like kids."

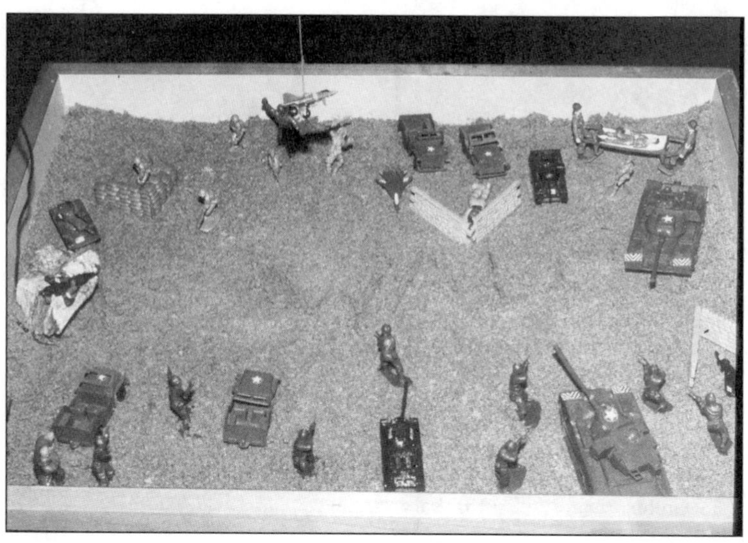

Aaron
Tray 13

Sandplay Record Form
AARON

Tray 14 ~ 2 Months Later
Dry Tray
Wet Tray X

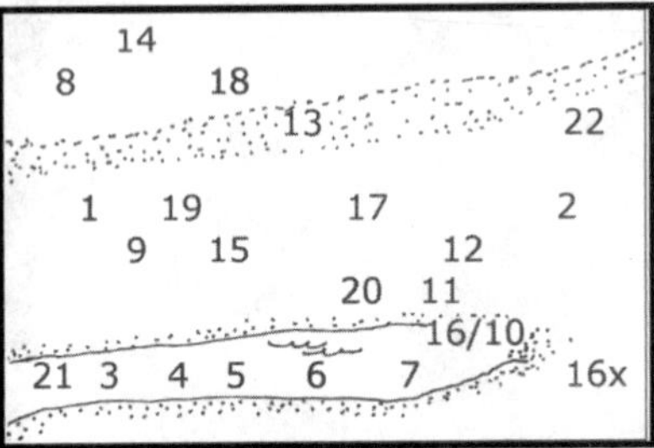

Initial Observations/Remarks ~ (Therapist) or "Client"
"I will make a golf course." (Playful, teasing mood)

Placement Sequence

1) Golfer
2) Flag and hole
3 – 7) Bicyclists
"This is going to be a funny picture, because the cyclists are riding in the water!"
8) Skier
9) Spy with looking glass
10) Bridge
(Shapes a road with his hand)
11 – 12) Cars
13) Large train
(Laughs)
14) Snow flakes
15) Well
16) Diver
"Ha, deep sea diver!"
17) Cow "Ha" Moo!"
18) Polar bear
"He (skier) sees the bear and skis up hill!"
19) Dick Tracy
20) Gas pumps
21) Fish bone
"The dead fish is floating."
22) Space shuttle
(Moved out of the path of the train)

Client's Closing Remarks

"This is Crazy Land. This guy (cyclist) is riding his bike backwards in the river. The space shuttle is taking off. Everything is on a golf course. These guys (Spy/Clouseau and Tracy) are looking for the golf ball because they think there is a bomb in it. The skier is going up hill."

Therapist: Is this a safe place or scary?

"Not very safe. You cannot get hurt, but you can't count on things."

(Moves diver to top of bridge right before picture is taken)

"He is getting ready to dive in!"

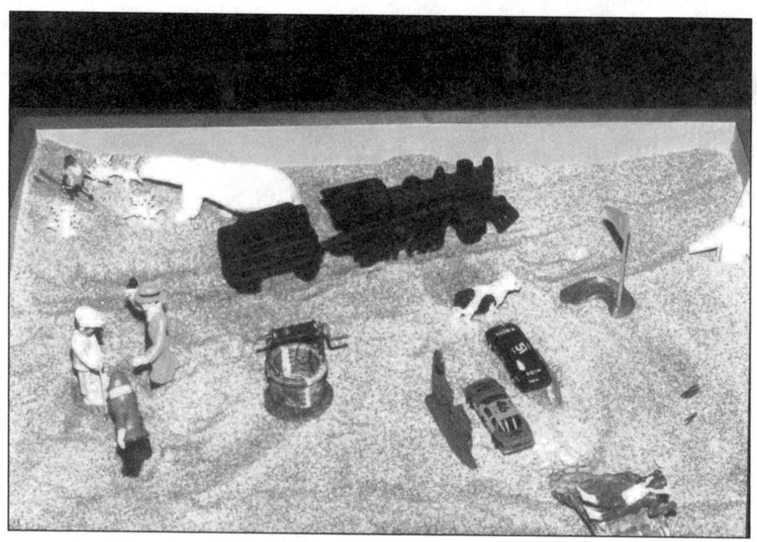

Aaron
Tray 14

Sandplay Record Form
AARON

Tray 15 ~ Final, 5 Mo. Later
1 Year 6 Mo. Since Tray 1
Wet Tray X

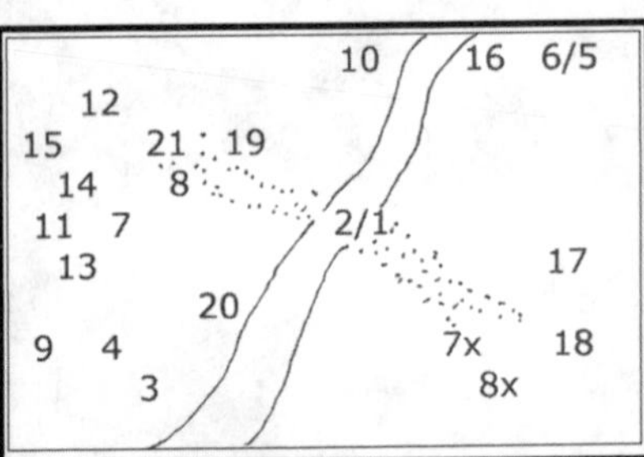

Initial Observations/Remarks ~ (Therapist) or "Client"
(Forms a river) "It's pretty hard to make a road."

Placement Sequence

1) Bridge (Traces a path over bridge, making road from far left corner to near right)
2) Car (On bridge)
3) Train tracks
4) Train engine
5) Bench
6) Lady (On bench)
7) Wrestler (Lays down)
8) Boxer
9) Napoleon statue
10) Rocket man (Suspends on hook above river, near bridge area)
11) Davy Crocket "I need all of the bad guys I had in the past."
12) Two headed dragon
13) Three headed dragon
14) Joker
15) Hitler
16 – 18) Oak trees
17 – 20) Small trees

Client's Closing Remarks

"This (the boxer) is me and these are all the bad guys that I killed, or are about to die. This (#9) is a statue of me. This is a train with me leaving the battle. This is a lake and people are driving. This is the Rocketeer, helping me kill all the bad guys. This (#6) is a lady watching the fight. She is my mom. (#9) This is the trophy I get."

(Adds #21)

21) Silver trophy (Stands beside boxer #8)
"It's as tall as me!"

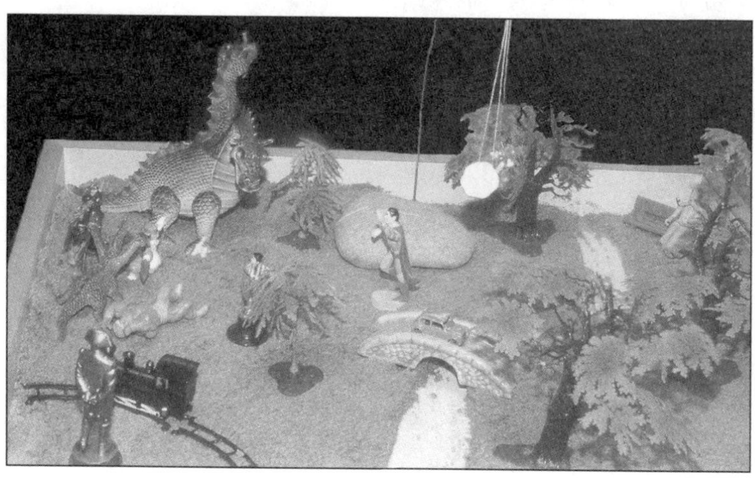

Aaron
Tray 15a

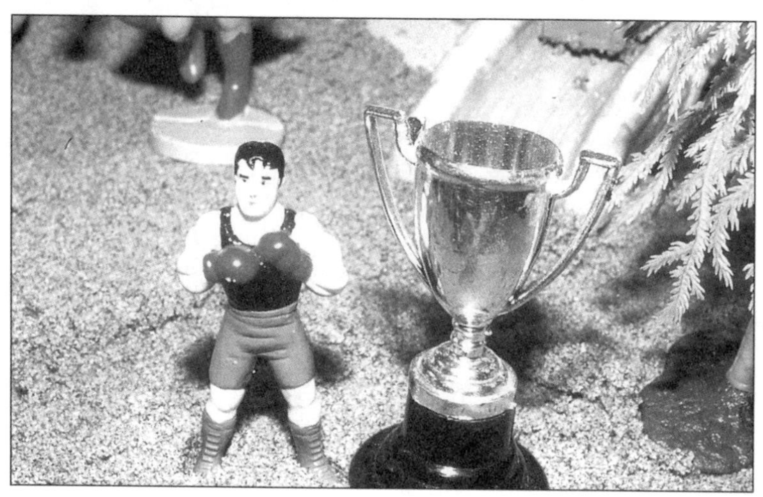

Aaron
Tray 15b ~ Detail

Client Profile
ADRIENNE

32 year-old female
Married
Two years of college
No children - Wants children
Describes being neglected by mother and father
One older brother
Jewish family, but not religious
Few memories before age 8 or 9
Father died of cancer when Adrienne was 16
Hates her mother - wants to deal with this so she does not repeat pattern with future children

Sandplay	Discussed on Page Number
Tray 1	384
Tray 10	27
Tray 11	27, 66
Tray 12	27
Tray 20	66, 68
Tray 26	66, 169
Tray 42	

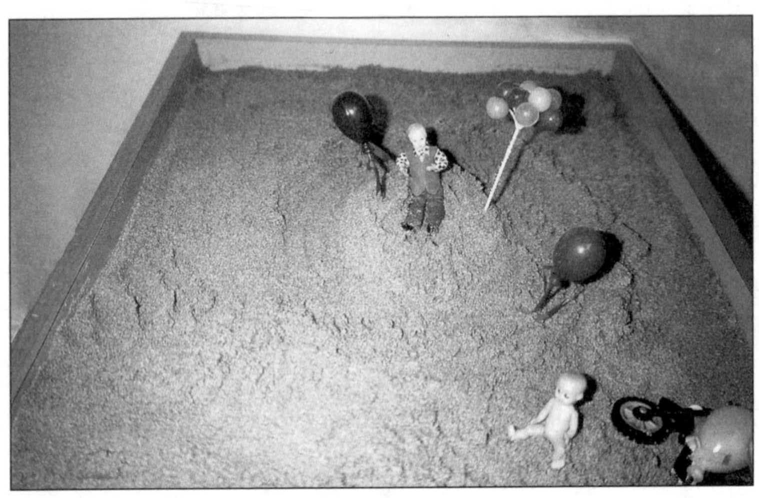

Adrienne
Tray 1 ~ 8 Months into Therapy

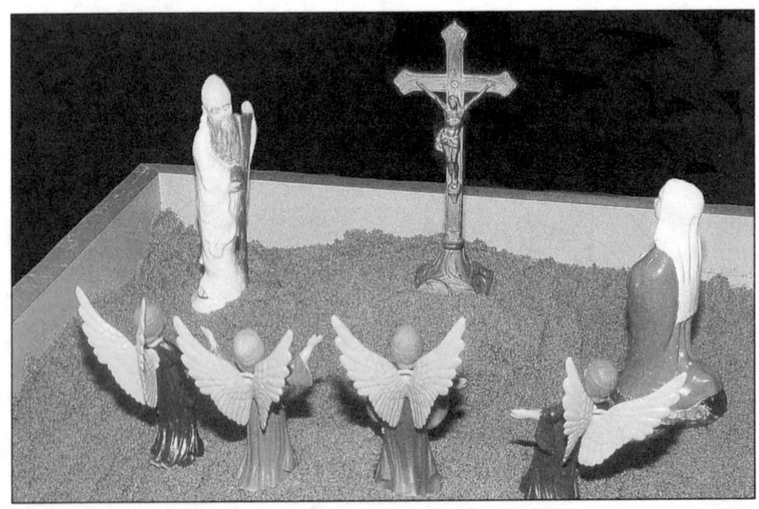

Adrienne
Tray 10 ~ 1 Year 10 Months Later

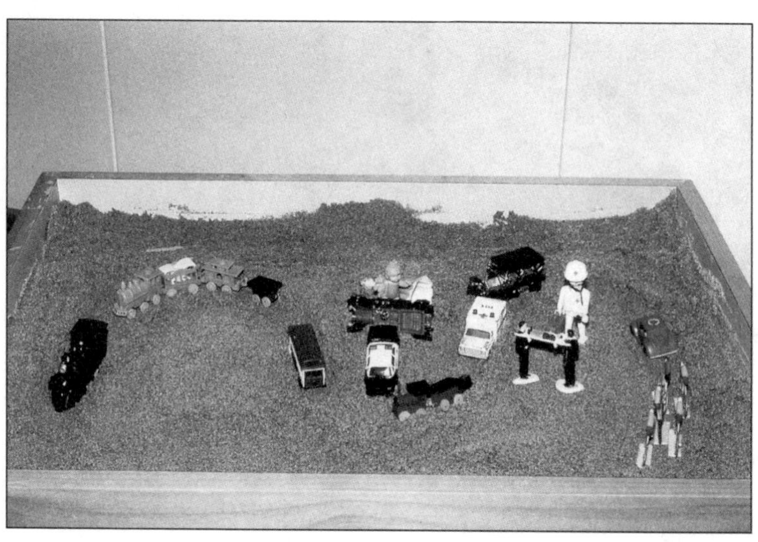

Adrienne
Tray 11 ~ 1 Week Later

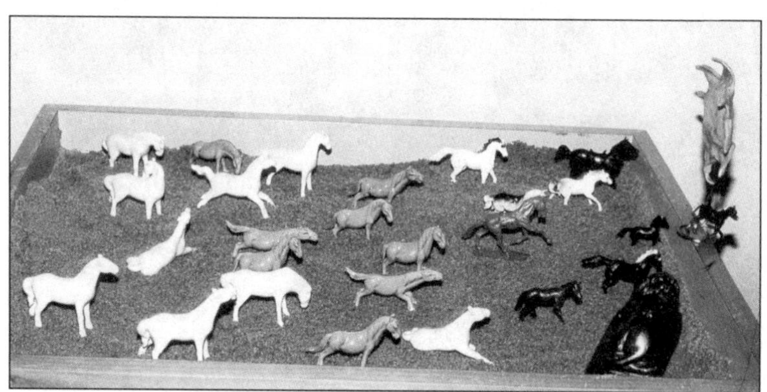

Adrienne
Tray 12 ~ 2 Weeks Later

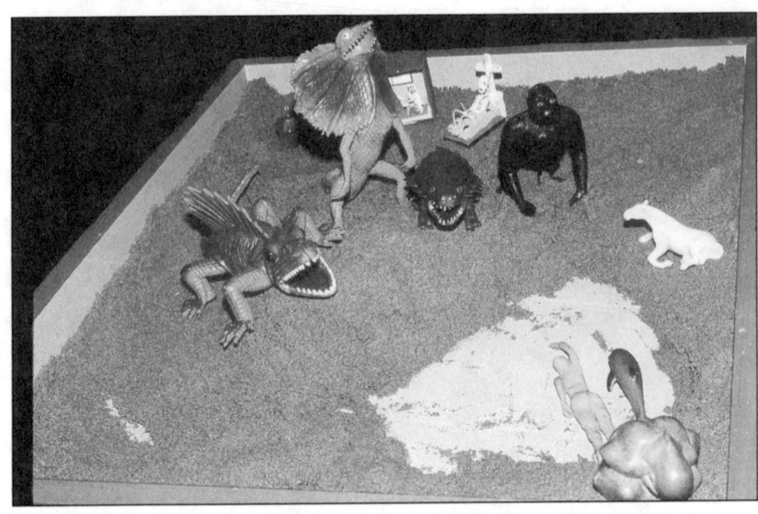

Adrienne
Tray 20 ~ 5 Months Later

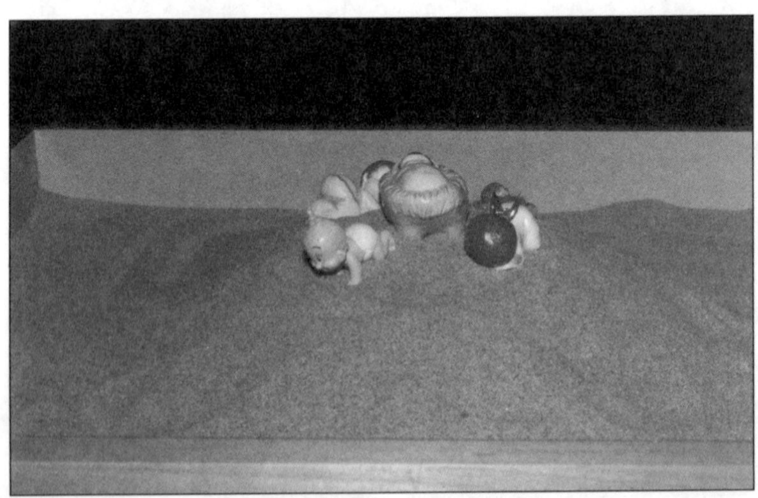

Adrienne
Tray 26a ~ 4 Months Later

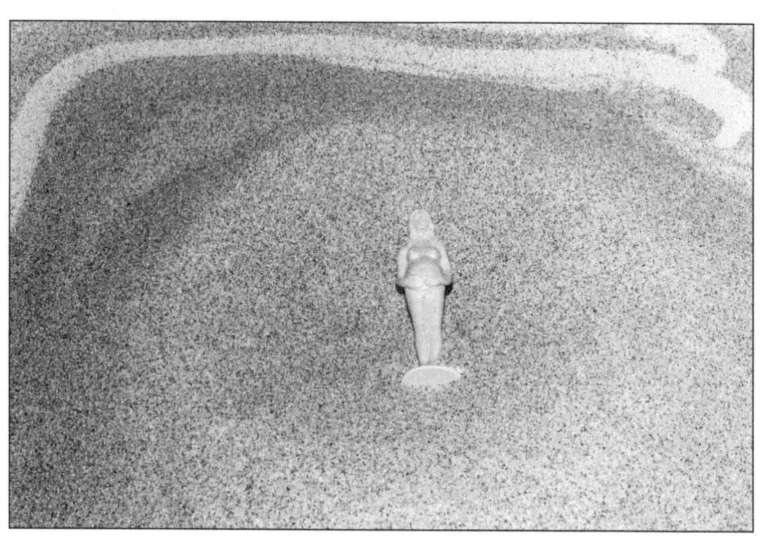

Adrienne 26b ~ Detail

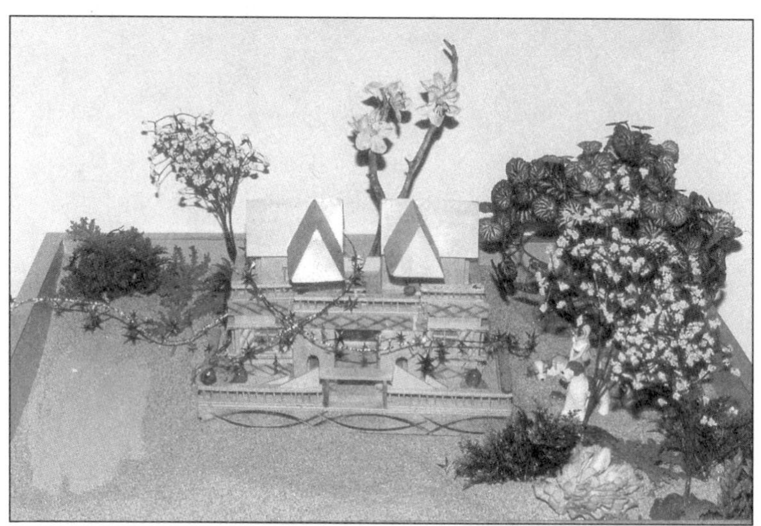

Adrienne
Tray 42 ~ Final ~ 4 Years 5 Months Later
7 Years Since Tray 1

Client Profile
ANNIE

11 year-old girl
Lives with Grandparents
Prenatal drug and alcohol involvement
Developmental delays, academic and social difficulties
Behavior problems
Bi-polar disorder
History of extensive sexual abuse

Sandplay	Discussed on Page Number
Tray 1	
Tray 2	
Tray 3	195
Tray 4	195
Tray 5	195
Tray 6	195

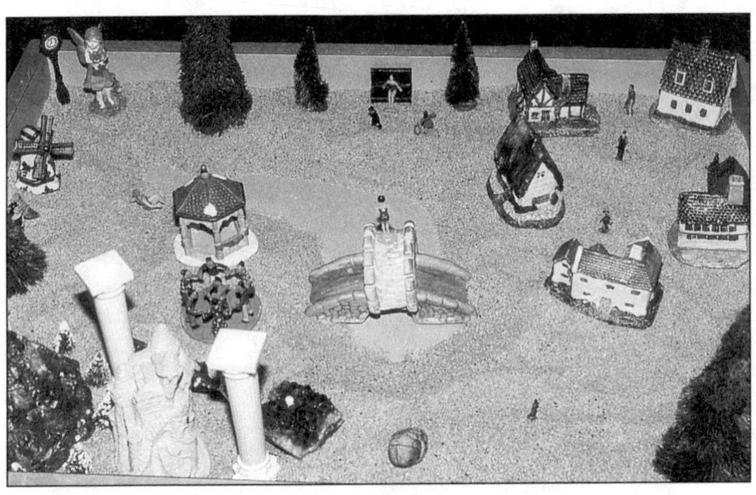

Annie
Tray 1 ~ Session 1

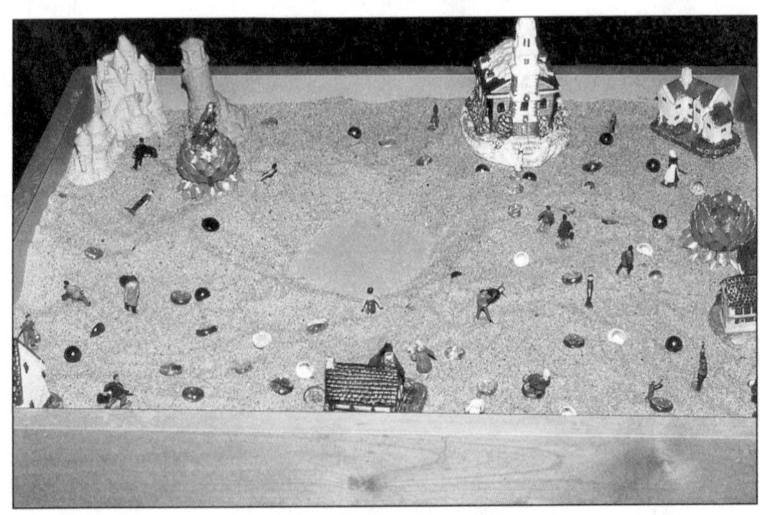

Annie
Tray 2~ 2 Weeks Later

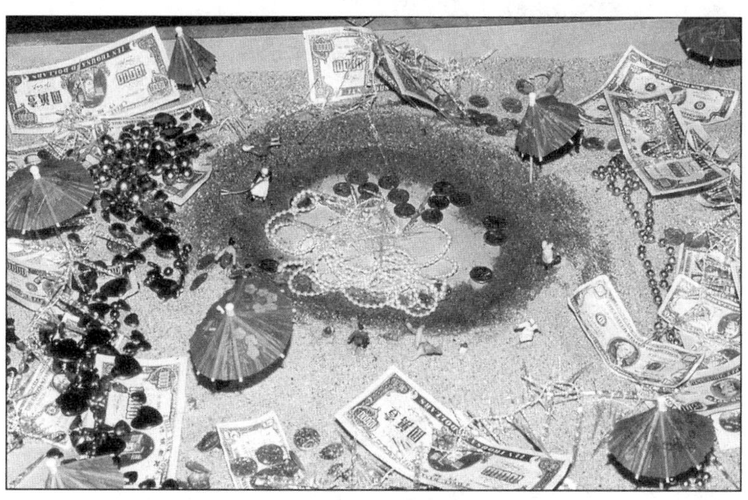

Annie
Tray 3 ~ 4 Weeks Later

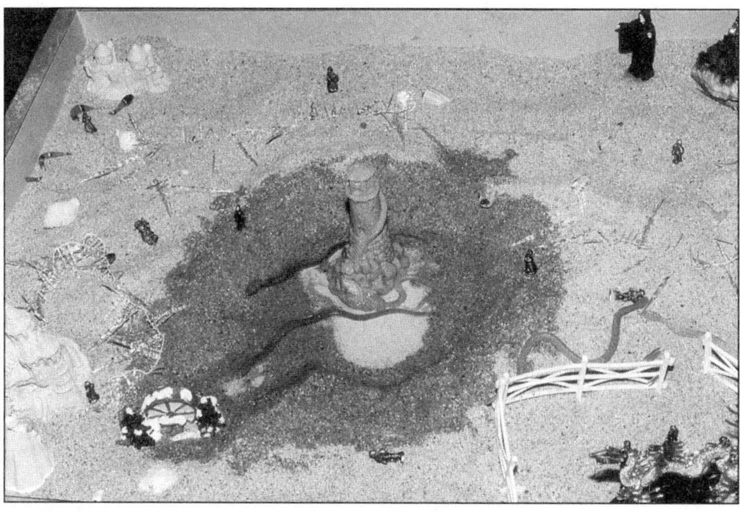

Annie
Tray 4a ~ 2 Months Later

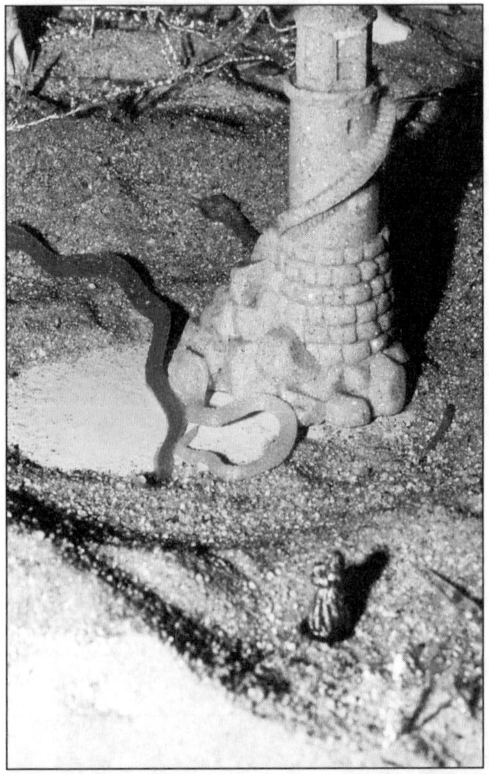

Annie
Tray 4b ~ Detail

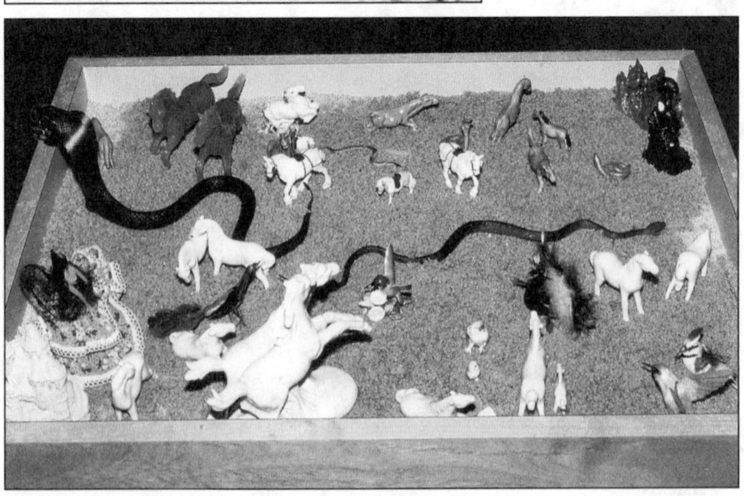

Annie Tray 5 ~ 3 Months Later

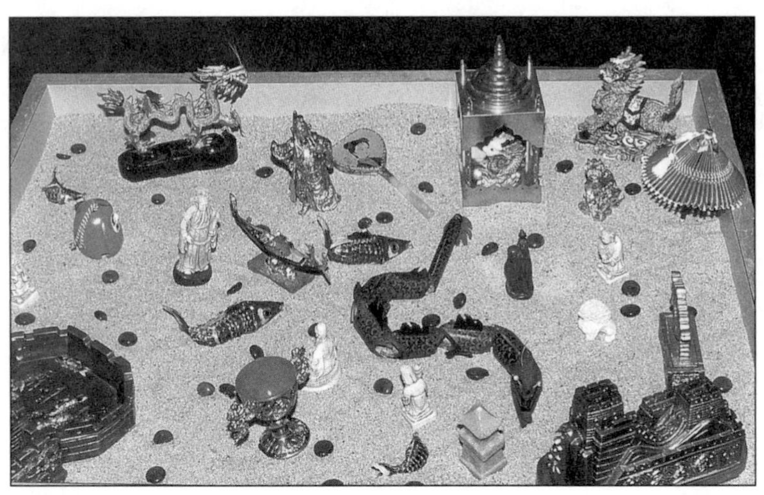

Annie
Tray 6~ Final ~ 7 Weeks Later
11 Months Since Tray 1

Client Profile
ARTIE

7 year-old boy
Parents in high conflict divorce process
Shared custody
Mother ill throughout pregnancy - normal delivery
Fear and anxiety, nightmares since he began school
Daily stomach aches, resistance to school
Highly active child
Several ADD evaluations, negative results

Sandplay	Discussed on Page Number
Tray 1	
Tray 12	228-9
Tray 13	229
Tray 18	229
Tray 28	225
Tray 29	225
Tray 30	225
Tray 41	229
Tray 42	229

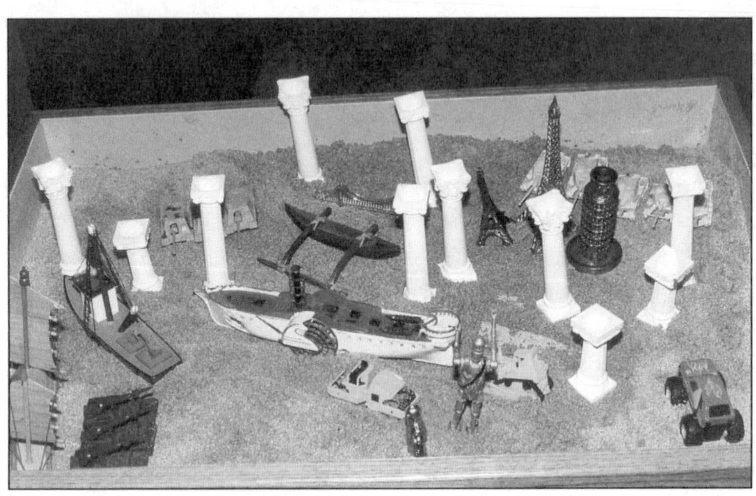

Artie
Tray 1 ~ Session 1

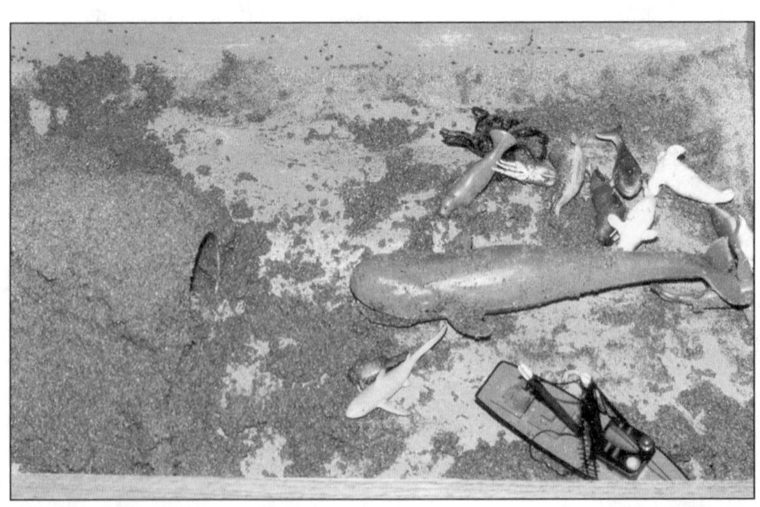

Artie
Tray 12a~ 10 Months Later

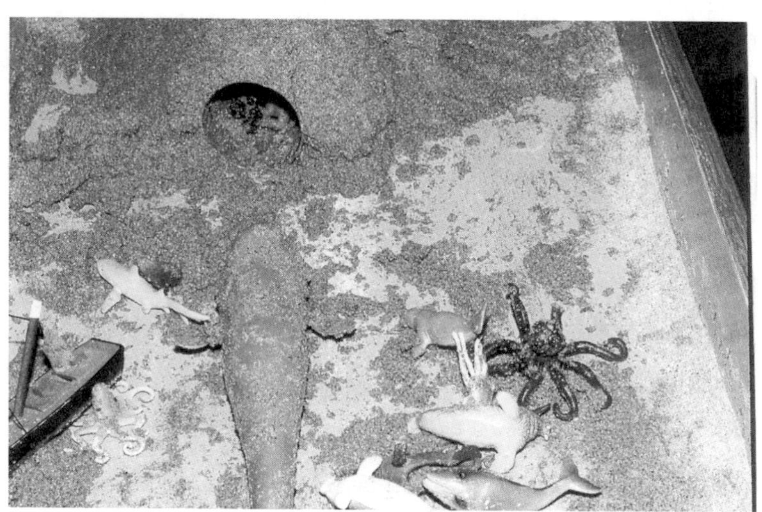

Artie
Tray 12b ~ Detail

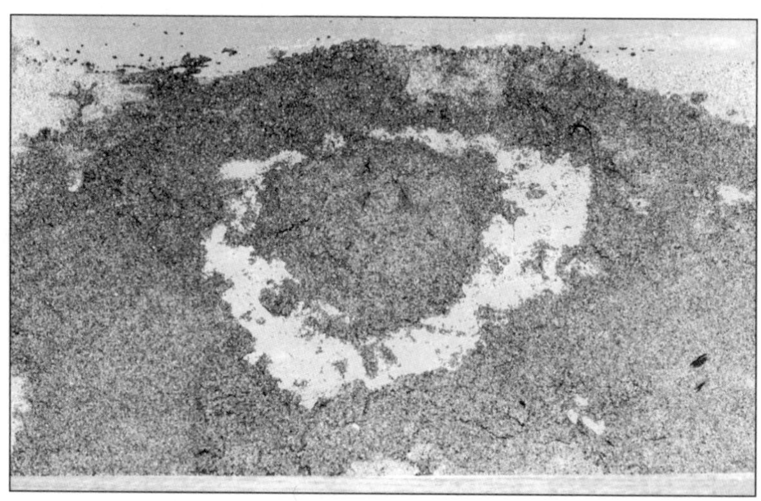

Artie
Tray 13 ~ 1 Week Later

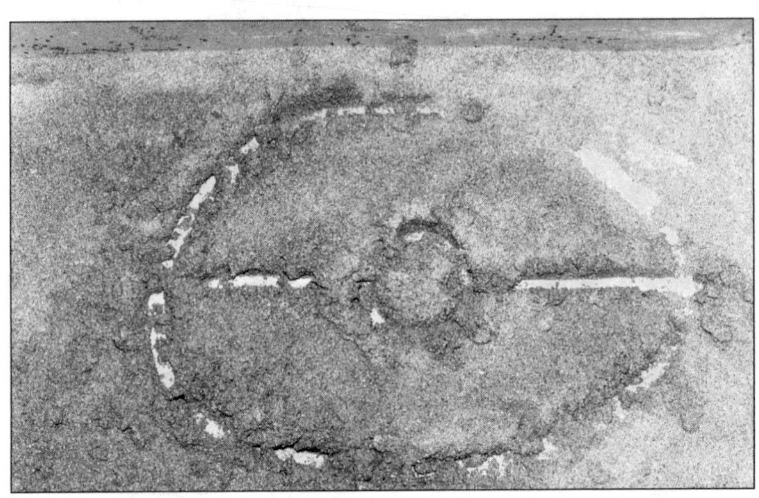

Artie
Tray 18 ~ 3 Weeks Later

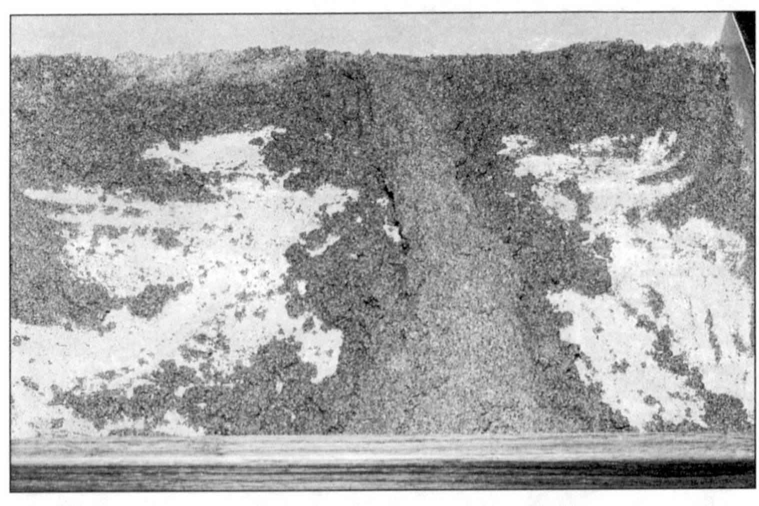

Artie
Tray 28a ~ 8 Months Later

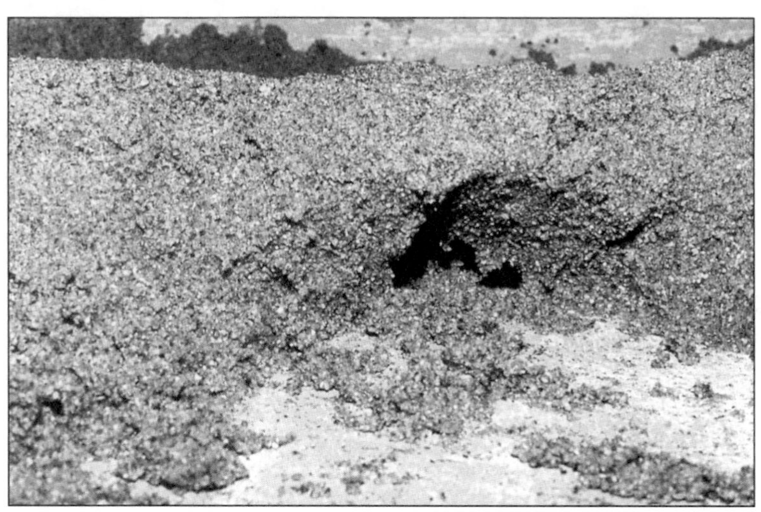

Artie
Tray 28b ~ Detail

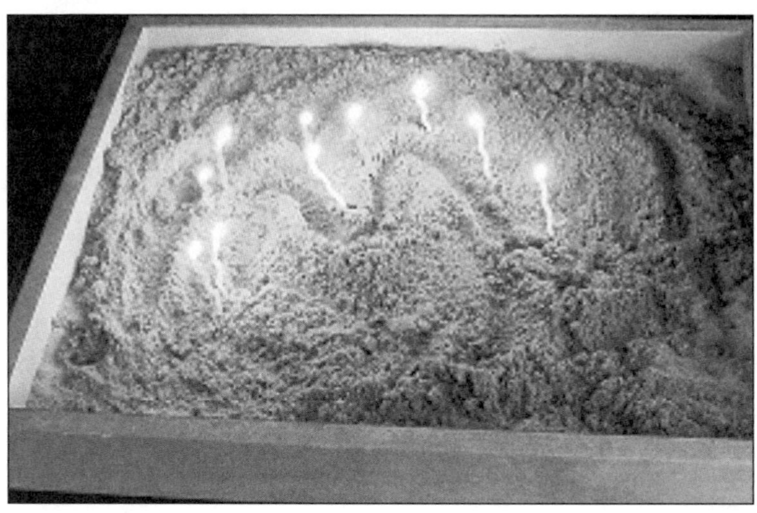

Artie
Tray 29 ~ 1 Week Later

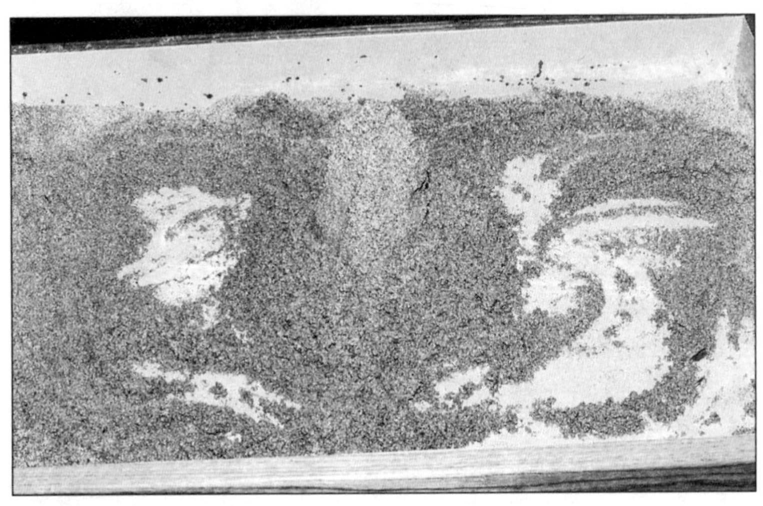

Artie
Tray 30 ~ Same Session

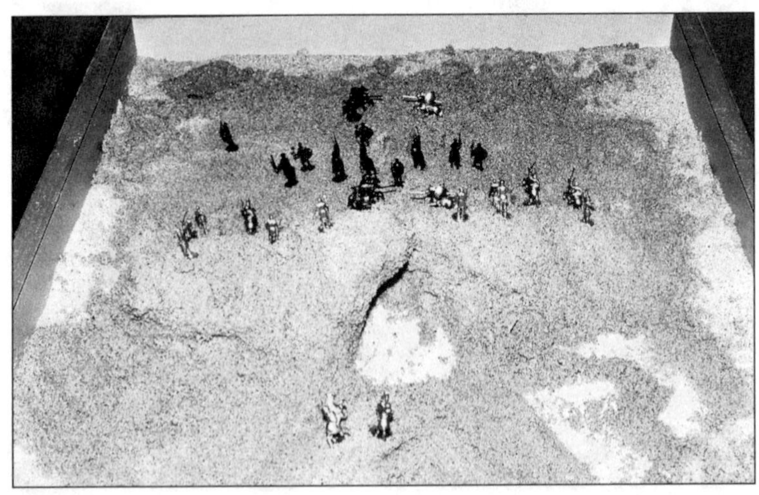

Artie
Tray 41 ~ 6 Months Later

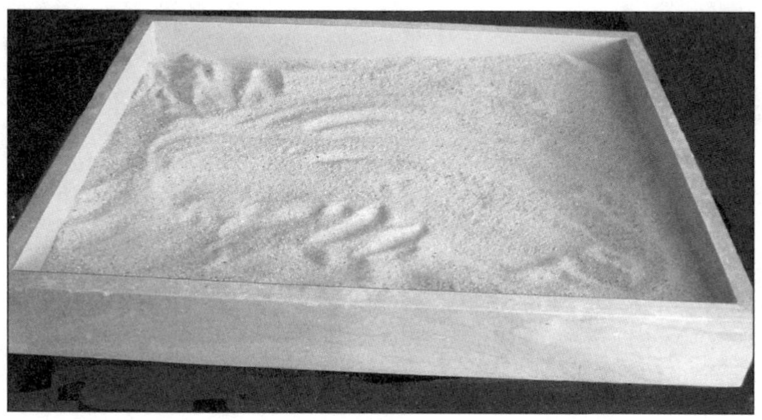

Artie
Tray 42 ~ Final ~ 3 Months Later
3 Years 5 Months Since Tray 1

Client Profile

BILLY

3 ½ year-old boy

Witnessed domestic abuse of Father's attack of Mother

Mother and Father divorcing - Doesn't see his dad

Mother reports frequent nightmares and fearful behavior

One brother, age 12

Sandplay	Discussed on Page Number
Tray 1	283-5
Tray 2	
Tray 3	
Tray 4	214, 284-5
Tray 5	284-5

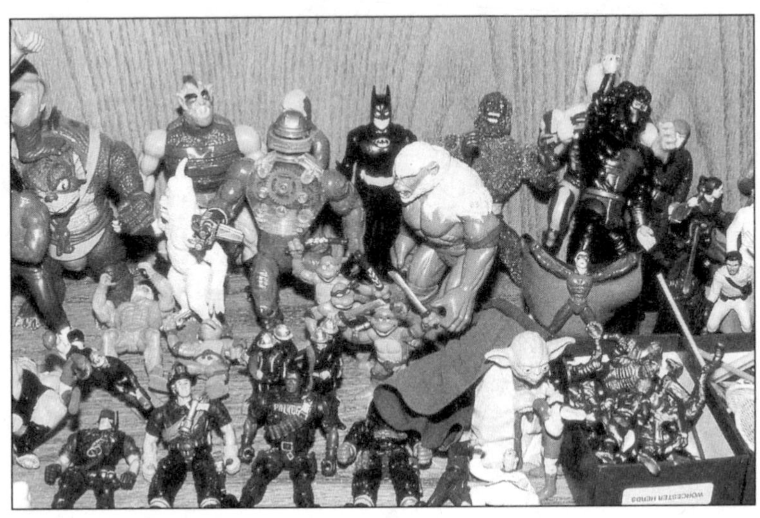

Billy
Tray 1 ~ Shelf ~ Session 1

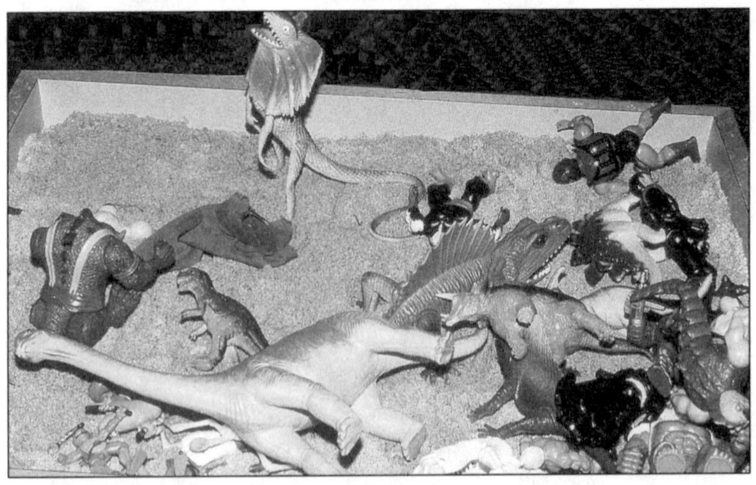

Billy
Tray 2a ~ 1 Week Later

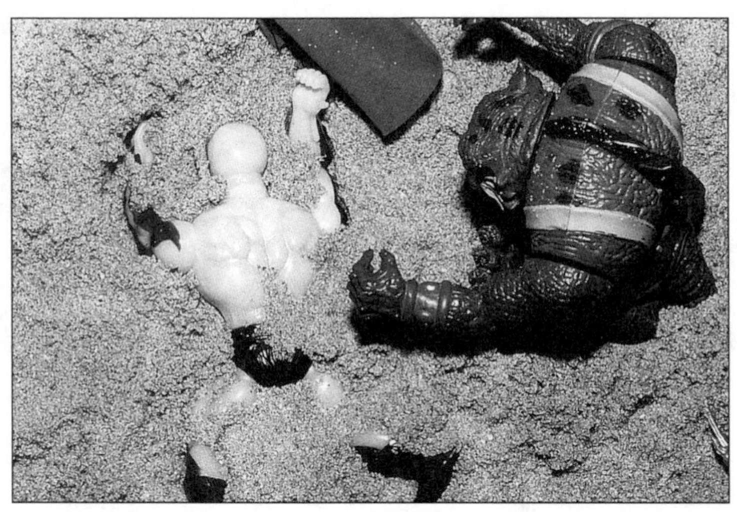

Billy
Tray 2b ~ Detail

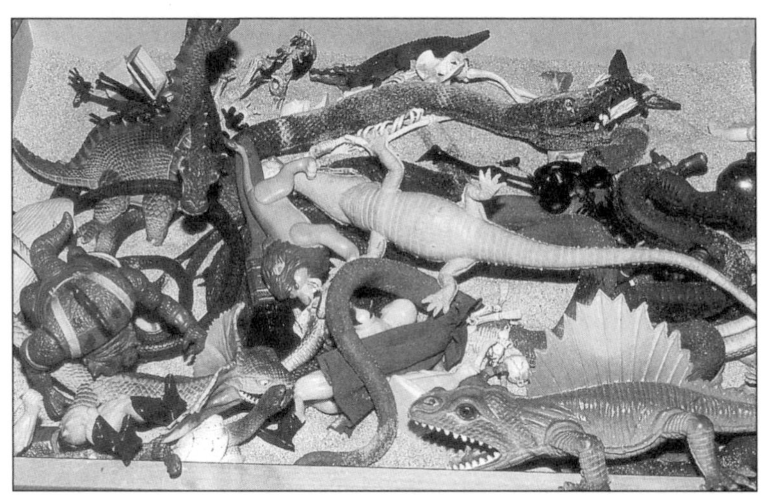

Billy
Tray 3a ~ 2 Weeks Later

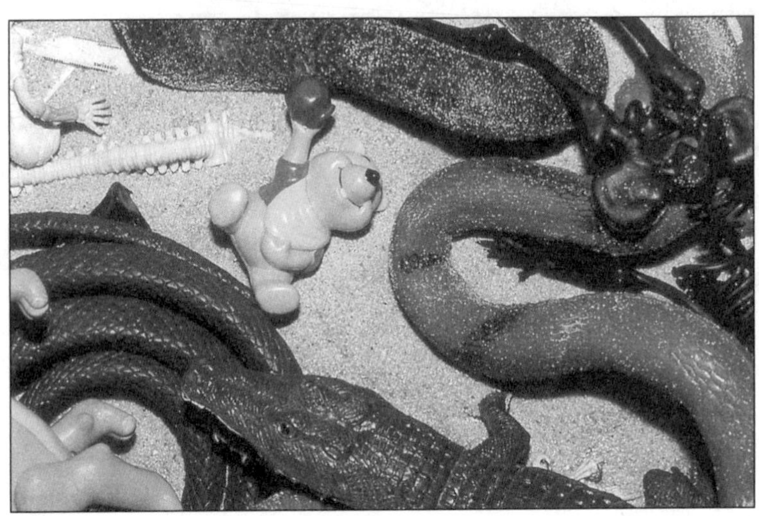

Billy
Tray 3b ~ Detail

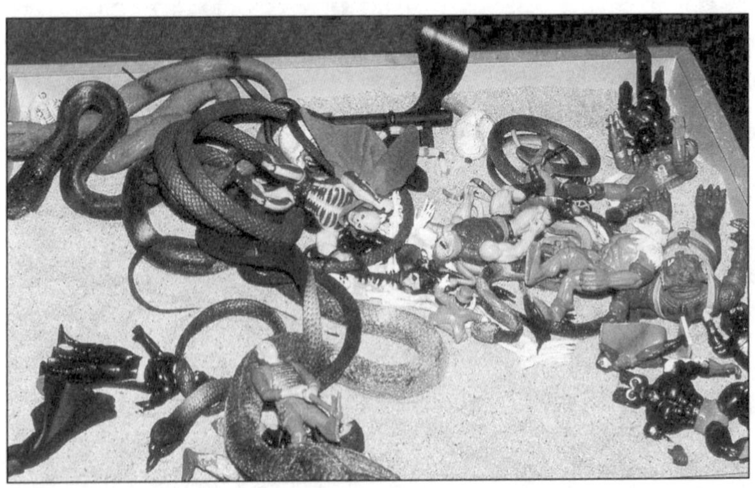

Billy
Tray 4 ~ 2 Weeks Later

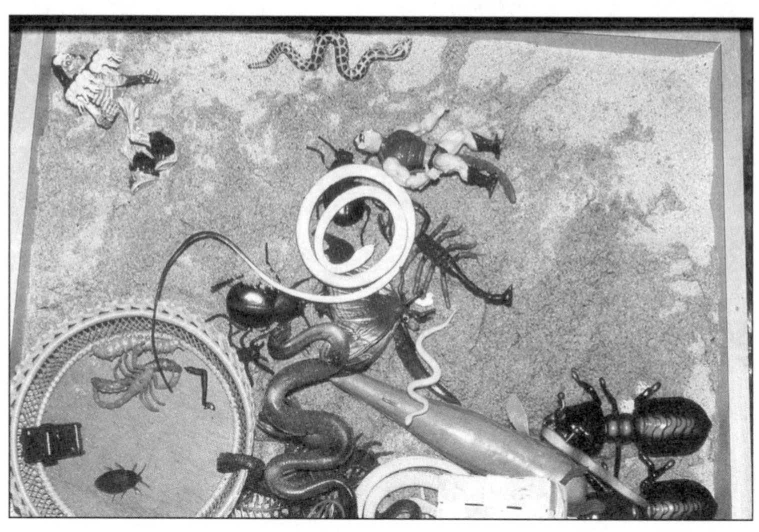

Billy
Tray 5a ~ Final ~ 3 Weeks Later
2 Months Since Tray 1

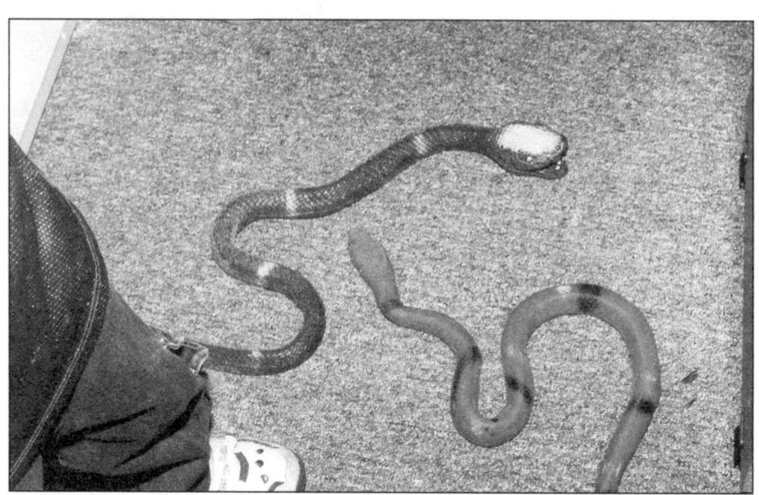

Billy
Tray 5b ~ Detail

Client Profile

CARY

Married woman, age 40
No children
1 Sister
High school education
Employed
Mother died of illness when Cary was 20
Cary has never had any feelings about Mother's death
Alcoholic father
Entered therapy to explore her family history and her feelings of repulsion and discomfort with her father

Sandplay	Discussed on Page Number
Tray 1	194
Tray 2	194
Tray 3	194
Tray 4	194
Tray 5	194
Tray 6	121, 194
Tray 7	115, 194
Tray 8	194
Tray 15	194
Tray 21	194
Tray 23	194
Tray 24	194
Tray 41	

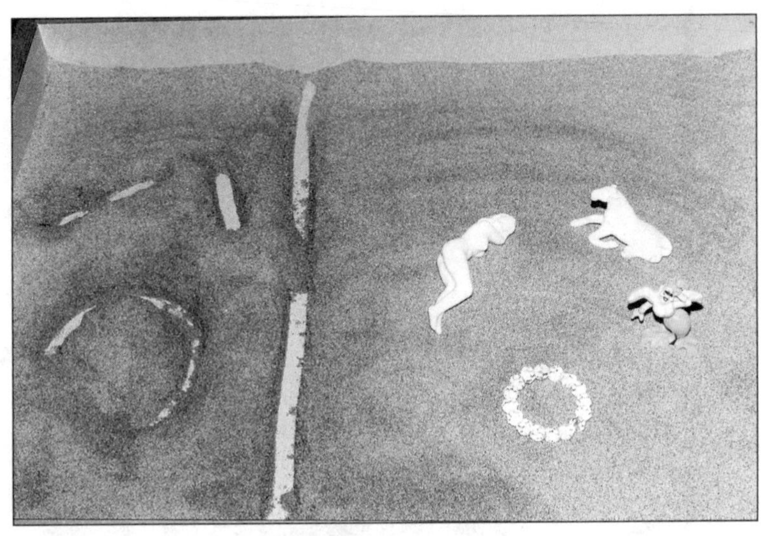

Cary
Tray 1 ~ Early in Treatment

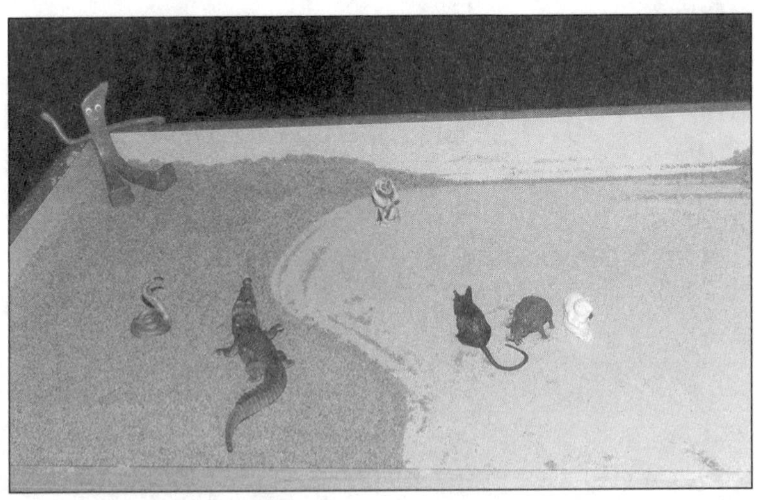

Cary
Tray 2 ~ 6 Weeks Later

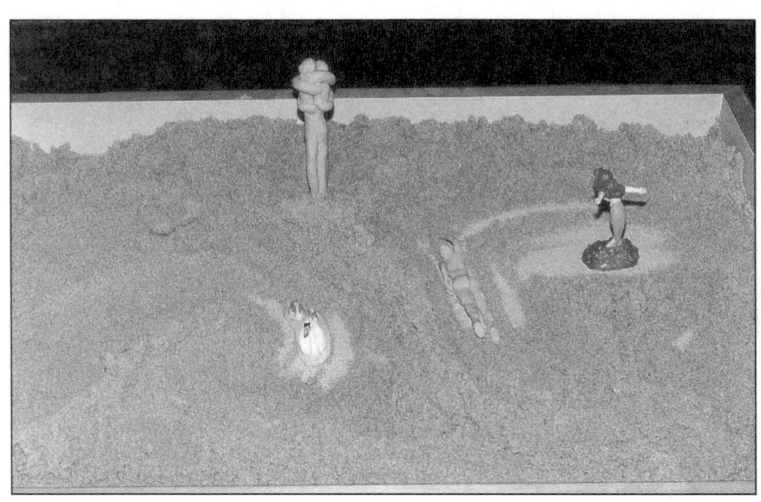

Cary
Tray 3 ~ 2 Weeks Later

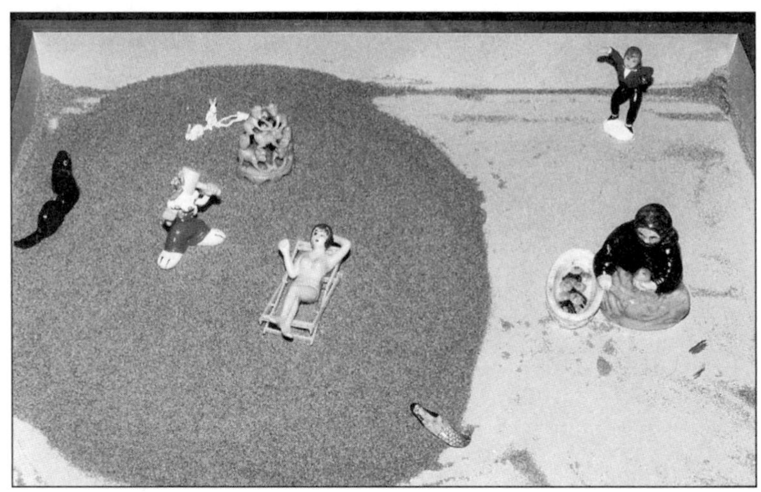

Cary
Tray 4 ~ 3 Weeks Later

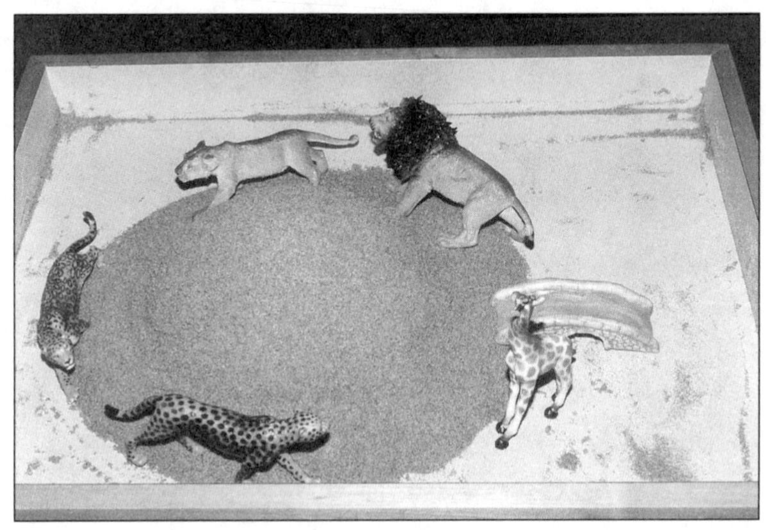

Cary
Tray 5 ~ 2 Weeks Later

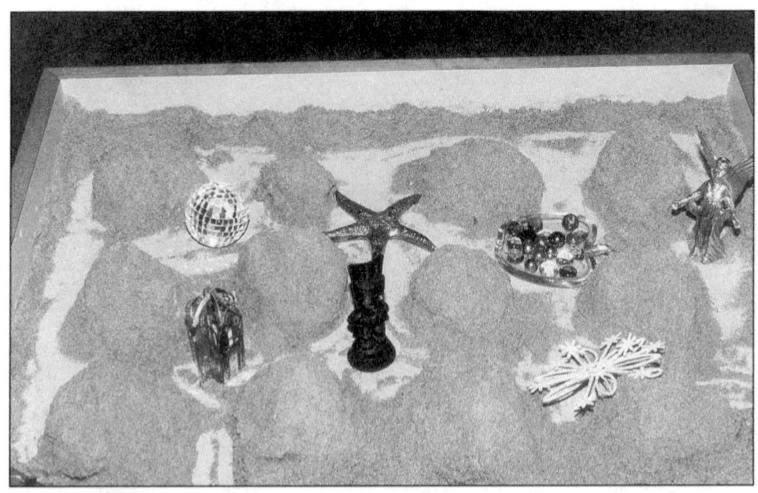

Cary
Tray 6a ~ 3 Weeks Later

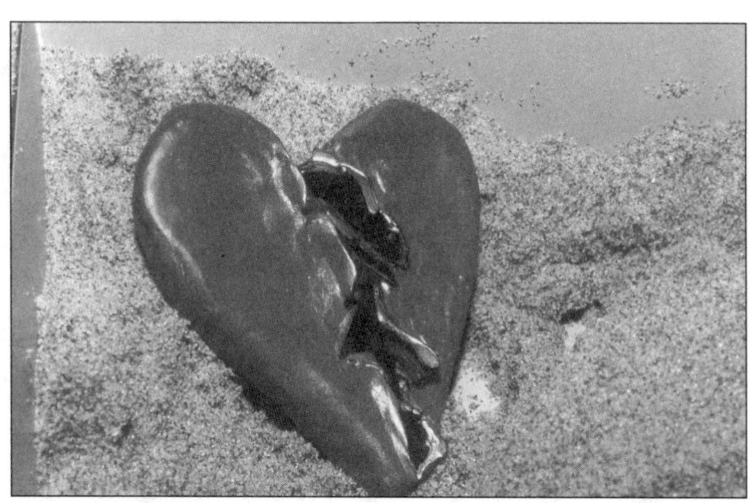

Cary
Tray 6b ~ Detail

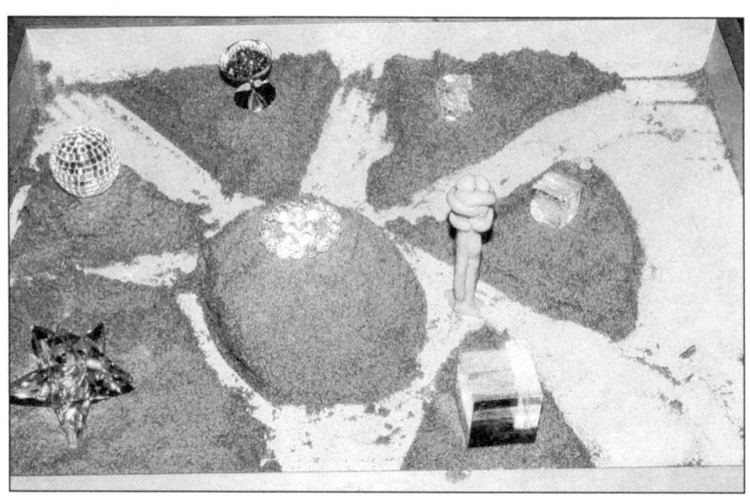

Cary
Tray 7 ~ 2 Weeks Later

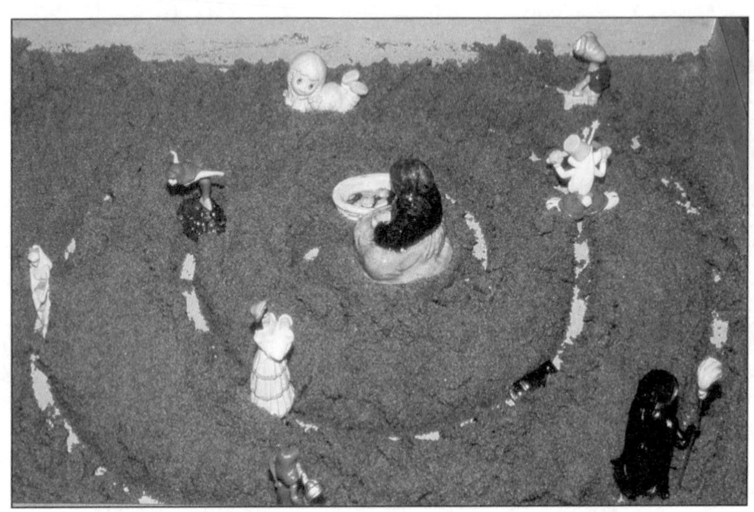

Cary
Tray 8 ~ 2 Weeks Later

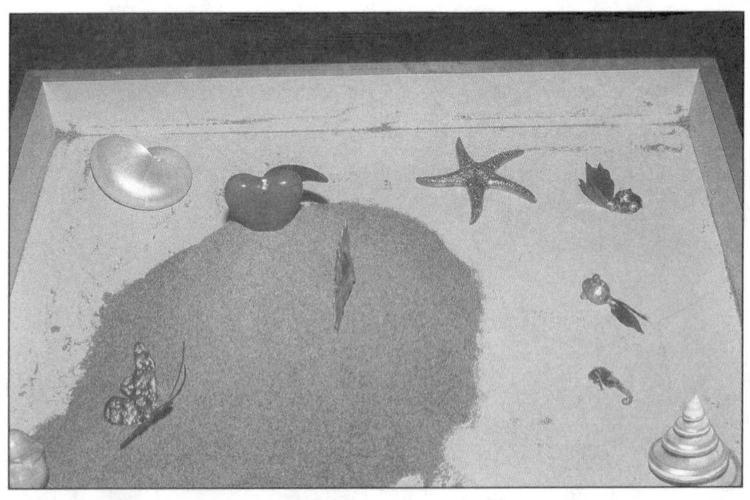

Cary
Tray 15 ~ 6 Months Later

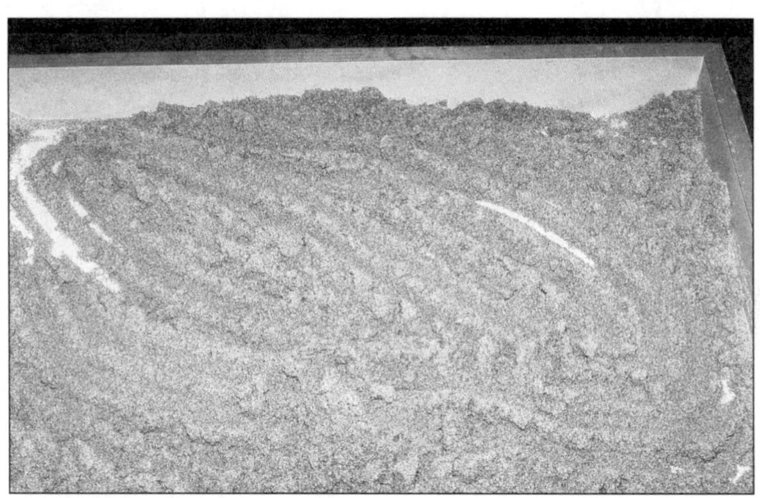

Cary
Tray 21 ~ 10 Months Later

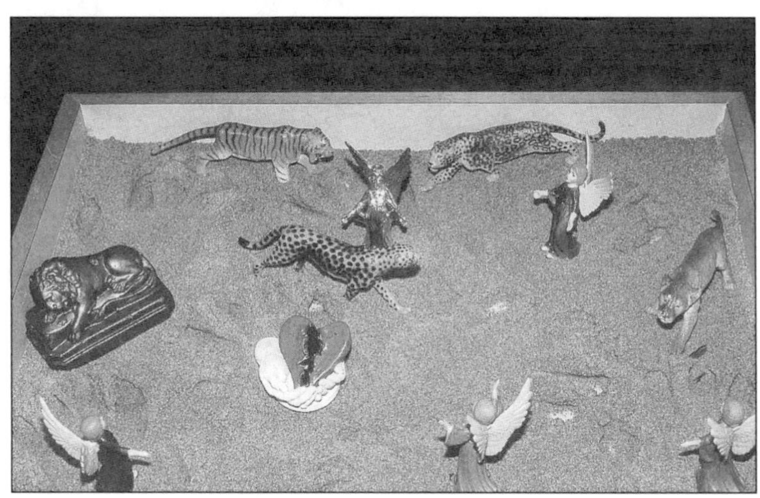

Cary
Tray 23 ~ 6 Weeks Later

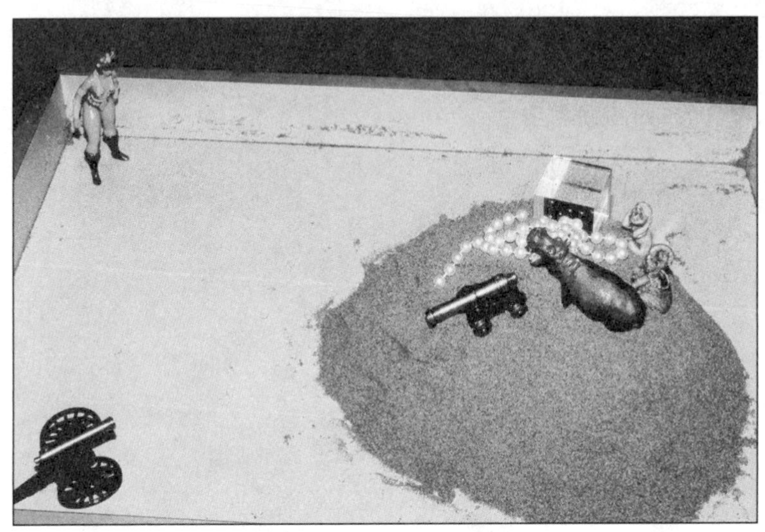

Cary
Tray 24 ~ 2 Months Later

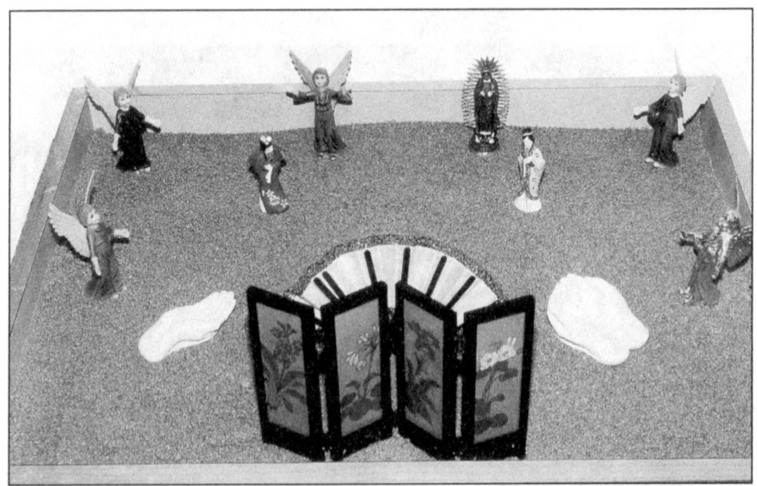

Cary
Tray 41a ~ Final ~ 5 Years Later
7 Years Since Tray 1

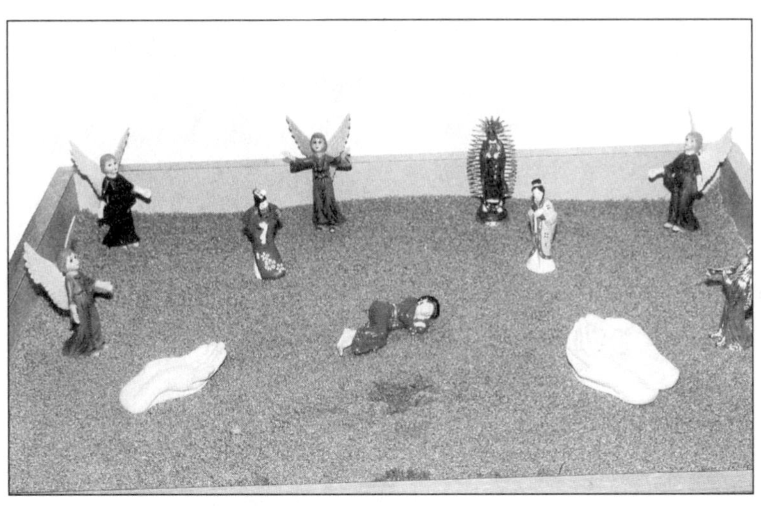

Cary
Tray 41b ~ Detail

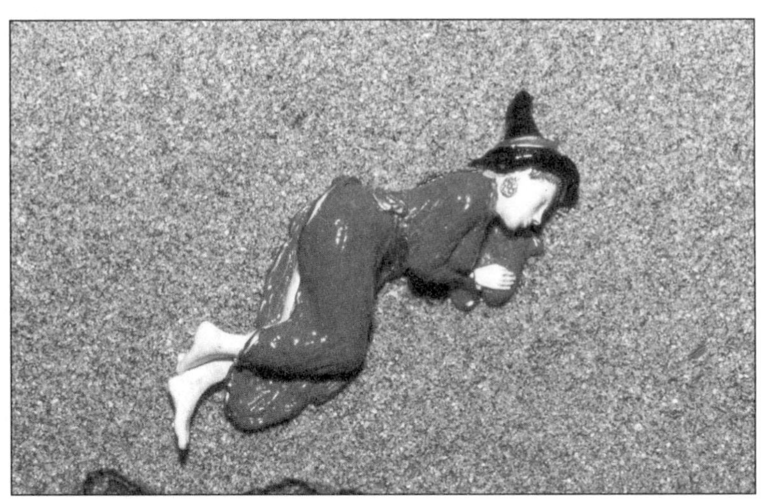

Cary
Tray 41c ~ Detail

Client Profile
CHARLIE

8 year-old boy
Immigrant parents, non-English speaking
Referred by pediatrician for Post Traumatic Stress Disorder
Nightmares and severe anxiety following recent motor vehicle accident

Sandplay	Discussed on Page Number
Tray 1	122
Tray 2	122
Tray 3	122
Tray 4	122
Tray 5	122
Tray 6	122
Tray 7	122

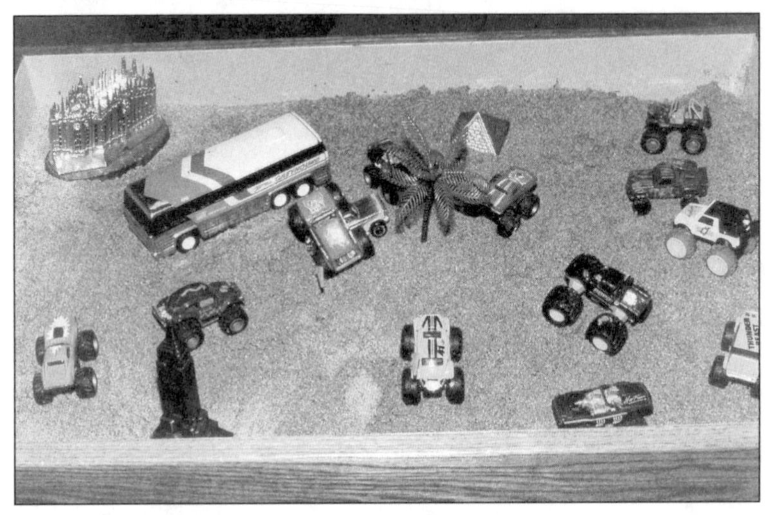

Charlie
Tray 1 ~ Session 1

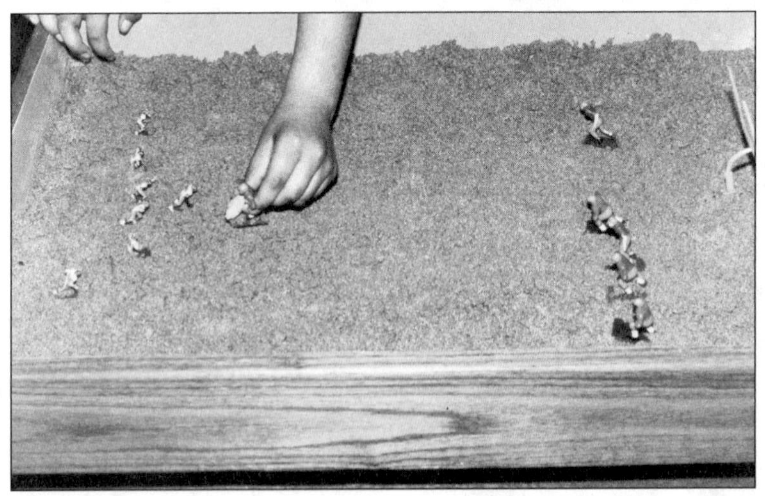

Charlie
Tray 2 ~ 1 Week Later

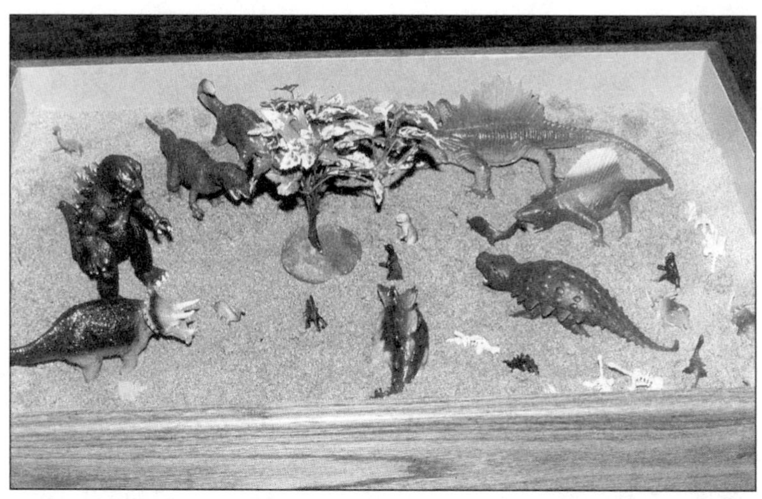

Charlie
Tray 3 ~ 1 Week Later

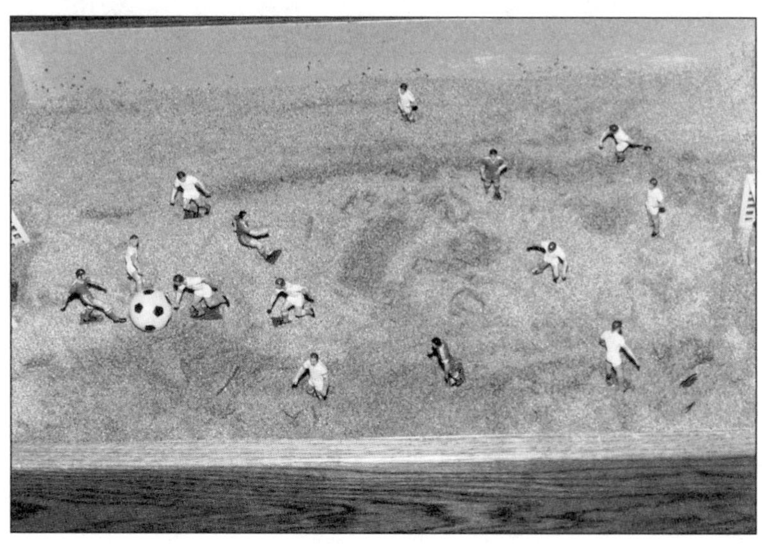

Charlie
Tray 4 ~ 2 Weeks Later

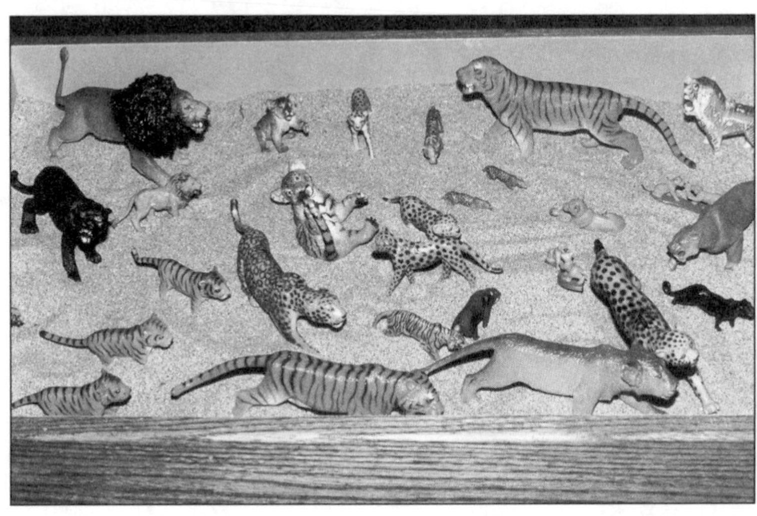

Charlie
Tray 5 ~ 1 Week Later

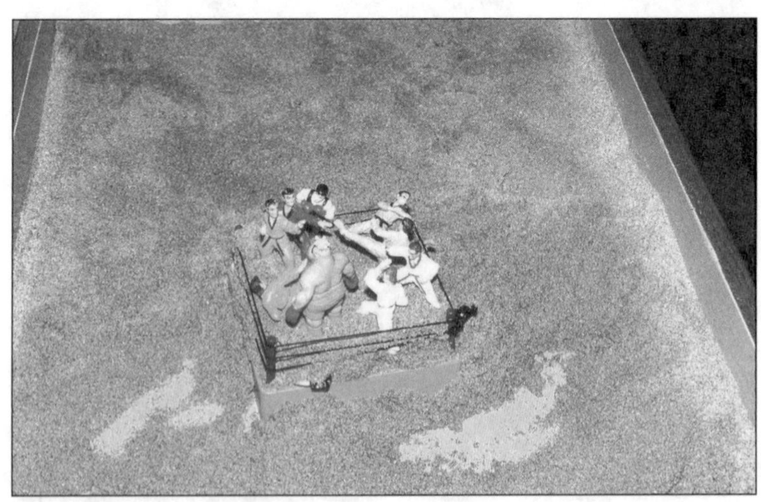

Charlie
Tray 6 ~ 2 Months Later

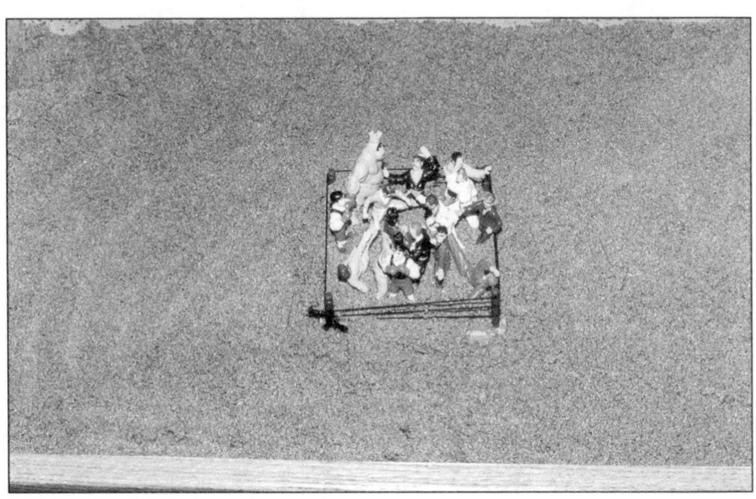

Charlie
Tray 7a ~ Final ~ 1 Month Later
4 Months Since Tray 1

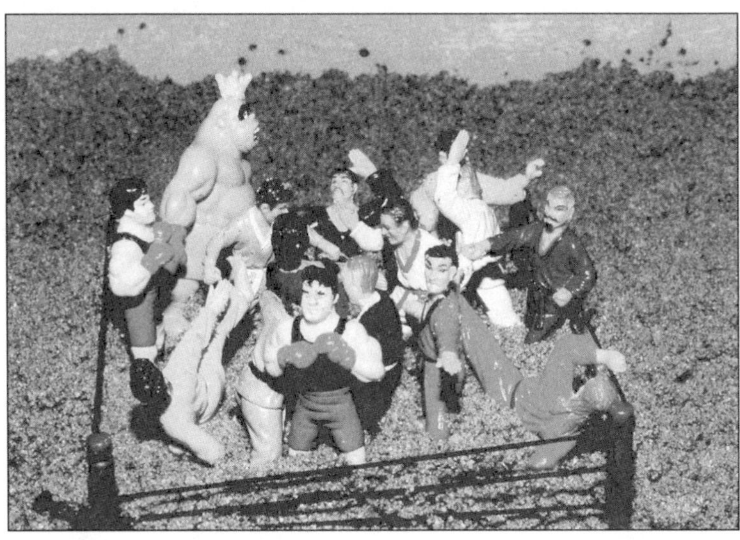

Charlie
Tray 7b ~ Detail

Client Profile
ELIZABETH

Woman, early 40's
Professional career, highly educated
Married, no children
Entered sandplay to, " …*Allow what is inside to appear and be heard* "

Sandplay	Discussed on Page Number
Tray 1	255
Tray 2	173, 259-60
Tray 3	173
Tray 4	
Tray 5	203
Tray 6	121
Tray 7	
Tray 8	
Tray 9	
Tray 10	129-30, 267
Tray 11	196-7, 255

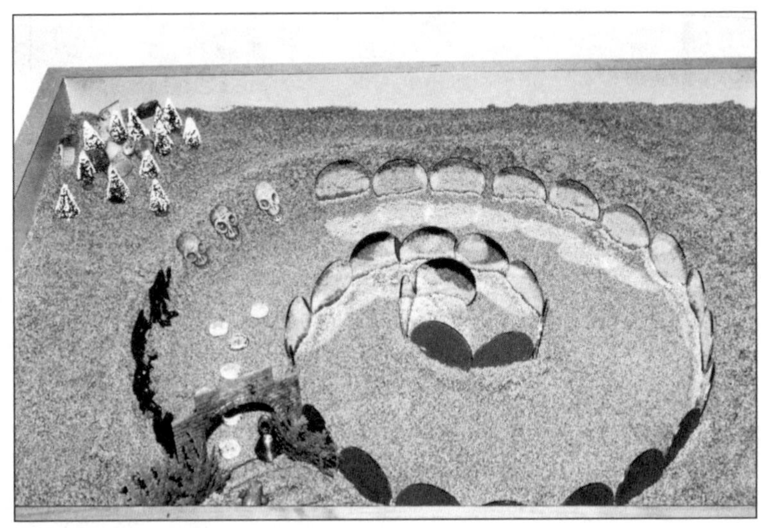

Elizabeth
Tray 1a ~ Session 1

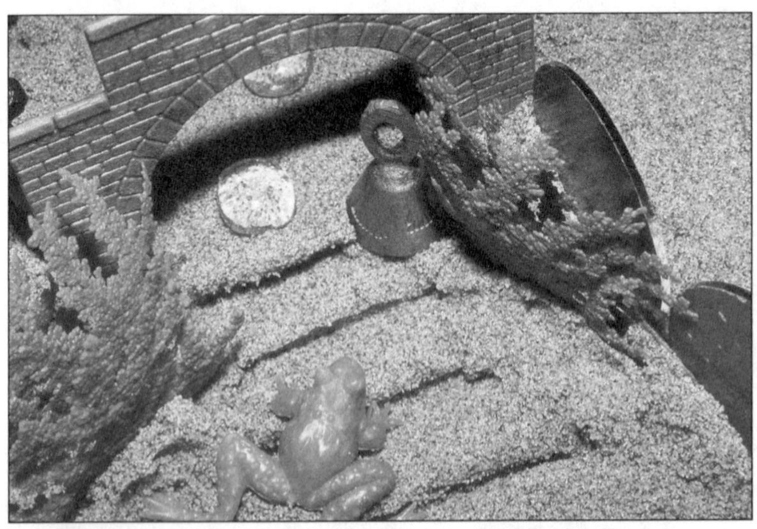

Elizabeth
Tray 1b ~ Detail

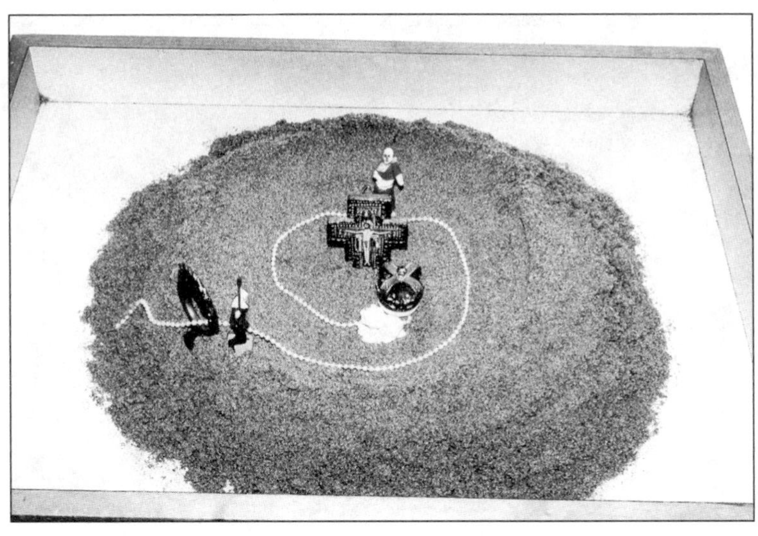

Elizabeth
Tray 2 ~ 1 Week Later

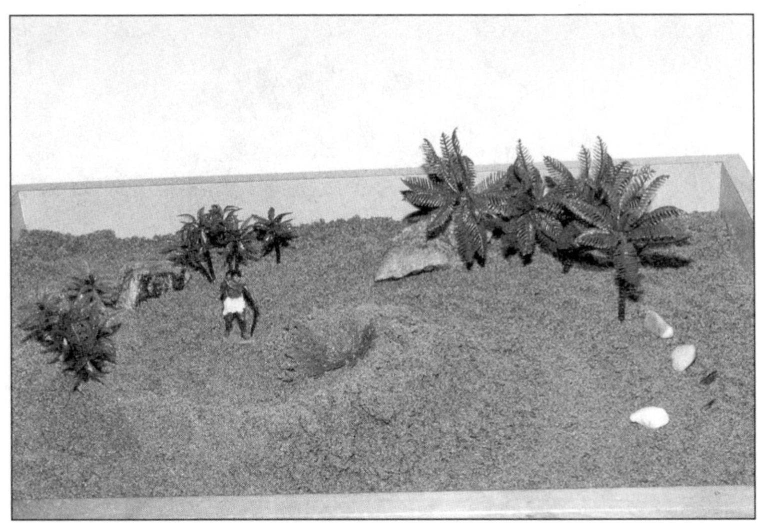

Elizabeth
Tray 3 ~ 1 Month Later

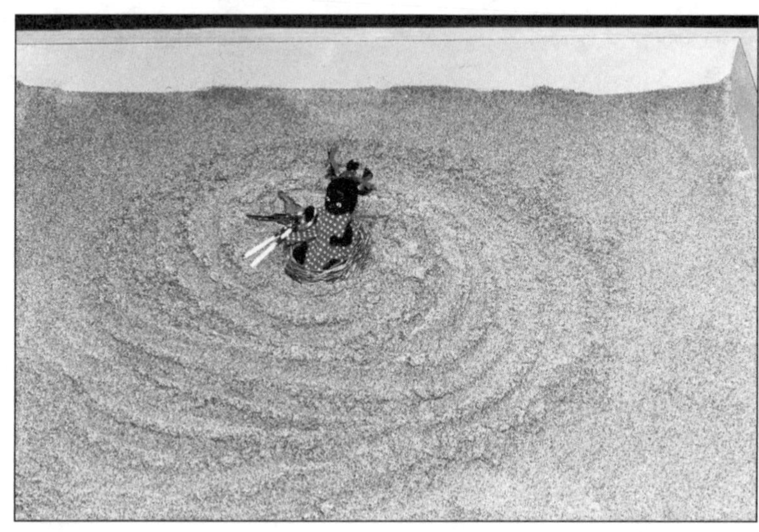

Elizabeth
Tray 4 ~ 2 Weeks Later

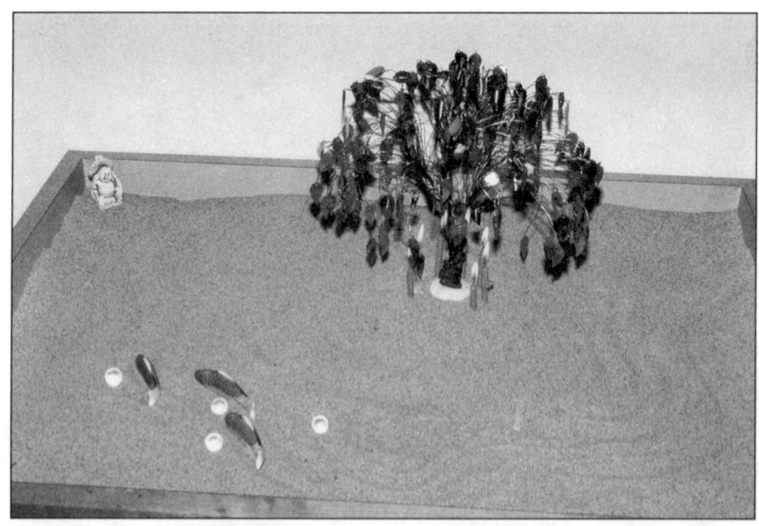

Elizabeth
Tray 5 ~ 2 Weeks Later

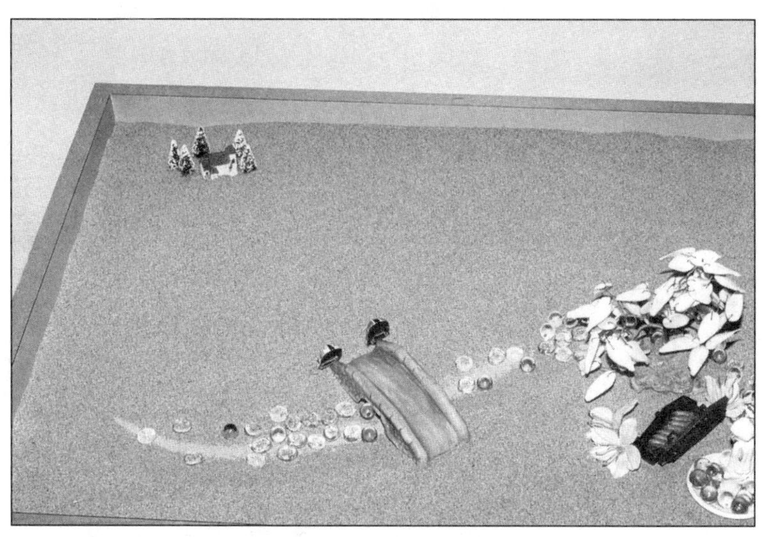

Elizabeth
Tray 6a ~ 2 Weeks Later

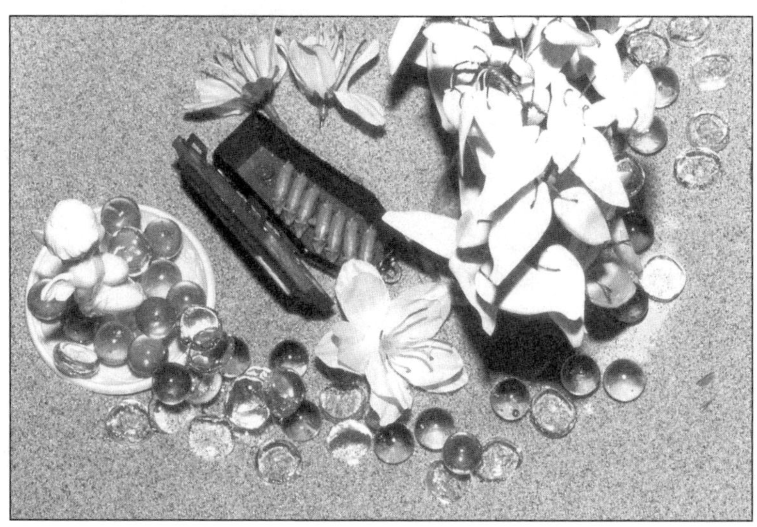

Elizabeth
Tray 6b ~ Detail

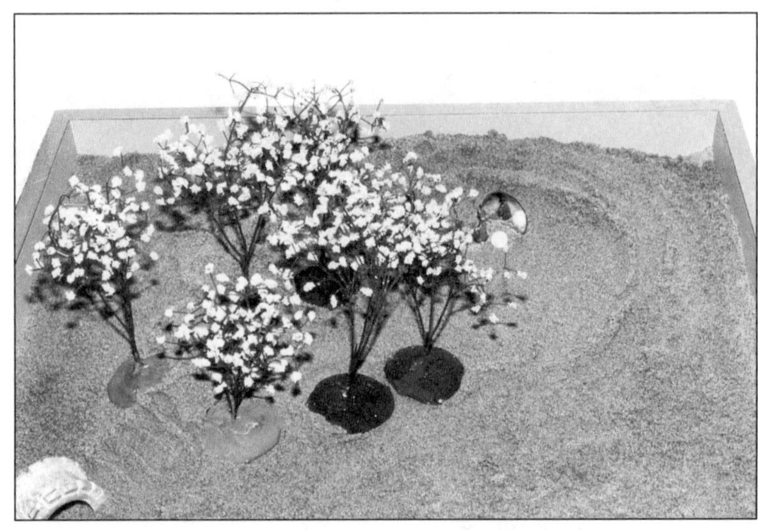

Elizabeth
Tray 7 ~ 5 Months Later

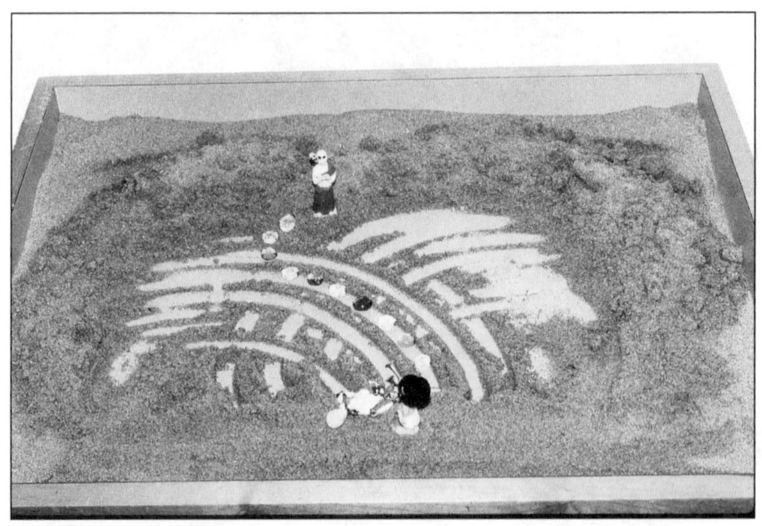

Elizabeth
Tray 8 ~ 1 Month Later

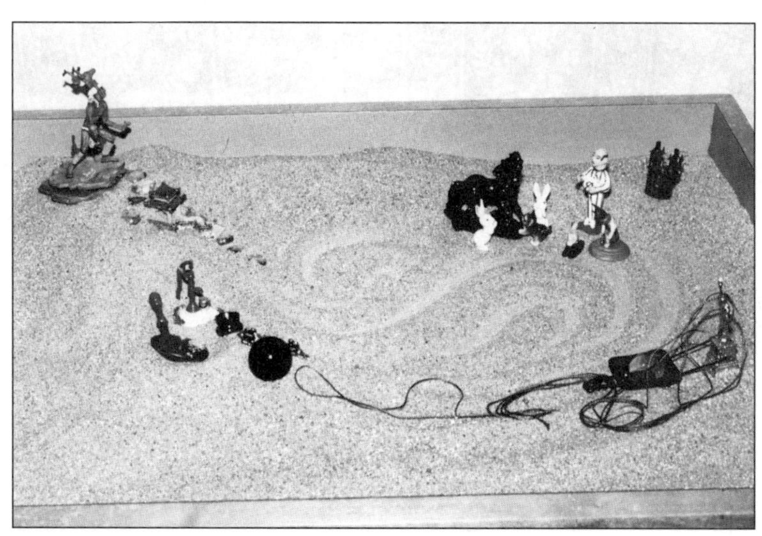

Elizabeth
Tray 9 ~ 7 Years Later

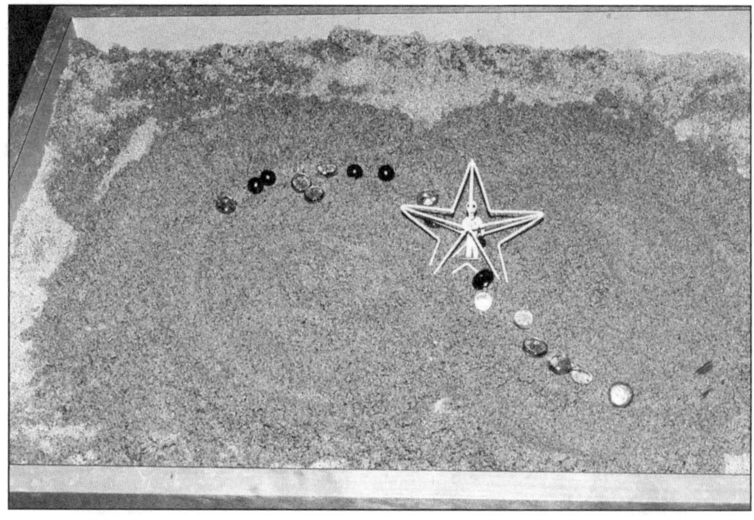

Elizabeth
Tray 10 ~ 1 Year Later

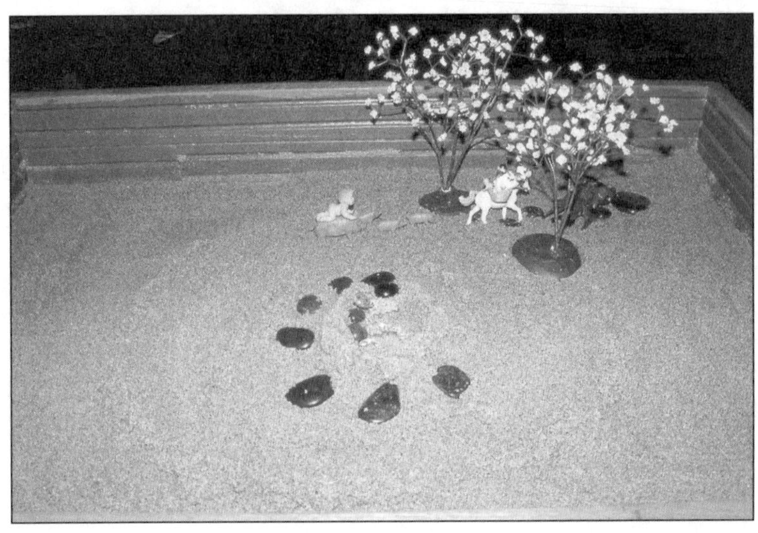

Elizabeth
Tray 11a ~ Final ~ 1 Year 4 Months Later

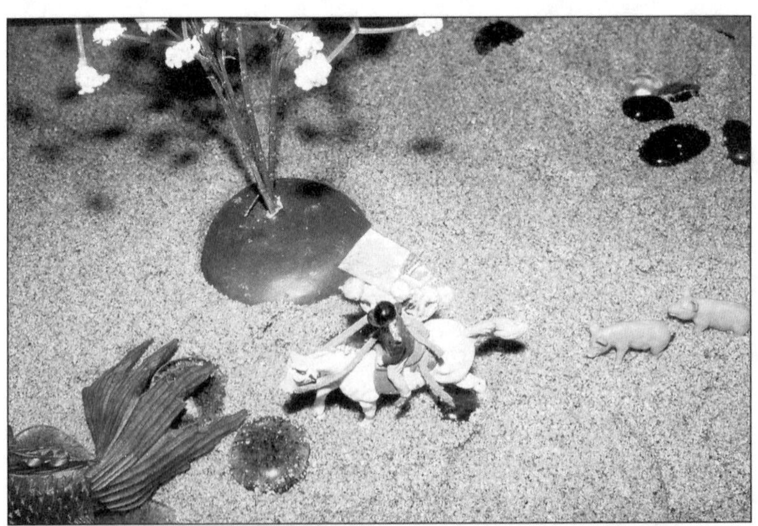

Elizabeth
Tray 11b ~ Detail

Elizabeth
Trays 11a - 11b

ELIZABETH

Client Profile

HAROLD

Male, 60's
Entered therapy at his wife's direction
Violent angry outbursts
Third marriage, several children
Professional career, entered at direction of second wife
Mother still living; father unknown
Complains of his mother controlling him

Sandplay	Discussed on Page Number
Tray 1	65
Tray 2	65
Tray 3	65
Tray 4	65
Tray 5	65-6
Tray 6	372-3
Tray 7	
Tray 8	86

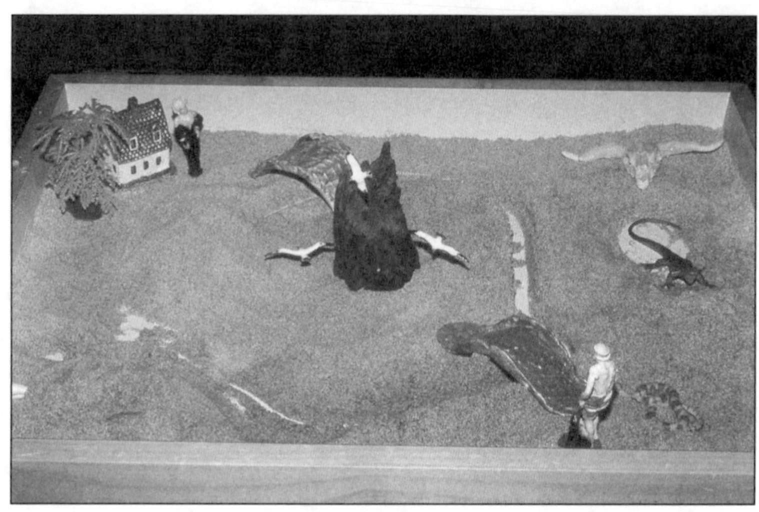

Harold
Tray 1 ~ Many Months into Treatment

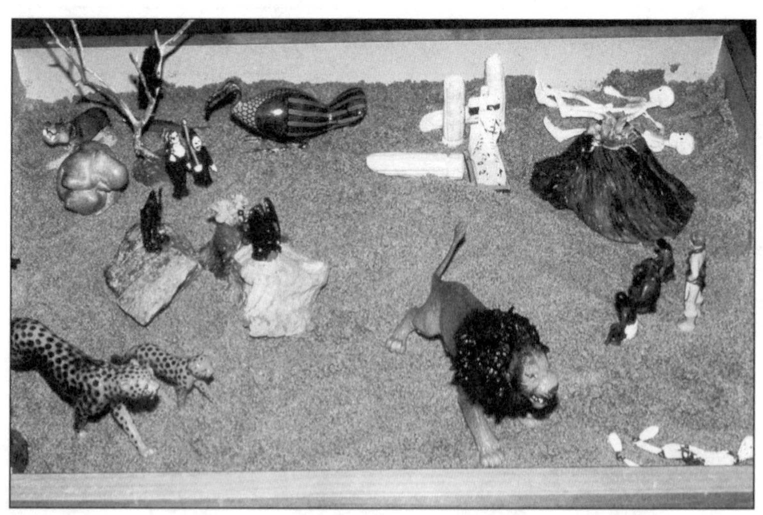

Harold
Tray 2 ~ 1 Week Later

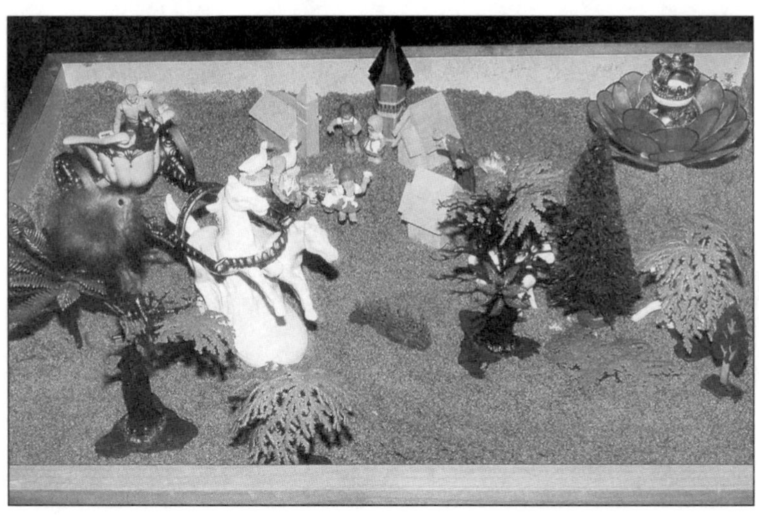

Harold
Tray 3 ~ 2 Weeks Later

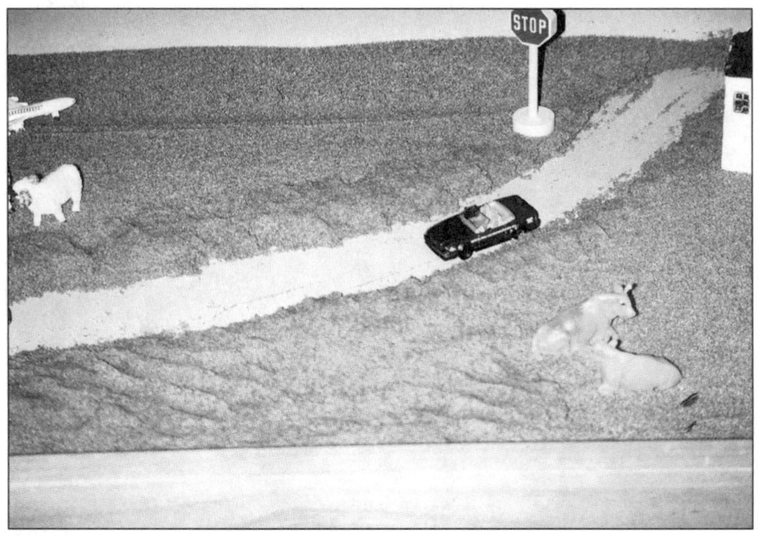

Harold
Tray 4 ~ 1 Month Later

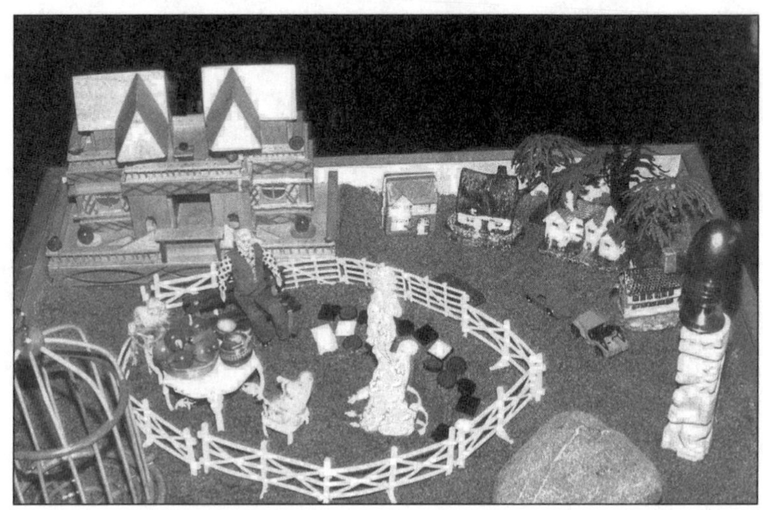

Harold
Tray 5 ~ 3 Weeks Later

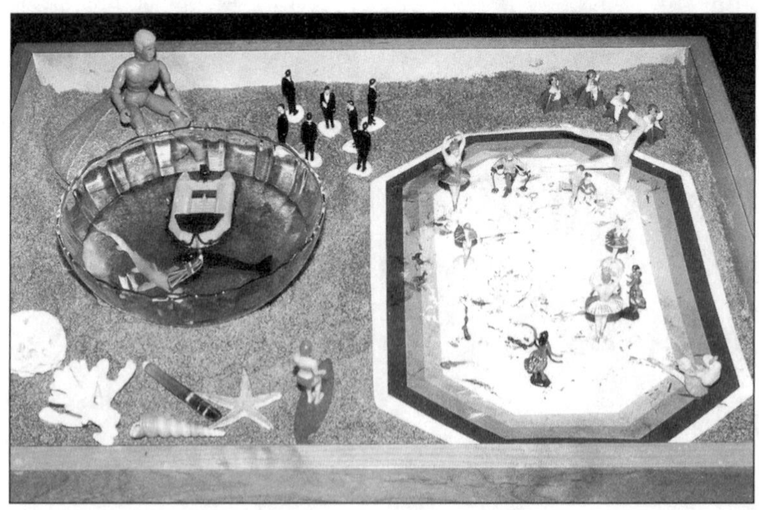

Harold
Tray 6 ~ 1 Month Later

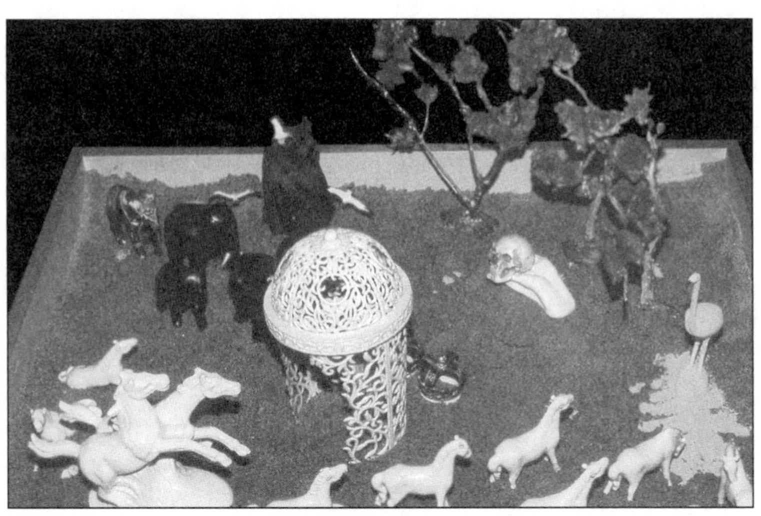

Harold
Tray 7 ~ 3 Months Later

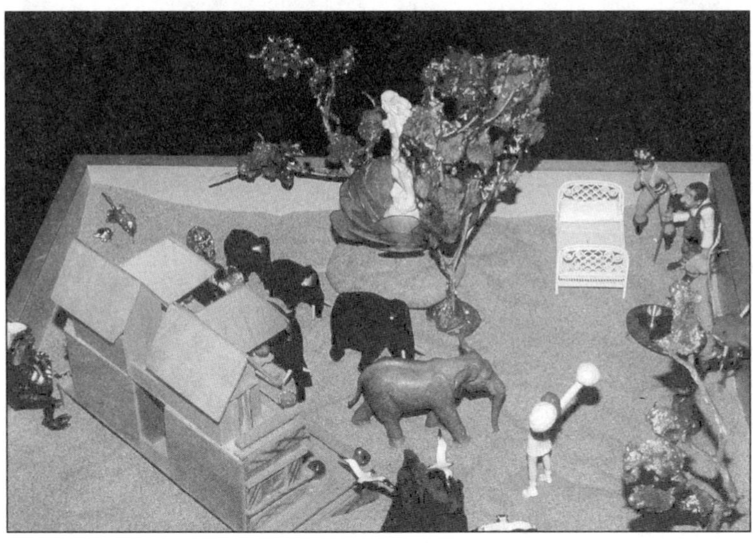

Harold
Tray 8 ~ Final ~ 5 Months Later
1 Year Since Tray 1

Client Profile
ISAAC

11 year-old boy
Entered therapy to address trauma and loss resulting from the recent murder of his favorite uncle by police, when being pursued for arrest

Sandplay	Discussed on Page Number
Tray 1	
Tray 6	
Tray 7	
Tray 8	
Tray 23	256
Tray 24	

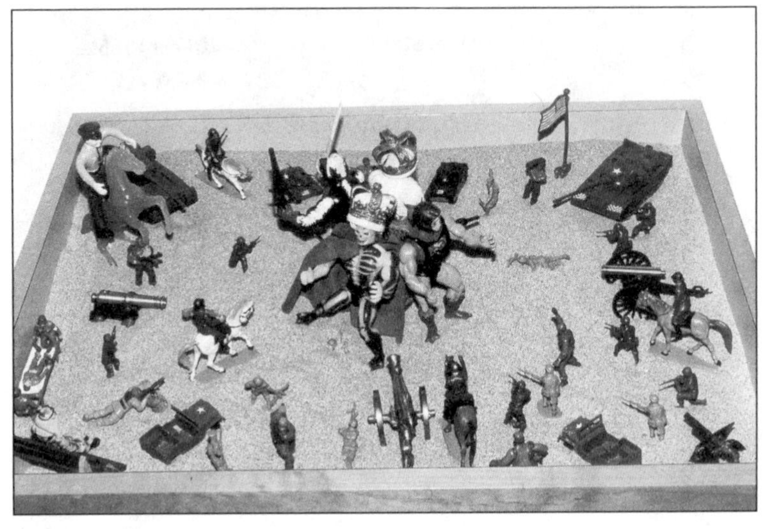

Isaac
Tray 1 ~ Session 1

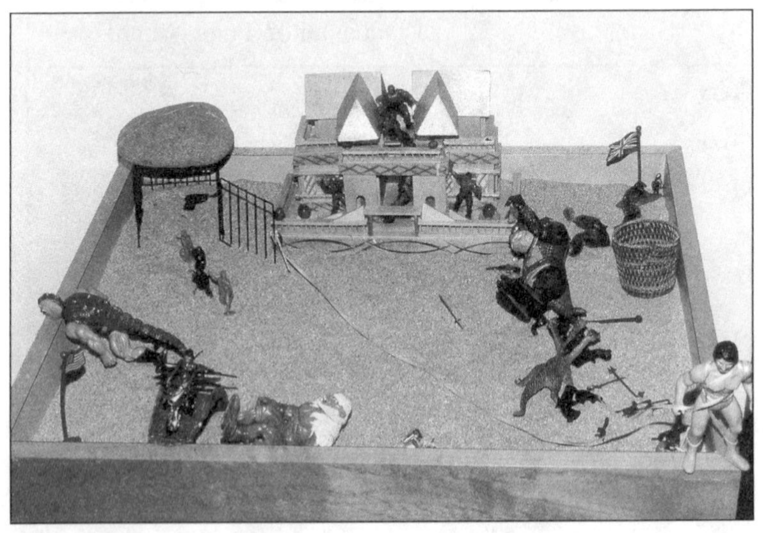

Isaac
Tray 6 ~ 4 Months 2 Weeks Later

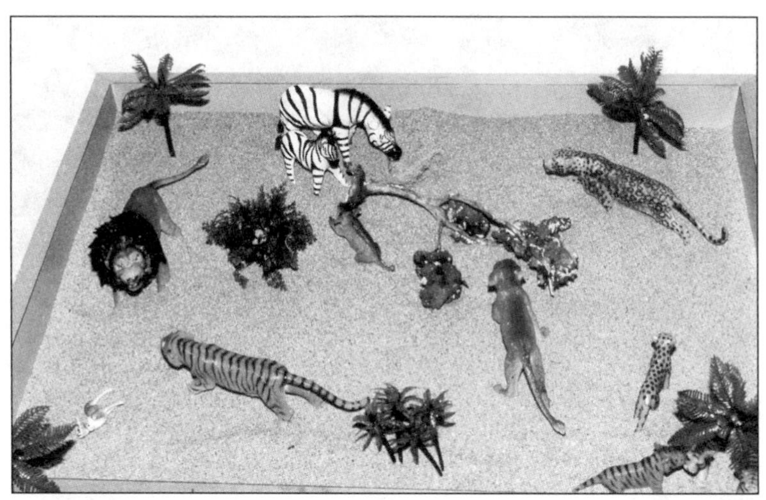

Isaac
Tray 7 ~ 4 Weeks Later

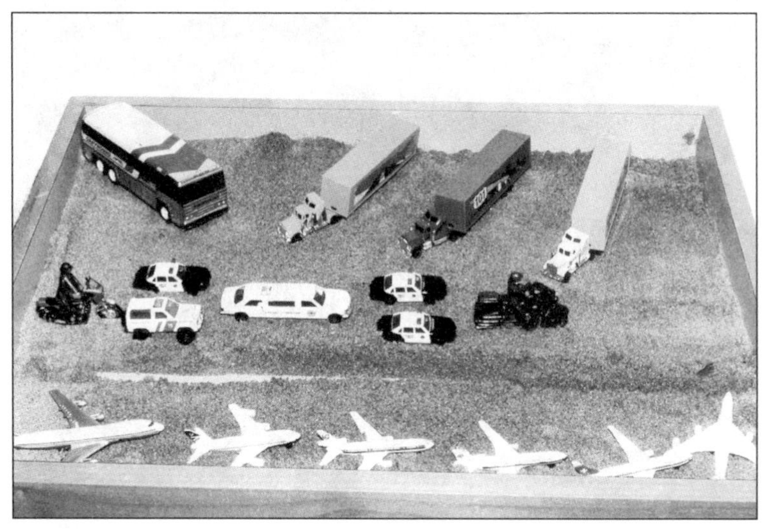

Isaac
Tray 8 ~ Same Session

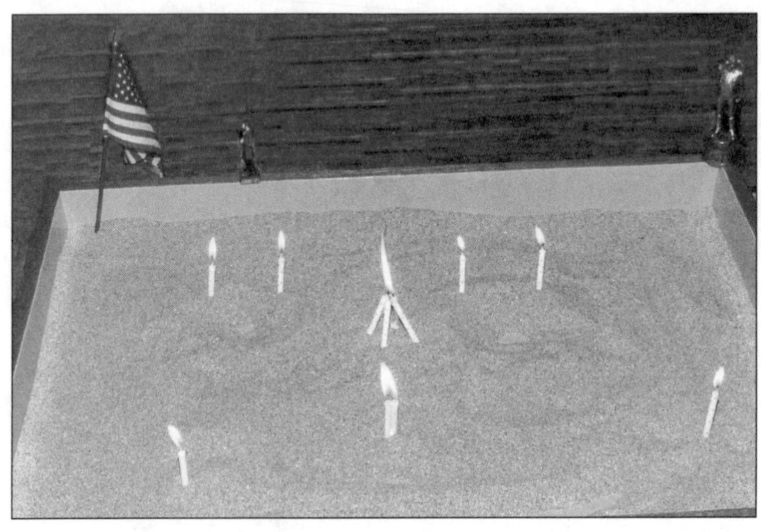

Isaac
Tray 23 ~ 1 Year 5 Months Later

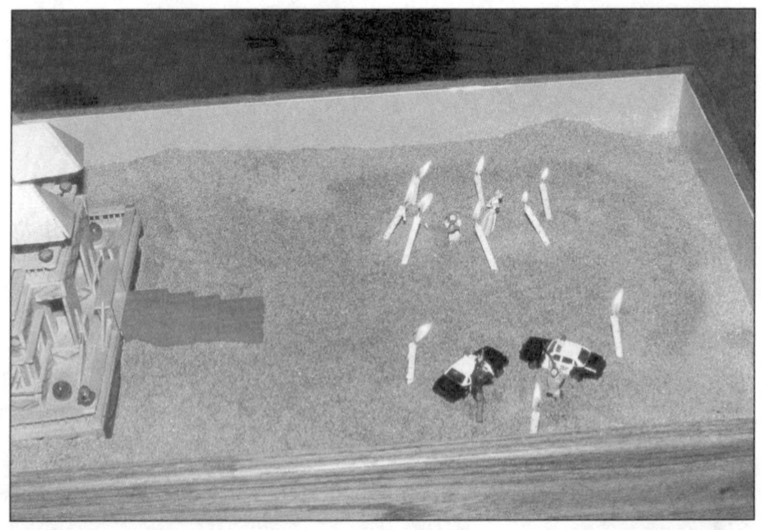

Isaac
Tray 24a ~ Final ~ 6 Weeks Later
2 Years Since Tray 1

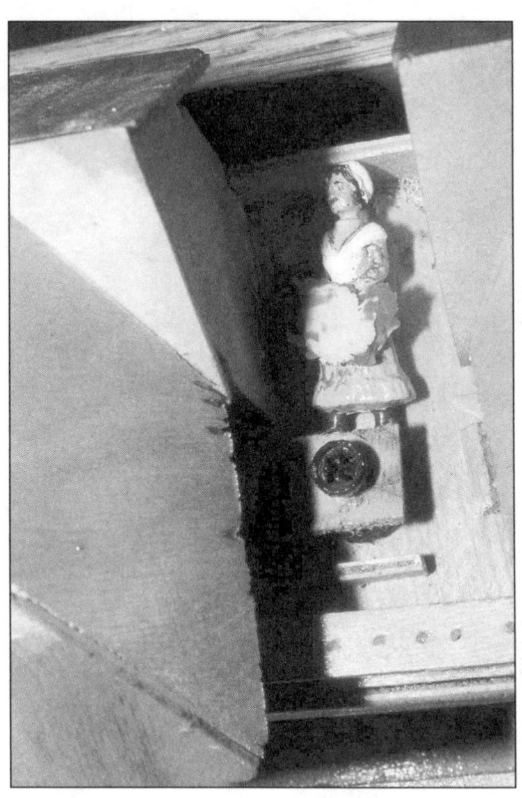

Isaac
Tray 24b ~
Detail

Client Profile

IVY

Nine year-old girl
Oldest of three children
New baby boy in family
Brought into therapy by her mother, who had concerns about her daughter's constant fighting with her seven year-old brother
On-going parental struggle
Father, alcoholic - In and out of the home

Sandplay	Discussed on Page Number
Tray 1	267, 367
Tray 2	67
Tray 3	
Tray 4	68, 176, 225-6
Tray 5	176, 225-6
Tray 6	
Tray 7	
Tray 8	159
Tray 9	81
Tray 10	77
Tray 11	77-8
Tray 12	77-8
Tray 13	85

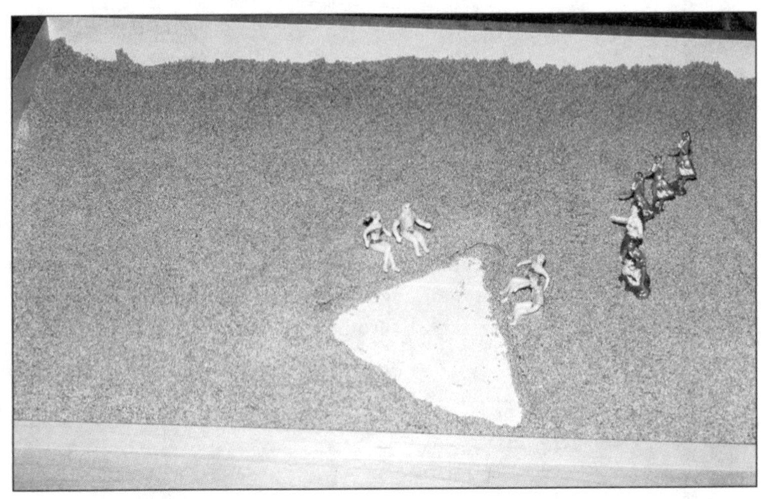

Ivy
Tray 1 ~ Session 1

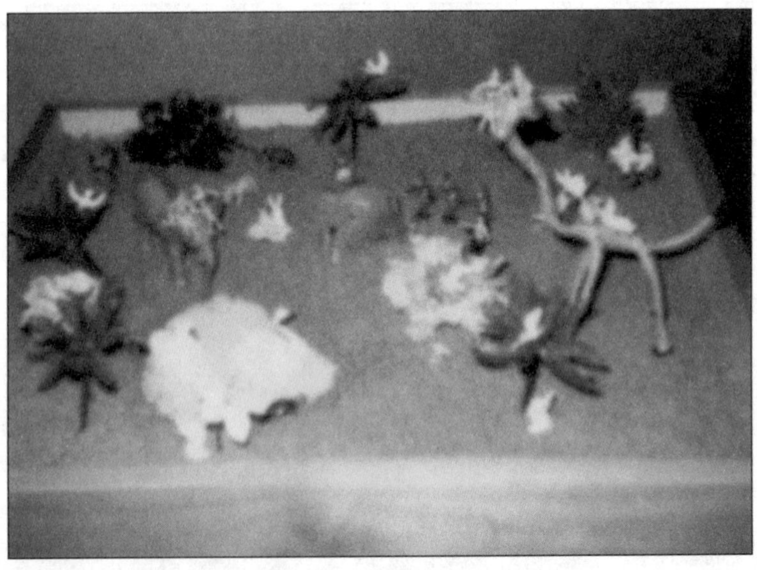

Ivy
Tray 2 ~ 1 Week Later

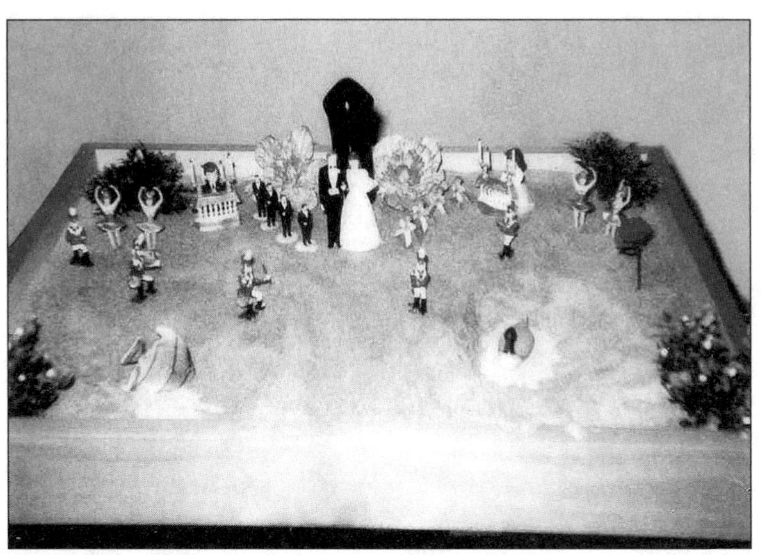

Ivy
Tray 3 ~ 1 Week Later

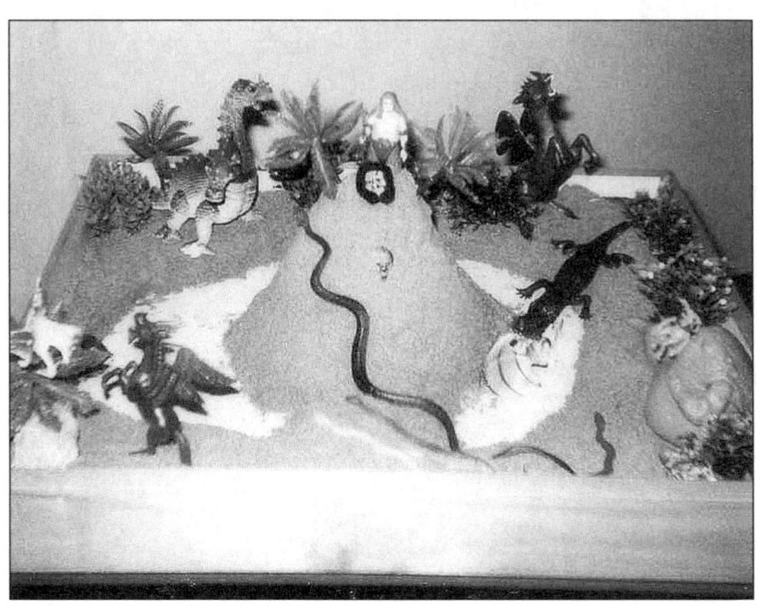

Ivy
Tray 4 ~ 2 Weeks Later

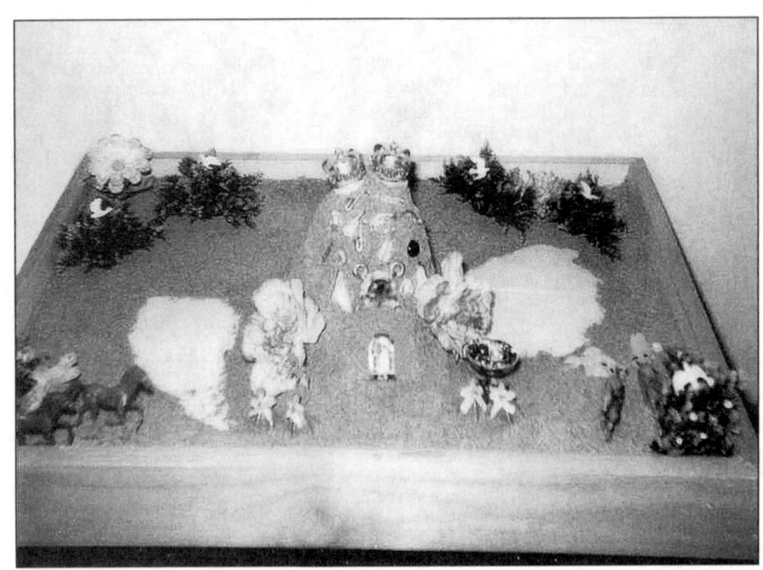

Ivy
Tray 5 ~ 1 Week Later

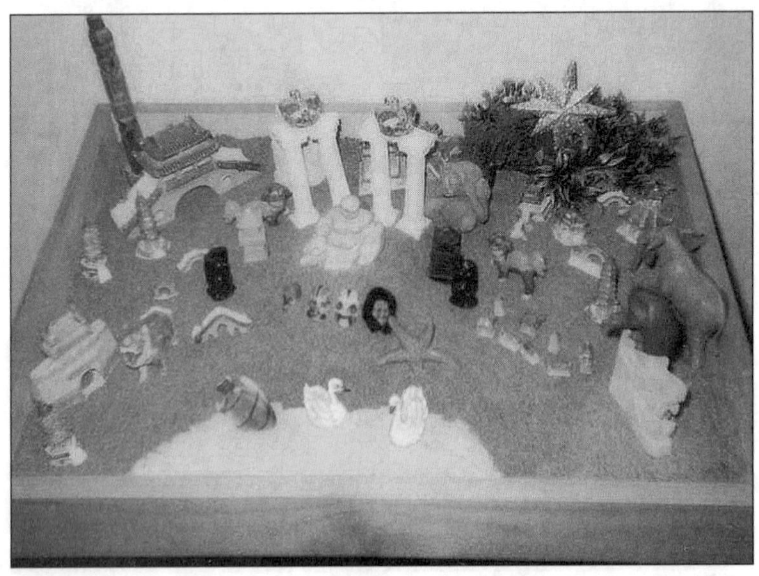

Ivy
Tray 6 ~ 4 Weeks Later

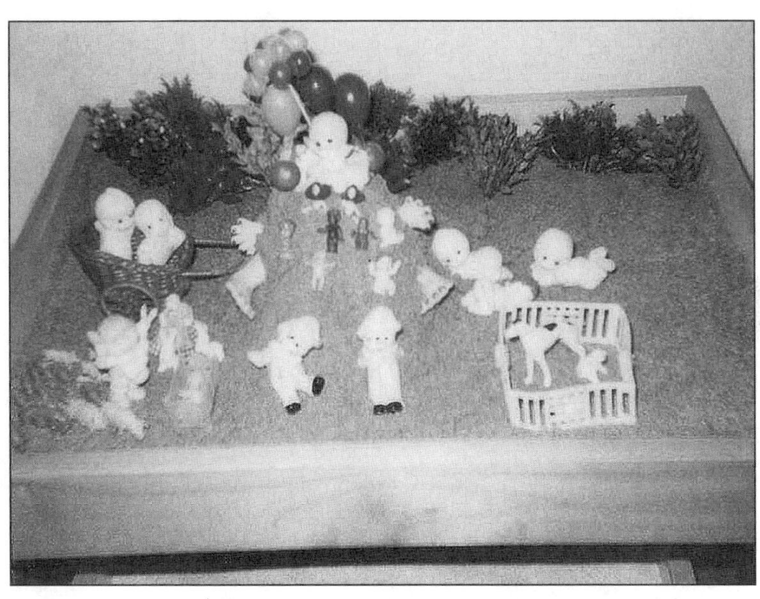

Ivy
Tray 7 ~ 1 Week Later

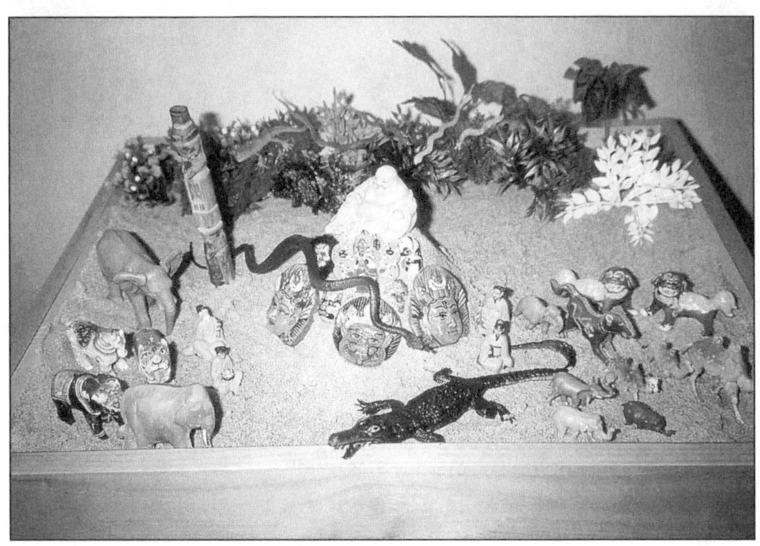

Ivy
Tray 8~ 2 Weeks Later

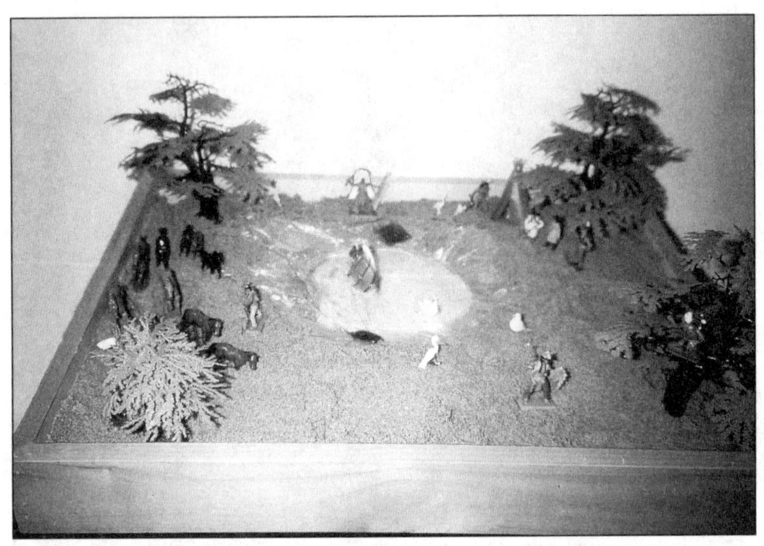

Ivy
Tray 9 ~ 5 Weeks Later

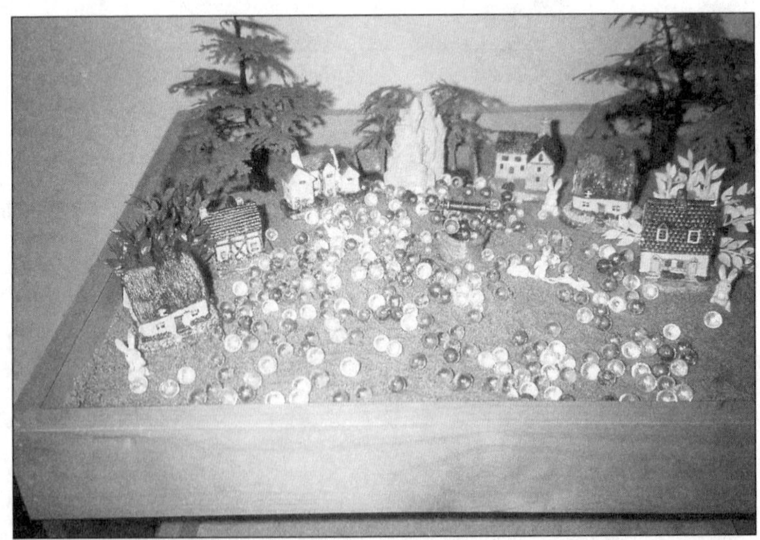

Ivy
Tray 10 ~ 1 Week Later

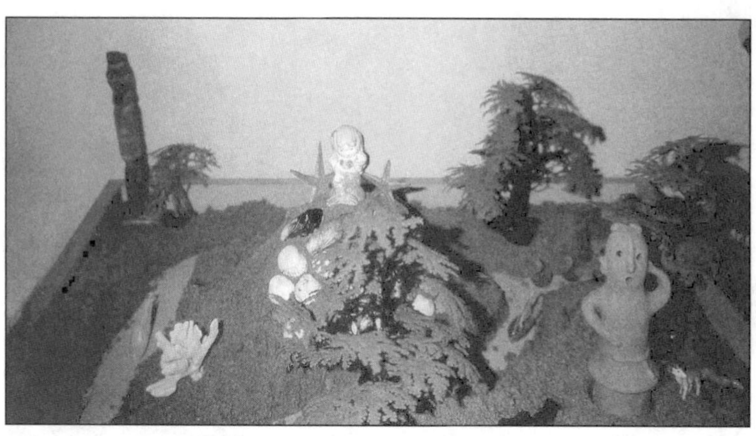

Ivy
Tray 11 ~ 2 Weeks Later

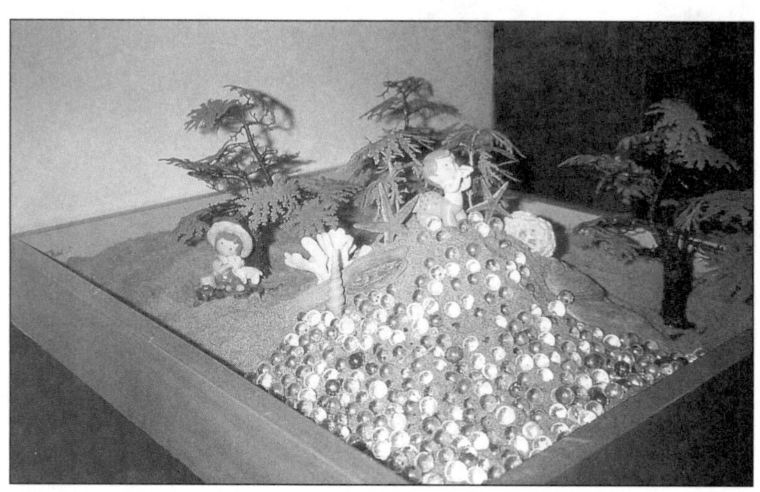

Ivy
Tray 12 ~ 1 Month Later

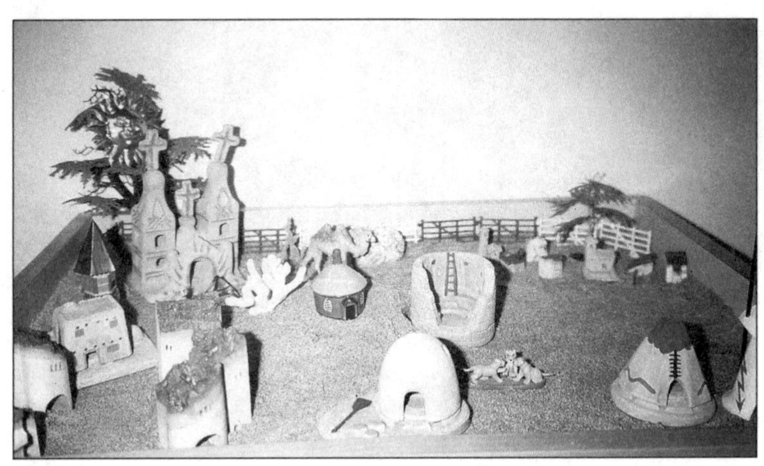

Ivy
Tray 13a ~ Final ~ 7 Months Later
1 Year 1 Month Since Tray 1

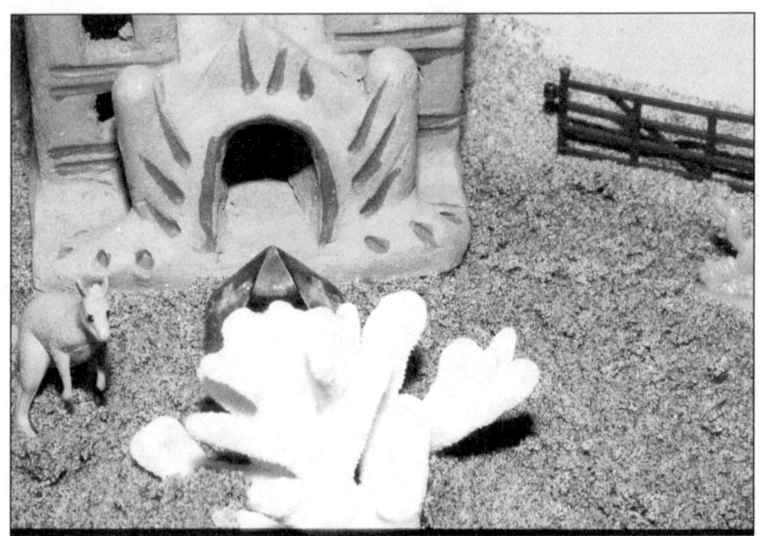

Ivy
Tray 13b ~ Detail

Client Profile
JASON

Male, 40's
Married, no children
Entered therapy to address chronic work dissatisfaction and health issues
Studied for the ministry
Works in management

Sandplay	Discussed on Page Number
Tray 1	
Tray 2	
Tray 19	246
Tray 20	246
Tray 21	246

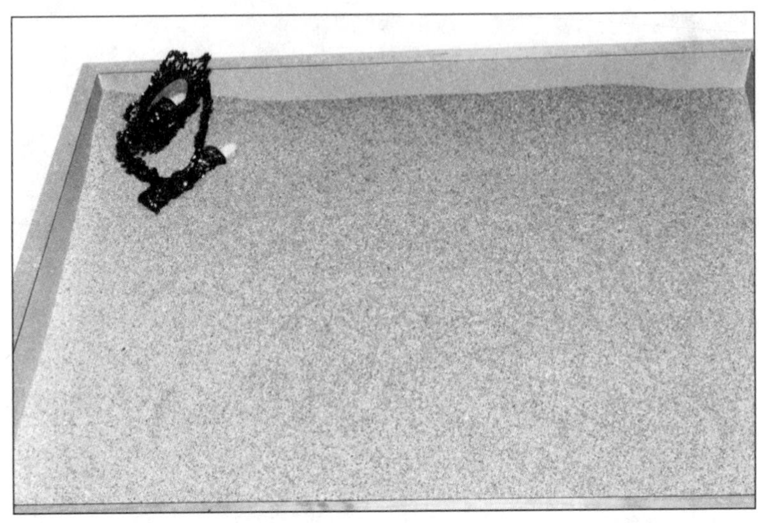

Jason
Tray 1 ~ Several Weeks into Treatment

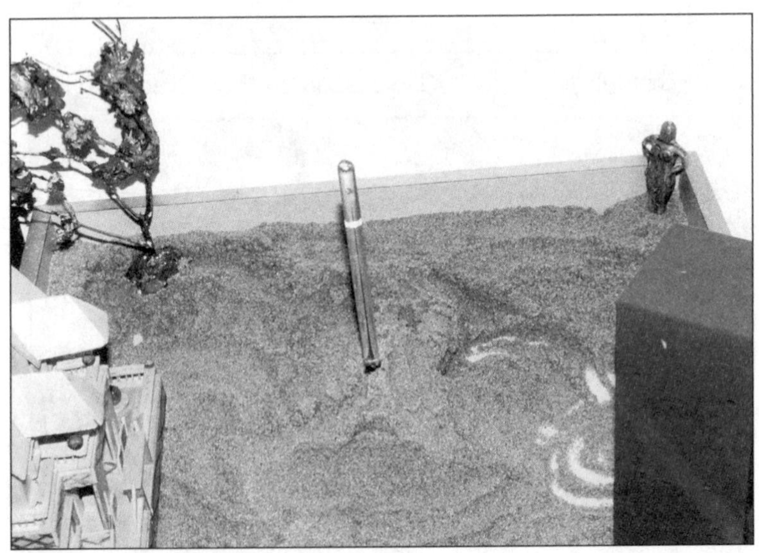

Jason
Tray 2~ Same Session

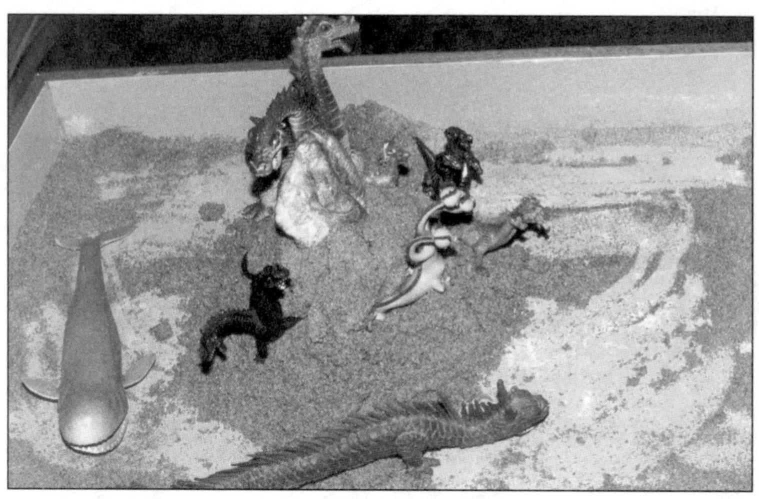

Jason
Tray 19 ~ 3 Years Later

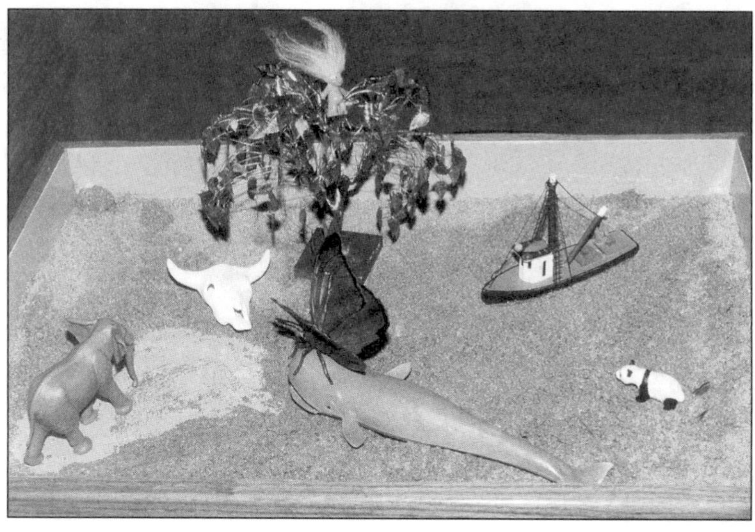

Jason
Tray 20 ~ 3 Weeks Later

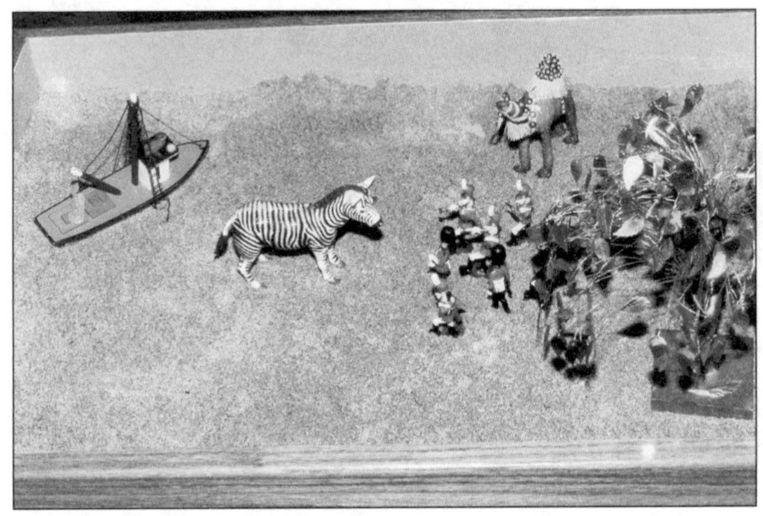

Jason
Tray 21 ~ Final ~ 2 Weeks Later
3 Years 1 Month Since Tray 1

Client Profile

KAILEIGH

Girl, 7 ½ years old
Second of four children in single parent (mother) family
Financial stress in family
Difficulty in school
Acting out, fighting with siblings

Sandplay	Discussed on Page Number
Tray 1	255, 273-5
Tray 2	255, 273-5
Tray 3	255
Tray 4	255
Tray 5	254-5
Tray 6	275
Tray 7	

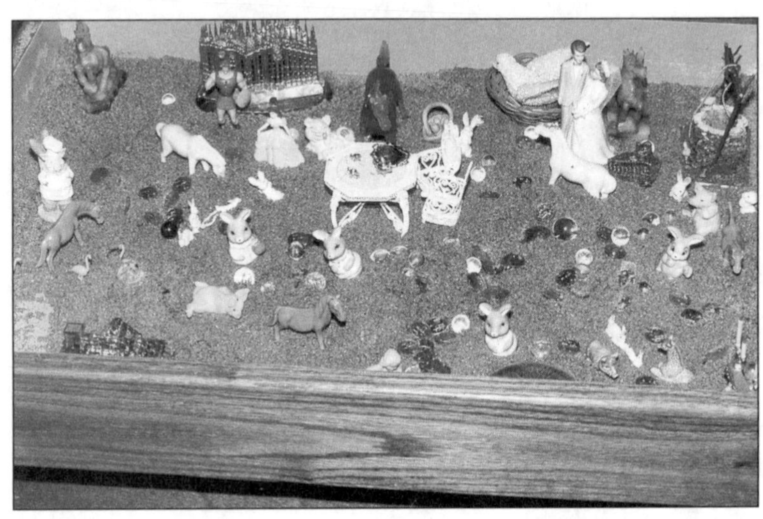

Kaileigh
Tray 1 ~ Session 1

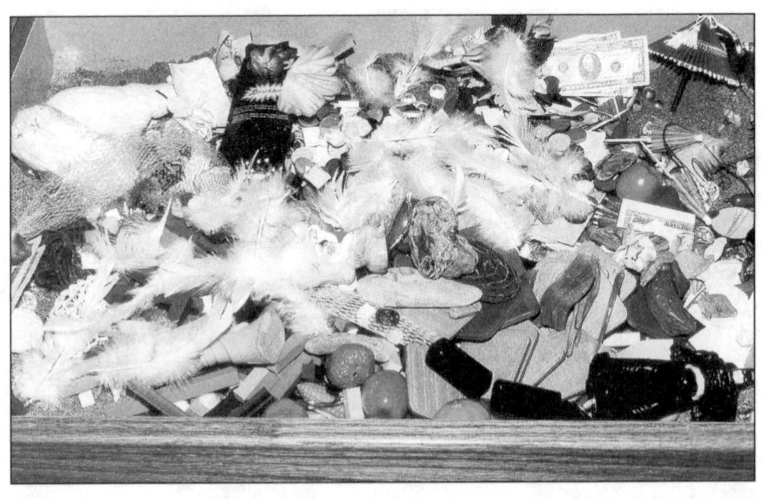

Kaileigh
Tray 2 ~ 3 Weeks Later

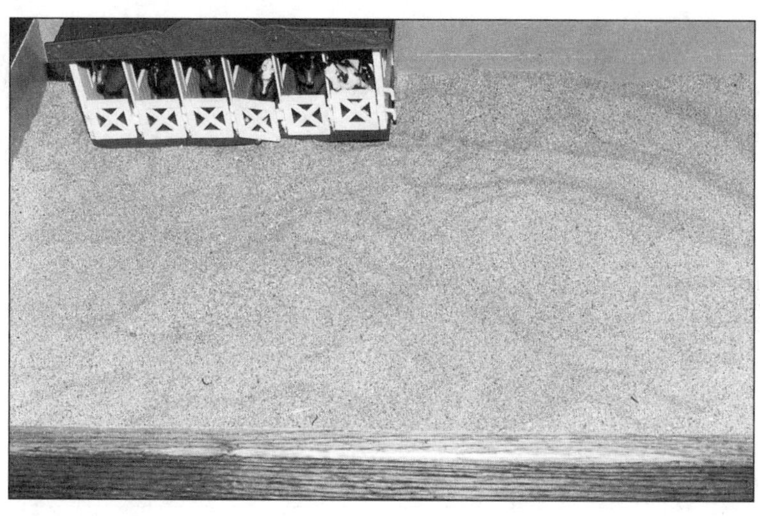

Kaileigh
Tray 3 ~ 2 Weeks Later

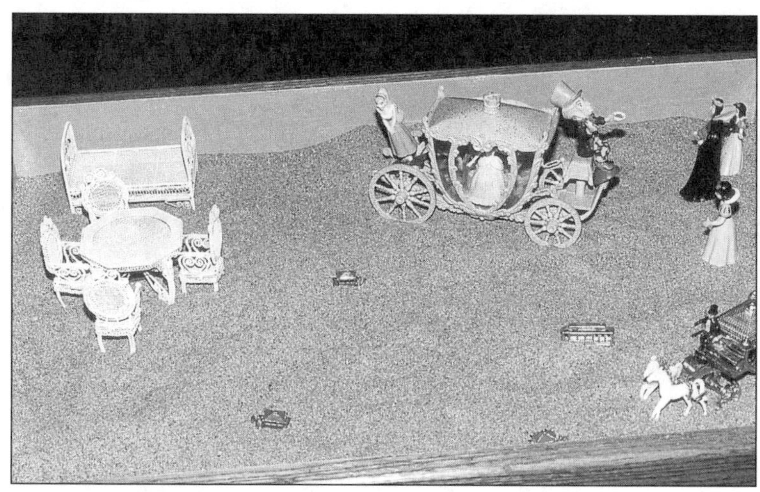

Kaileigh
Tray 4 ~ 4 Months Later

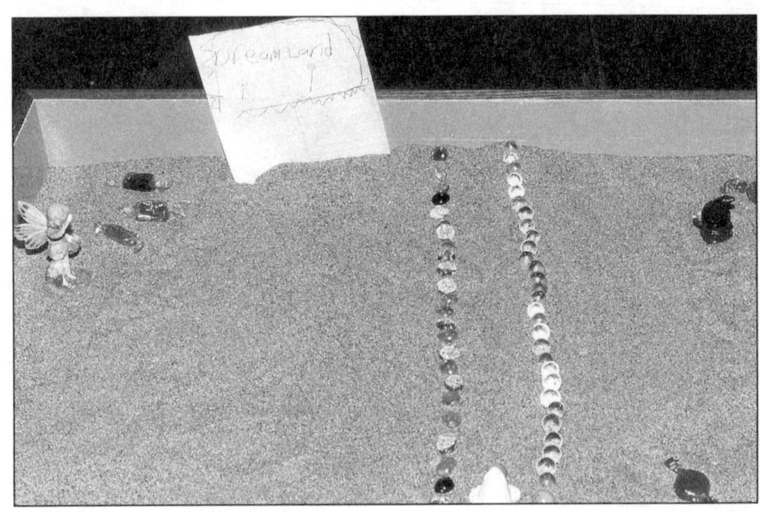

Kaileigh
Tray 5 ~ Same Session

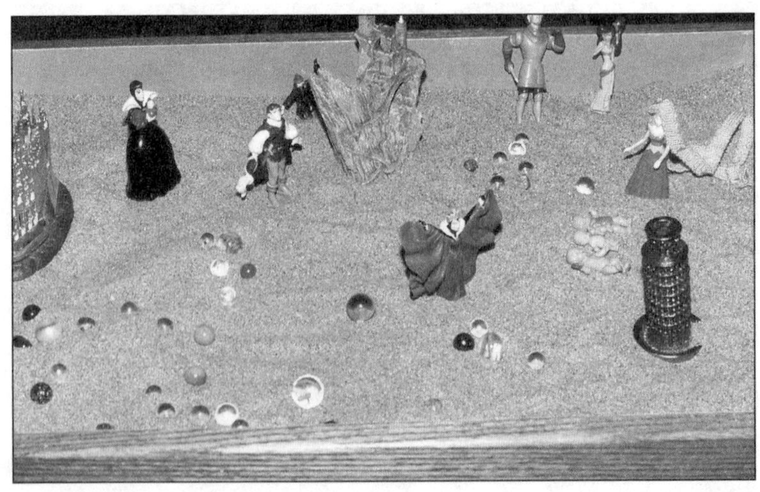

Kaileigh
Tray 6 ~ 4 Months Later

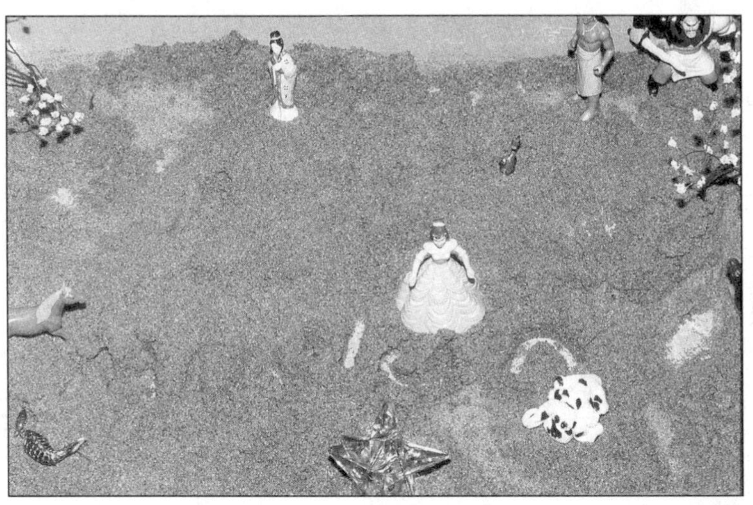

Kaileigh
Tray 7 ~ Final ~ 1 Month Later
10 Months Since Tray 1

Client Profile
LARRY

Boy, age 5
Brought to treatment by foster-adopt Mom and Dad for treatment of trauma
Third child of four siblings removed from family of origin
Extensive history of severe neglect and sexual abuse by birth parents
Possible fetal alcohol and/or drug impairment

Sandplay	Discussed on Page Number
Tray 1	165
Tray 2	165
Tray 3	165
Tray4	
Tray 5	165
Tray 7	
Tray 8	

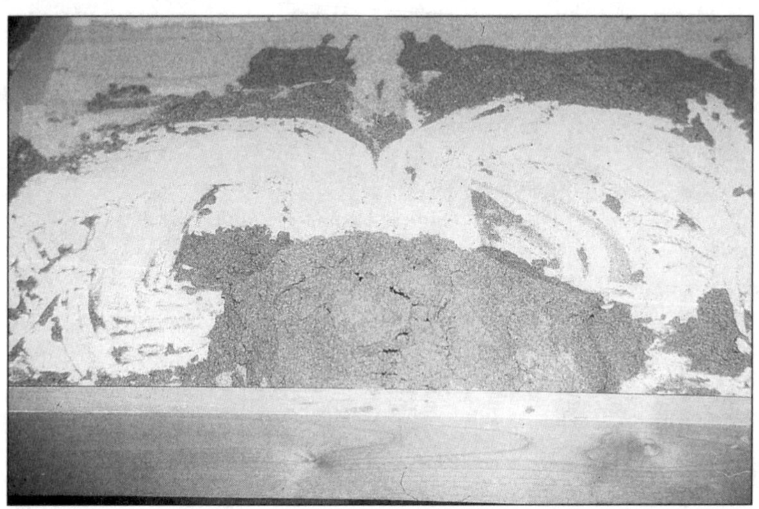

Larry
Tray 1 ~ 2 Months into Treatment

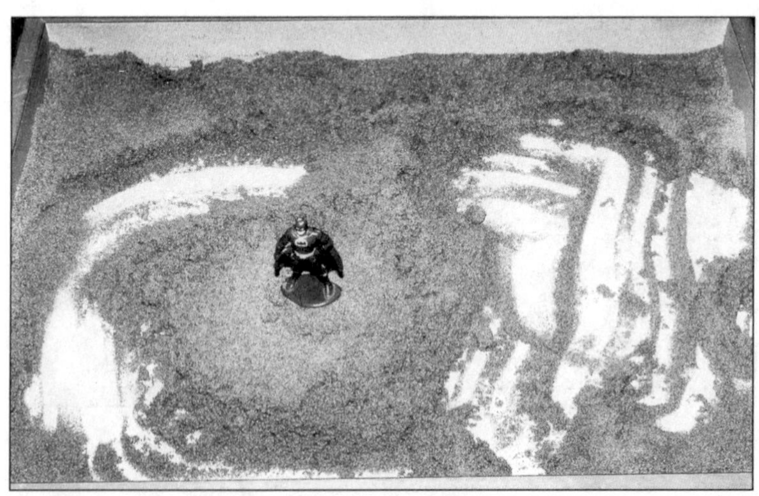

Larry
Tray 2 ~ 5 Months Later

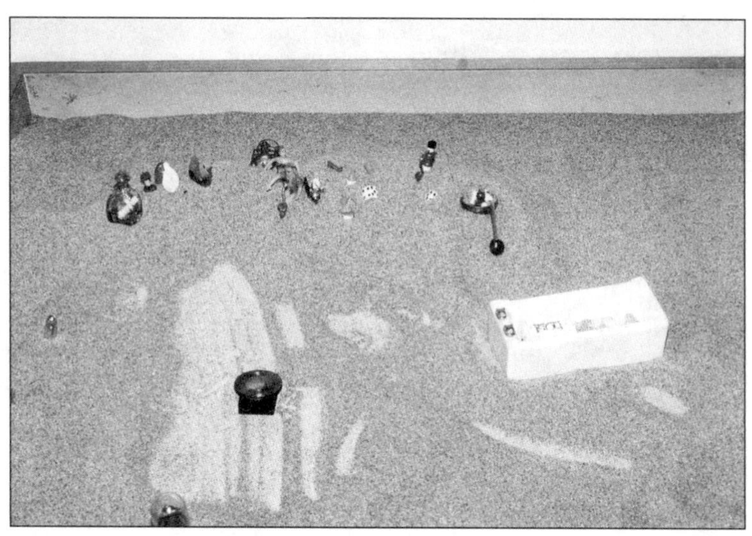

Larry
Tray 3 ~ 5 Months Later

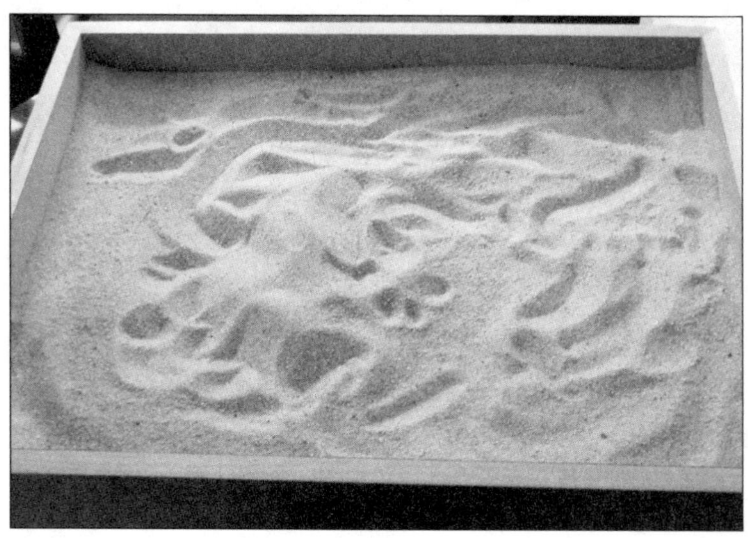

Larry
Tray 4 ~ 1 Week Later

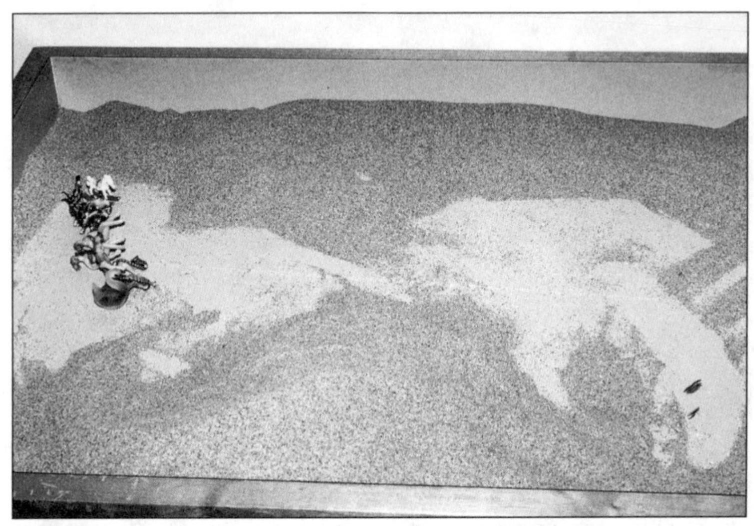

Larry
Tray 5a ~ 3 Months Later

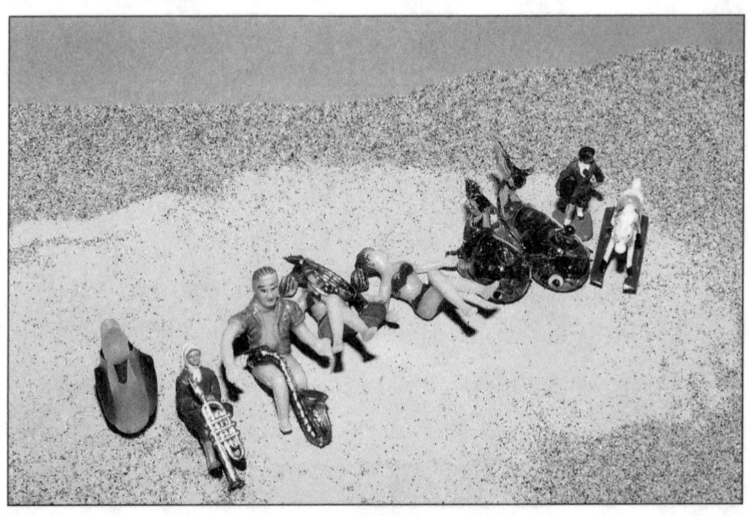

Larry
Tray 5b ~ Detail

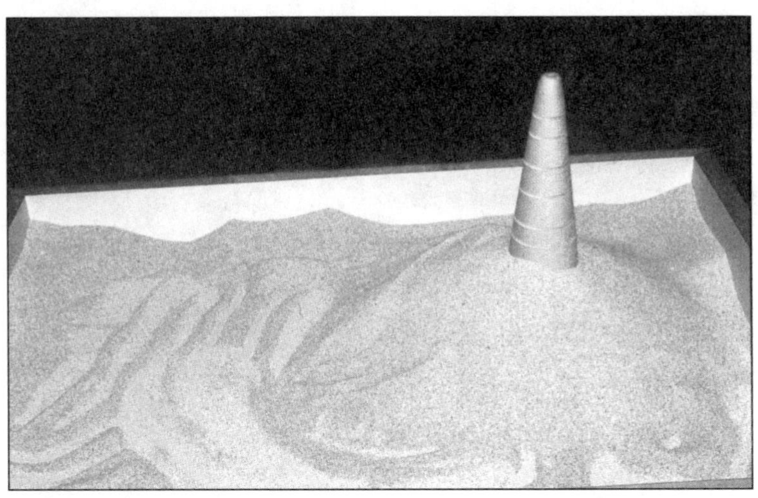

Larry
Tray 6 ~ 5 Months Later

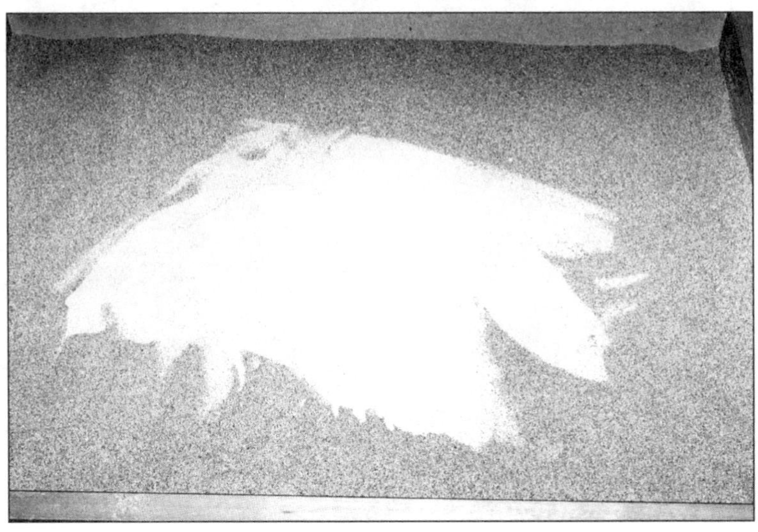

Larry
Tray 7 ~ 3 Weeks Later

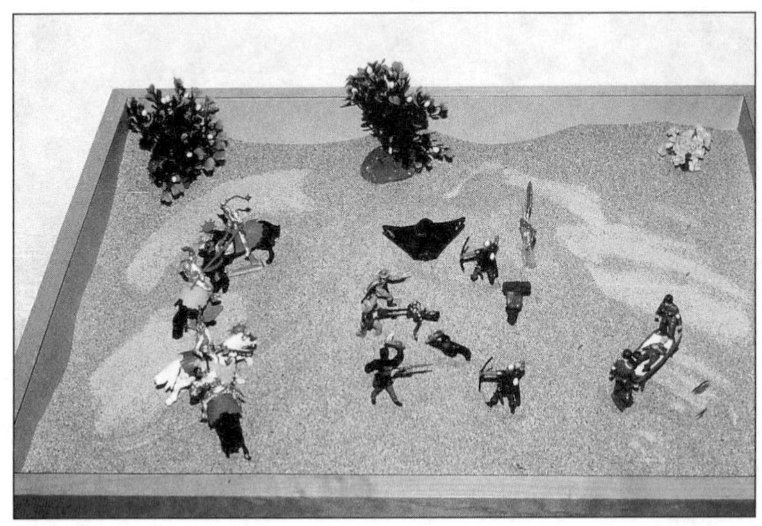

Larry
Tray 8 ~ Final ~ 2 Years 8 Months Later
4 Years 2 Months Since Tray 1

Client Profile
LEELA

Girl, 5 ½ years old
Brought to therapy to deal with anxieties stemming from parents' highly conflicted divorce
Child lives with Mother, visits Father weekly for a few hours
Parents have not spoken for years

Sandplay	Discussed on Page Number
Tray 1	
Tray 11	276
Tray 12	276

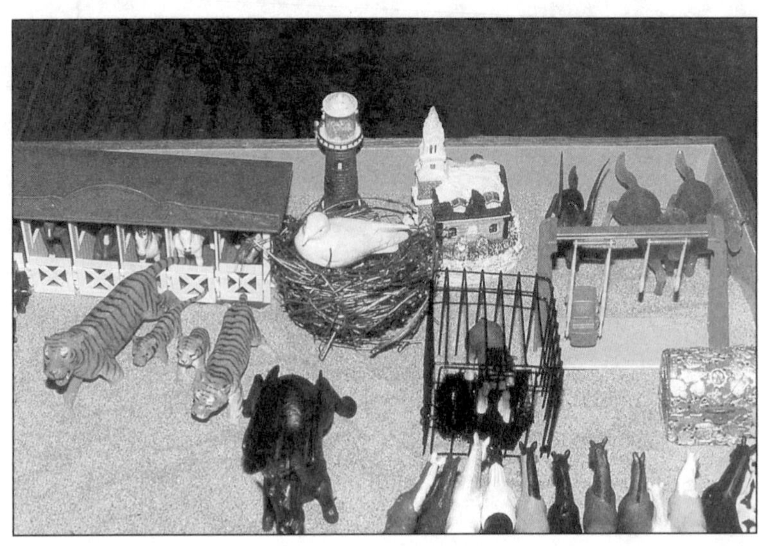

Leela
Tray 1a ~ Session 1

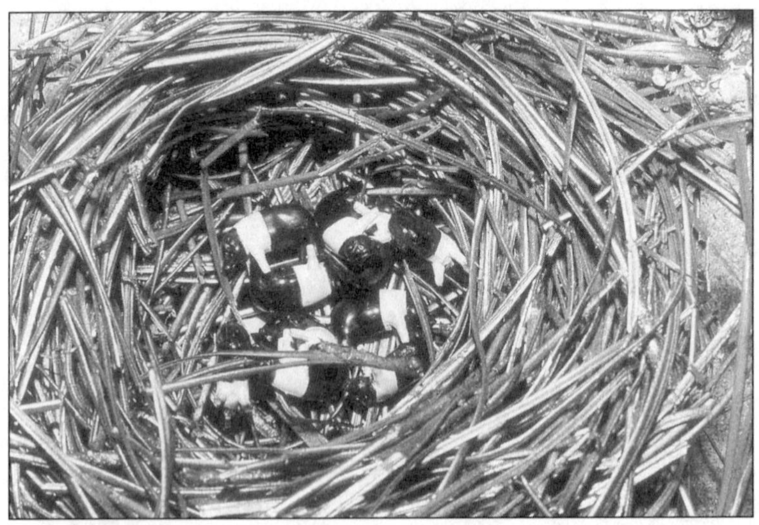

Leela
Tray 1b ~ Detail

Leela
Tray 11 ~ Final
1 Year Later ~
1 Year Since
Tray 1

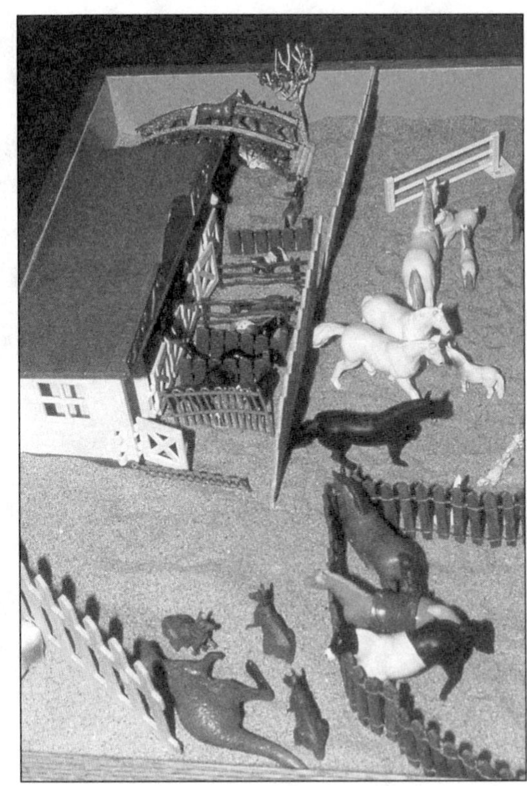

Leela
Tray 12 ~
Same Session

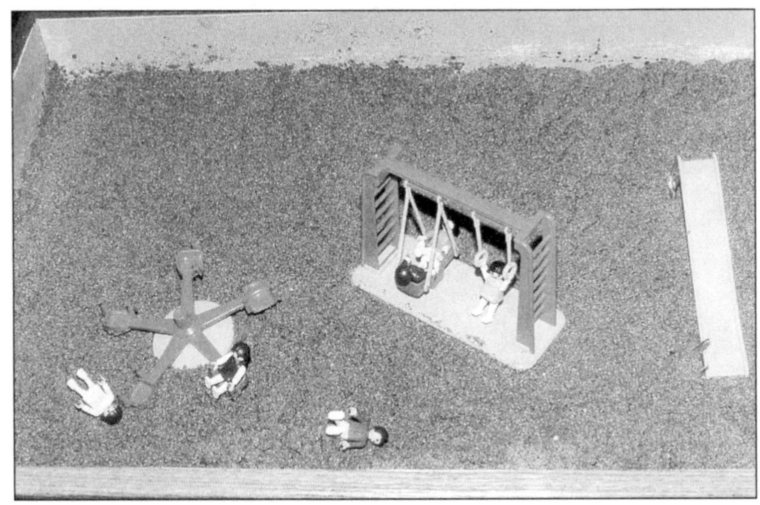

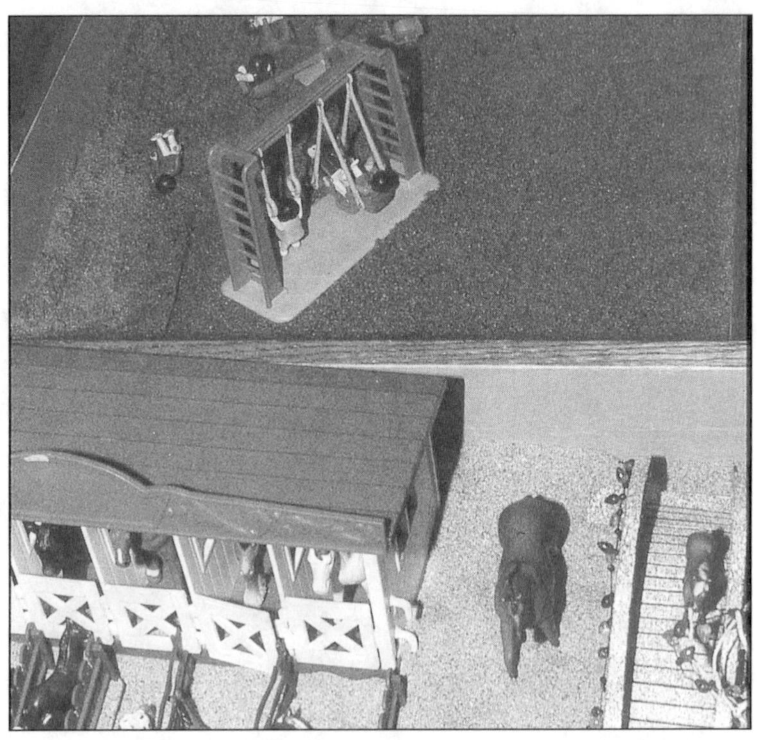

Leela
Trays 11 & 12 Together

Client Profile
LENAE

Girl, age 7
Youngest of two girls - Teen age sister
Mother and Father separated
Lives with Mother, visits father
Father alcoholic
Brought to treatment by Mother, who suspects sexual abuse by father following recent suspicious injuries to child

Sandplay	Discussed on Page Number
Tray 1	14, 234-5
Tray 6	14
Tray 14	77, 289
Tray 15	77
Tray 19	77
Tray 20	77
Tray 41	288-9
Tray 42	288-9
Tray 43	288-9
Tray 44	288-9
Tray 45	288-9, 302
Tray 46	289, 302
Tray 49	303
Tray 50	303
Tray 51	303

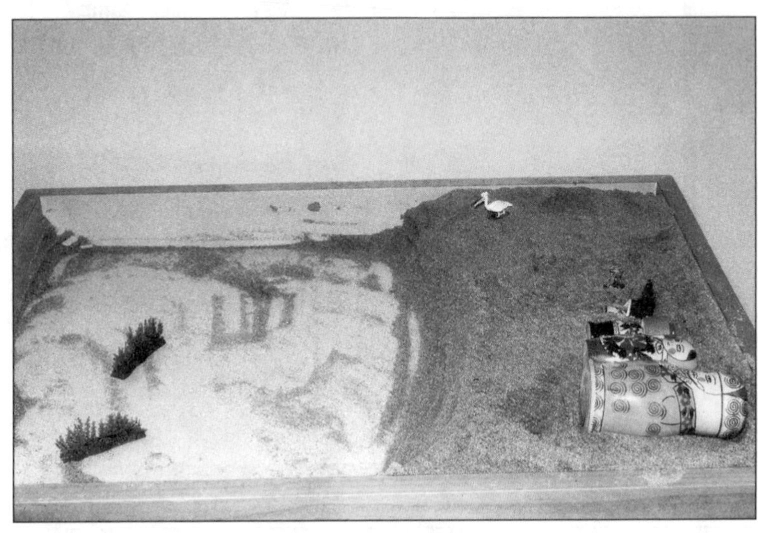

Lenae
Tray 1~ Session 1

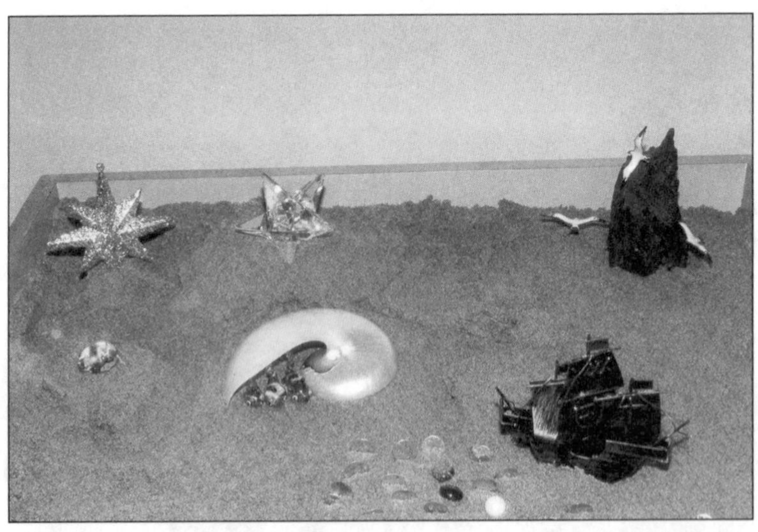

Lenae
Tray 6 ~ 1 Month Later

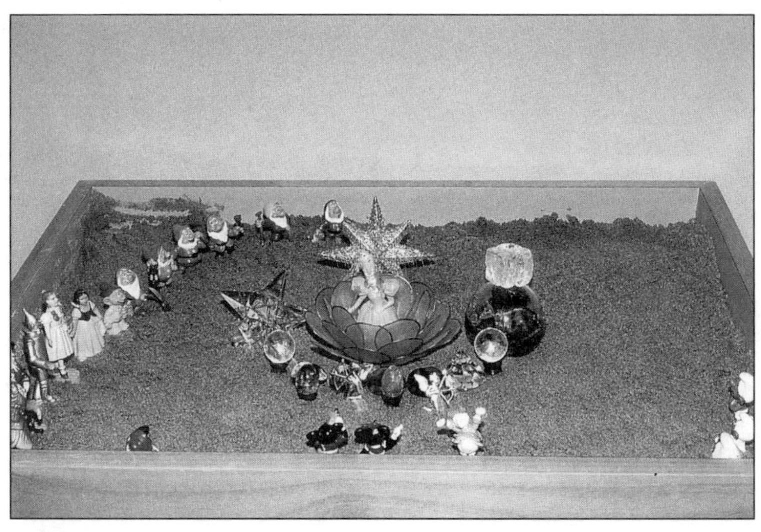

Lenae
Tray 14 ~ 2 Months 2 Weeks Later

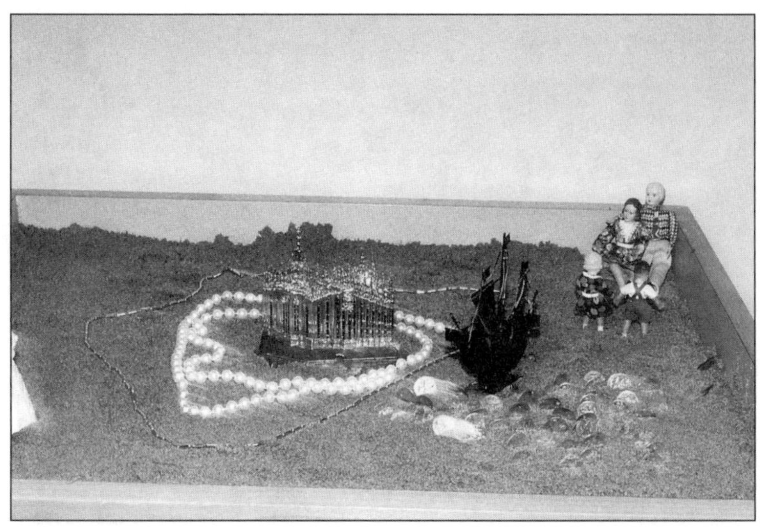

Lenae
Tray 15 ~ 1 Week Later

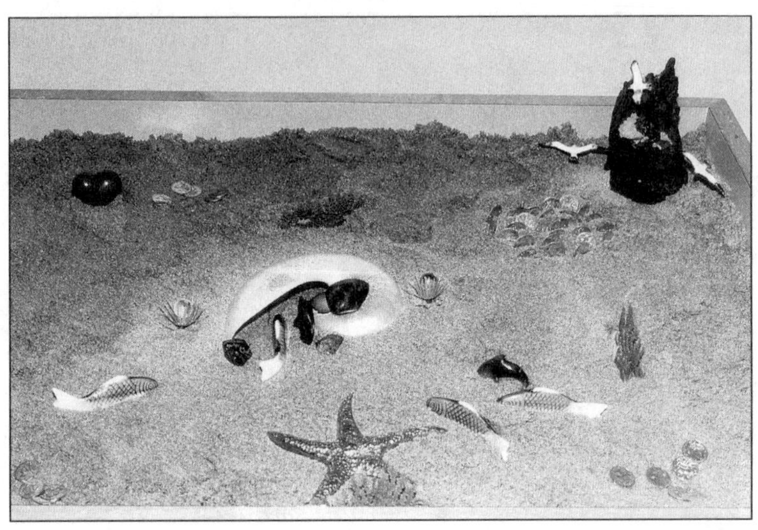

Lenae
Tray 19 ~ 1 Month Later

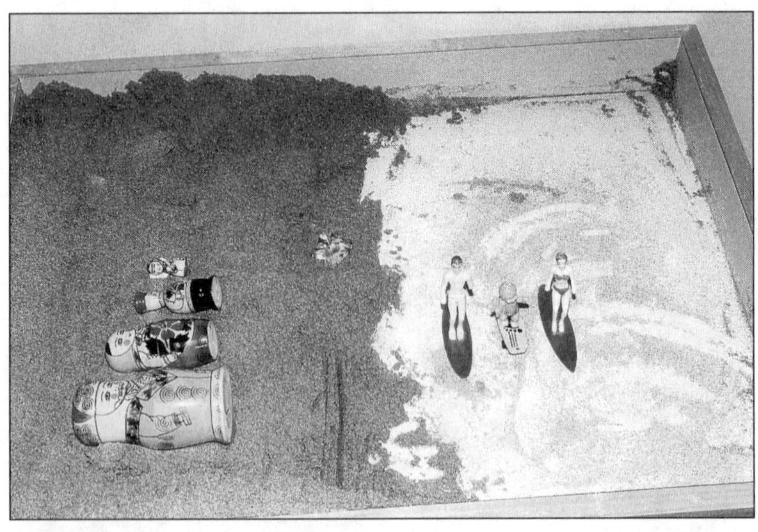

Lenae
Tray 20 ~ 2 Weeks Later

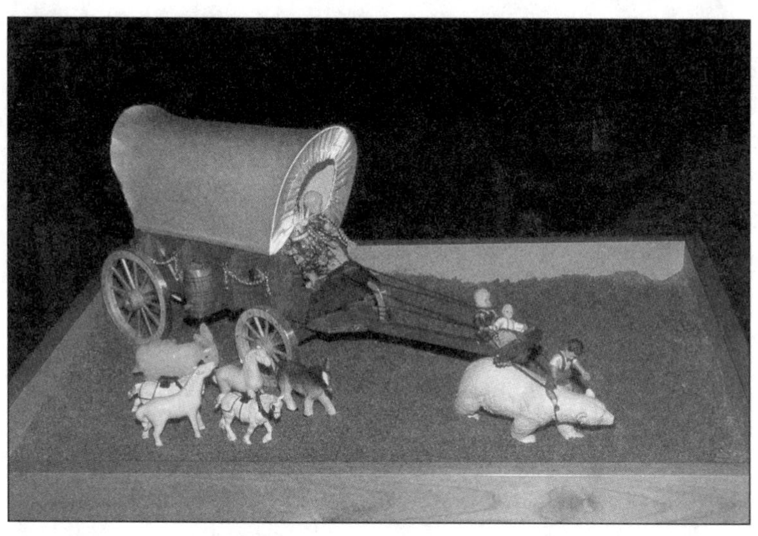

Lenae
Tray 41 ~ 6 Months 2 Weeks Later

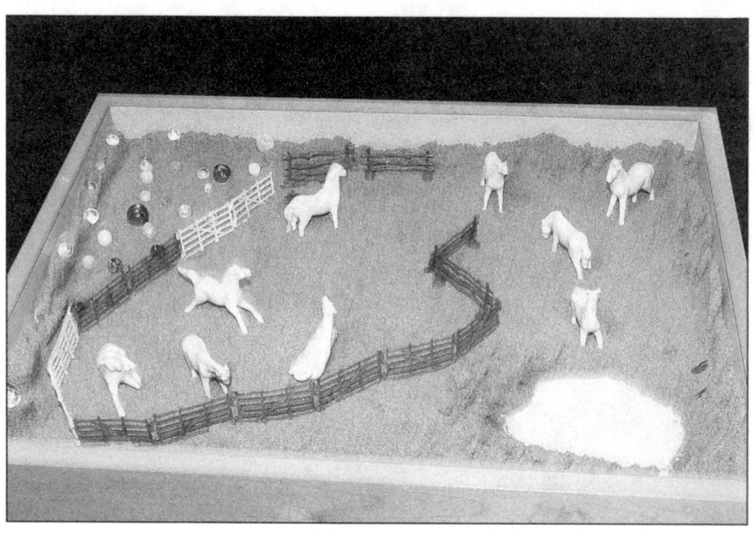

Lenae
Tray 42 ~ 1 Week Later

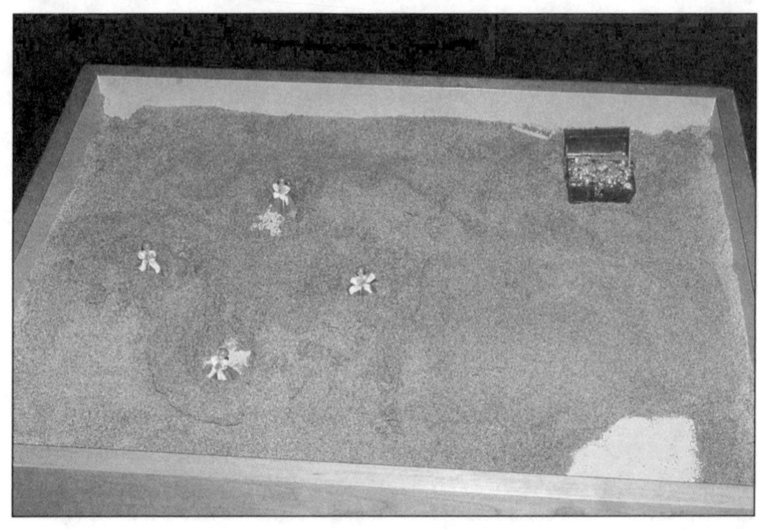

Lenae
Tray 43 ~ 2 Weeks Later

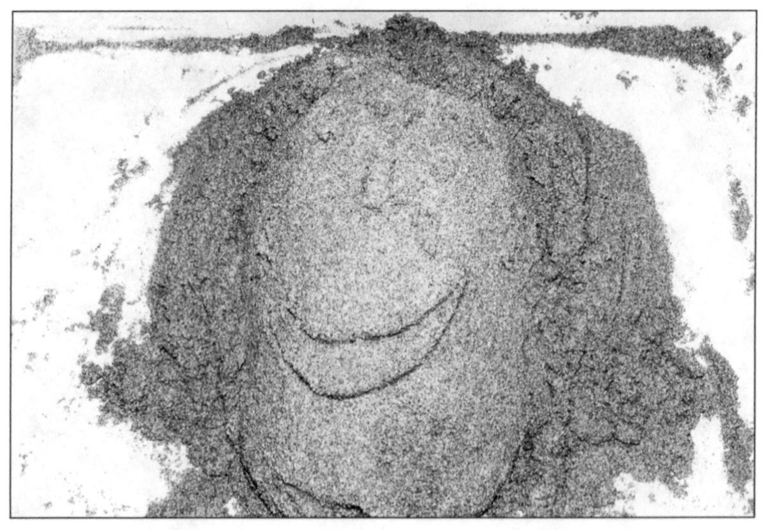

Lenae
Tray 44 ~ 2 Weeks Later

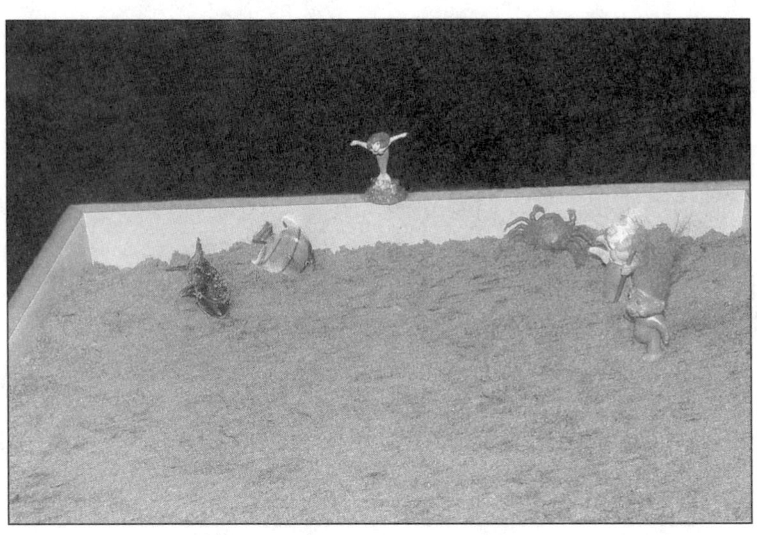

Lenae
Tray 45 ~ 1 Week Later

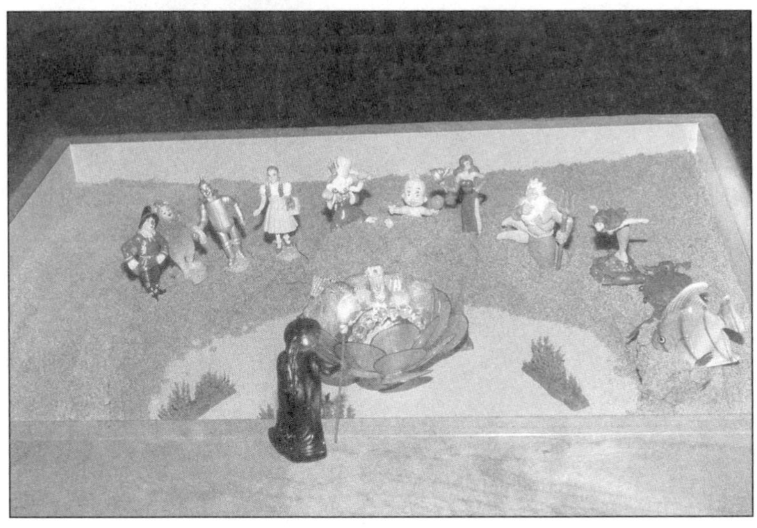

Lenae
Tray 46 ~ 2 Months 1 Week Later

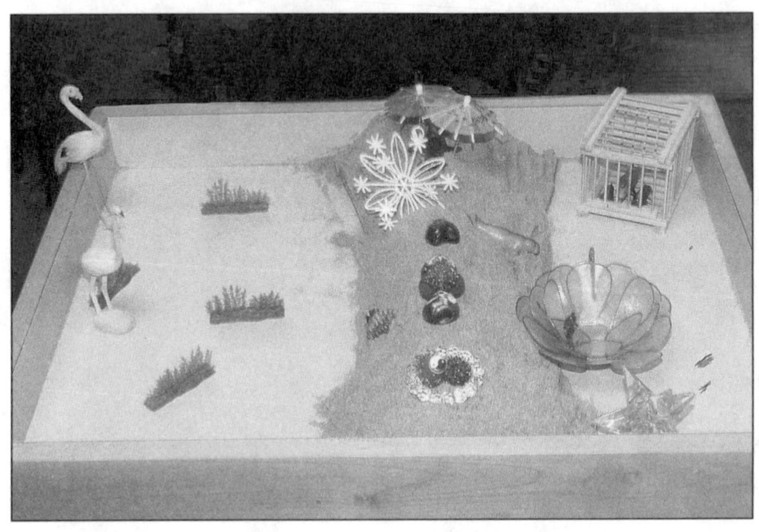

Lenae
Tray 49a ~ 2 Months 2 Weeks Later

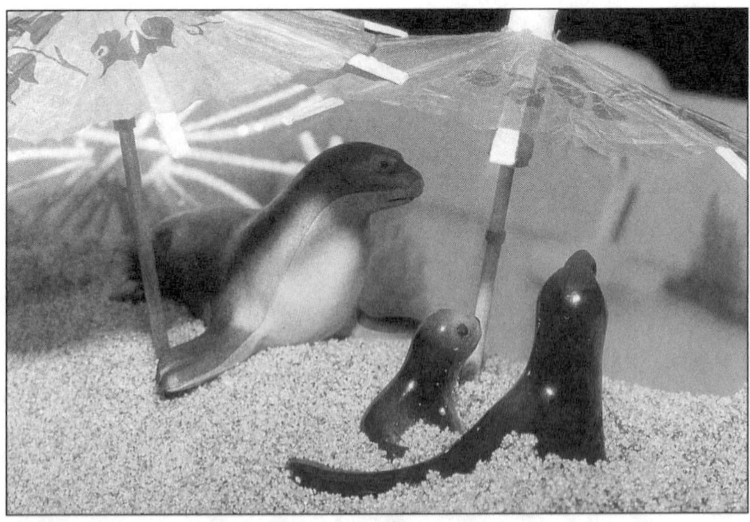

Lenae
Tray 49b ~ Detail

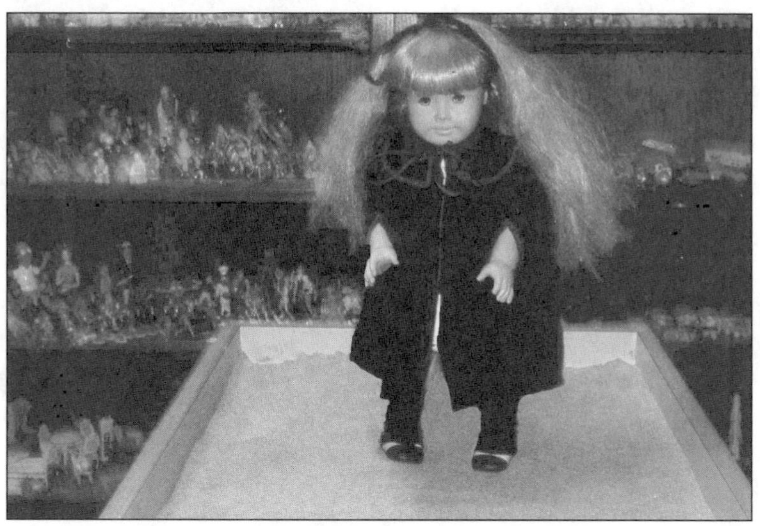

Lenae
Tray 50 ~ 10 Months Later

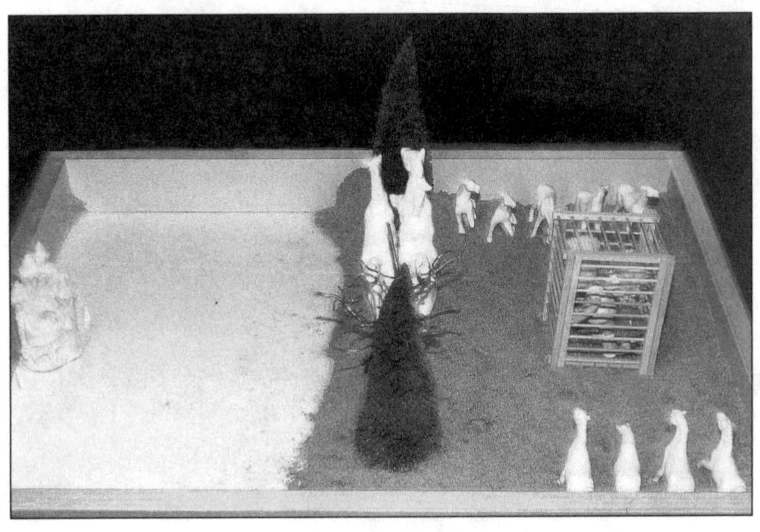

Lenae
Tray 51 ~ Final ~ 3 Months Later
2 Years 6 Months Since Tray 1

Client Profile

LEO

Boy, age eight
Chronic parental discord
Father left family
Chaotic life circumstances

Sandplay	Discussed on Page Number
Tray 1	19
Tray 4	19
Tray 6	19

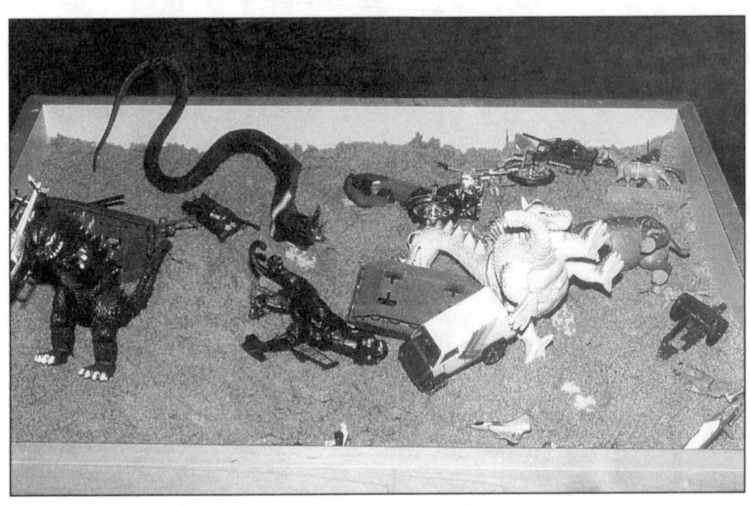

Leo
Tray 1 ~ Session 1

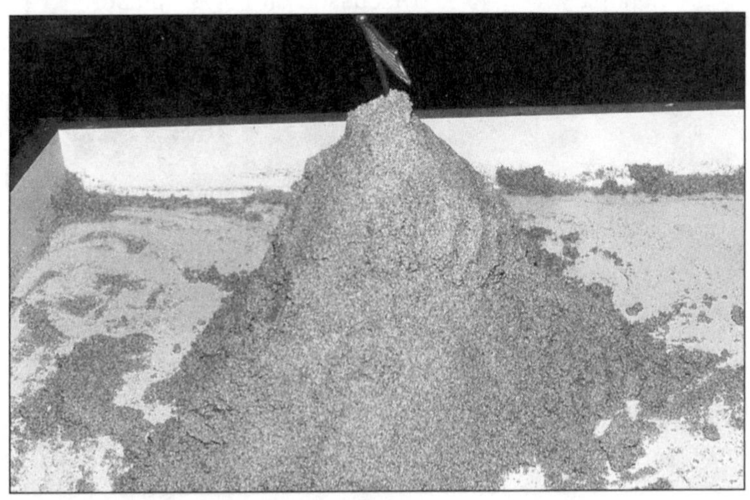

Leo
Tray 4 ~ 6 Weeks Later

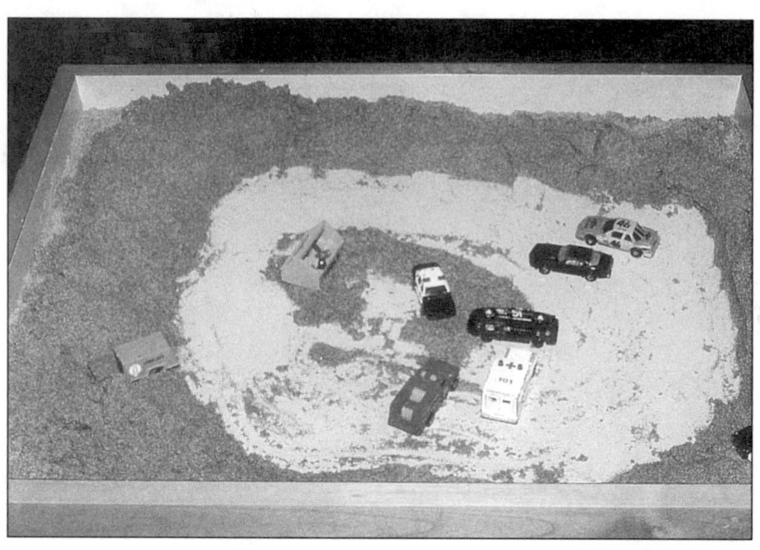

Leo
Tray 6 ~ Final ~ 3 Weeks Later
2 Months 1 Week Since Tray 1

Client Profile
LILLY

Girl, age seven
Oldest of two children
Abandoned by her drug addicted mother
Brought to therapy by stepfather to address loss and traumas

Sandplay	Discussed on Page Number
Tray 1	
Tray 2	148
Tray 5	34
Tray 10	34, 148
Tray 11	

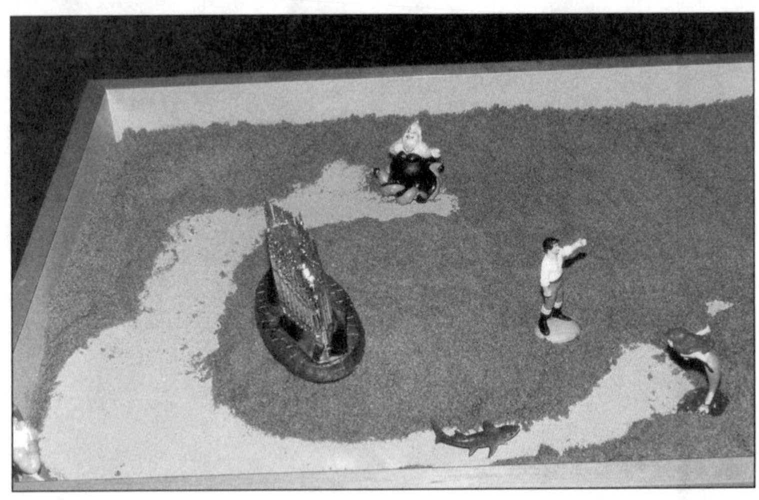

Lilly
Tray 1 ~ Session 1

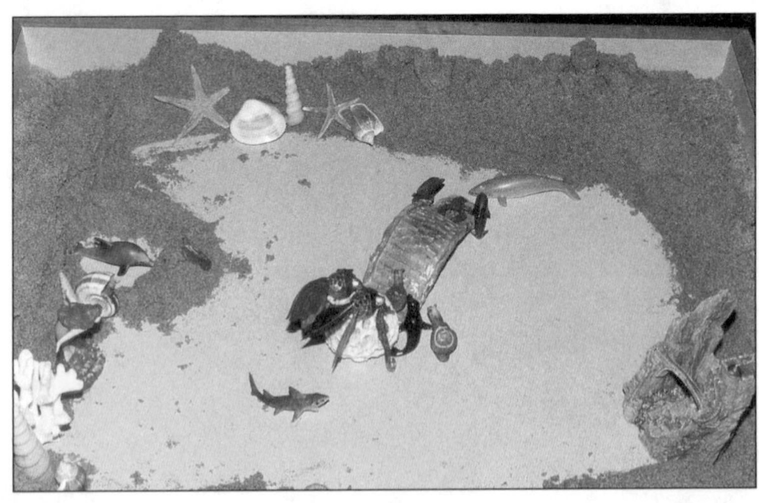

Lilly
Tray 2a ~ 1 Week Later

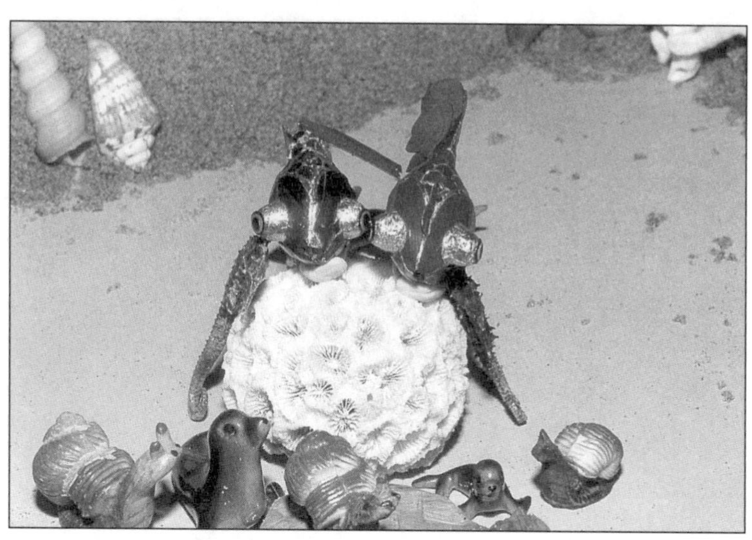

Lilly
Tray 2 b ~ Detail

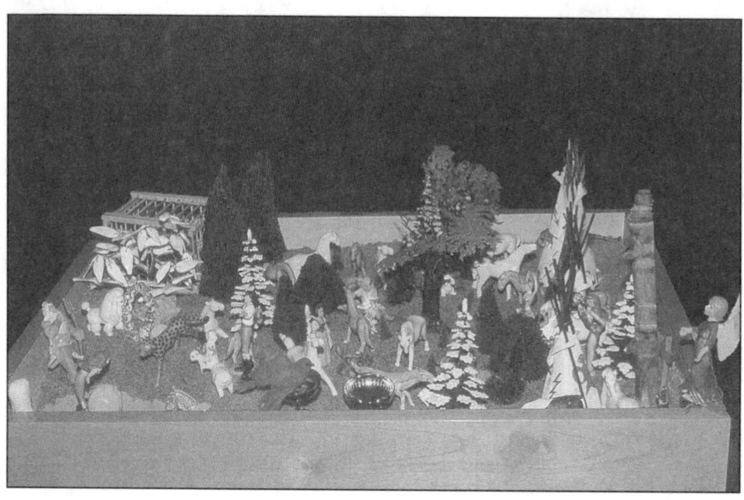

Lilly
Tray 5 ~ 3 Weeks Later

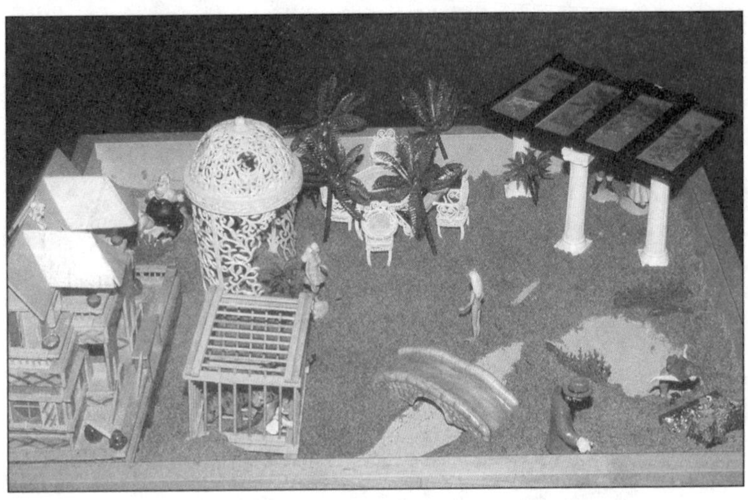

Lilly
Tray 10a ~ 4 Months Later

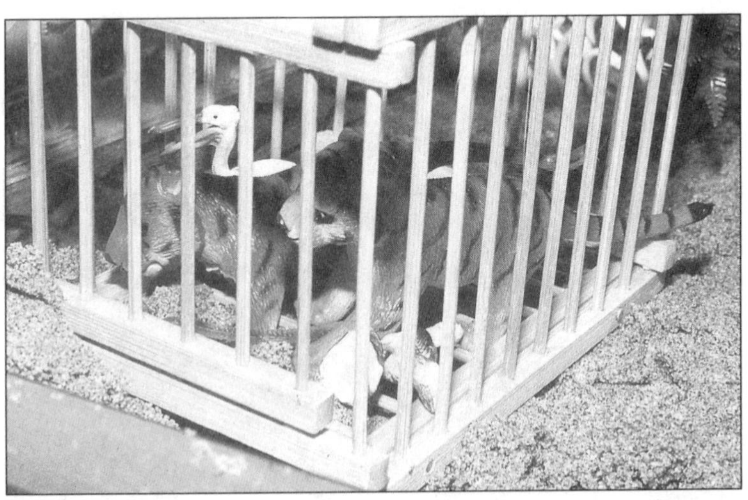

Lilly
Tray 10b ~ Detail

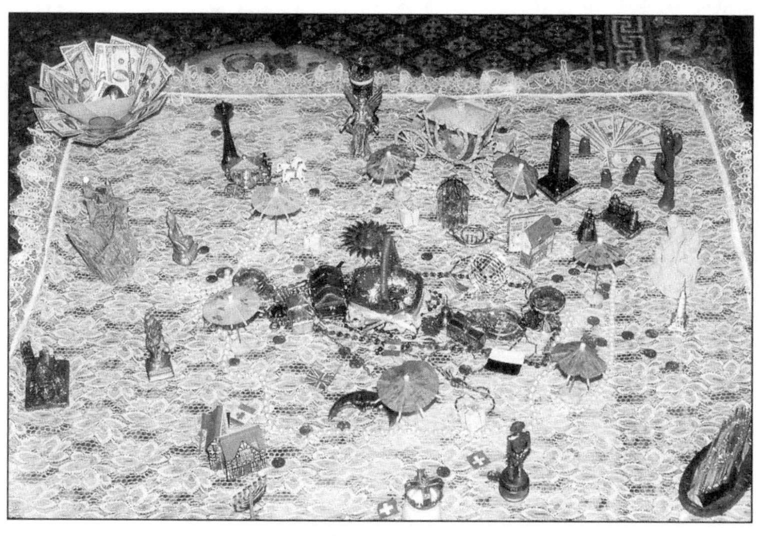

Lilly
Tray 10c ~ Floor Play ~ Same Session

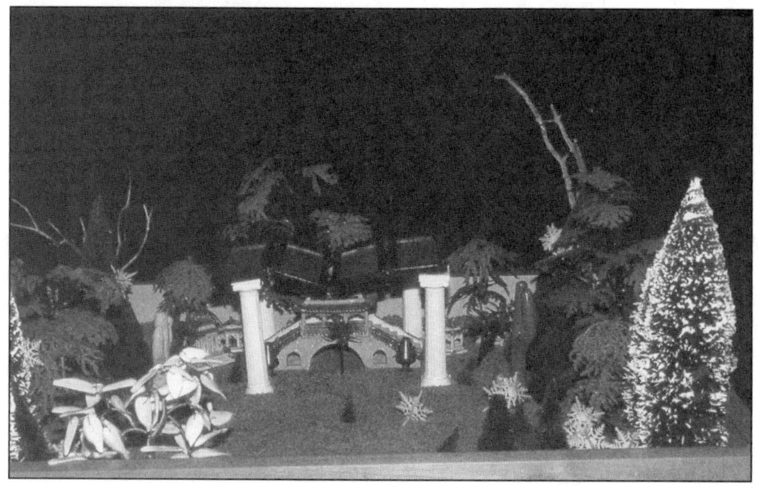

Lilly
Tray 11 ~ Final ~ 3 Weeks Later
7 Months Since Tray 1

Client Profile
MAIZIE

Girl, age 8
Estranged from birth mother following conflicted divorce and allegations of substance abuse
Father remarried
Child adjusting to blended family and new siblings
Anxiety symptoms

Sandplay	Discussed on Page Number
Tray 1	230
Tray 9	35
Tray 10	35

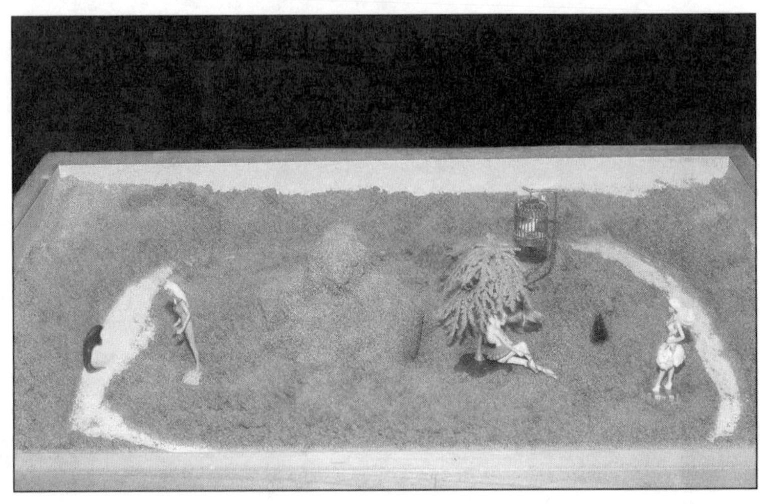

Maizie
Tray 1a ~ Session 1

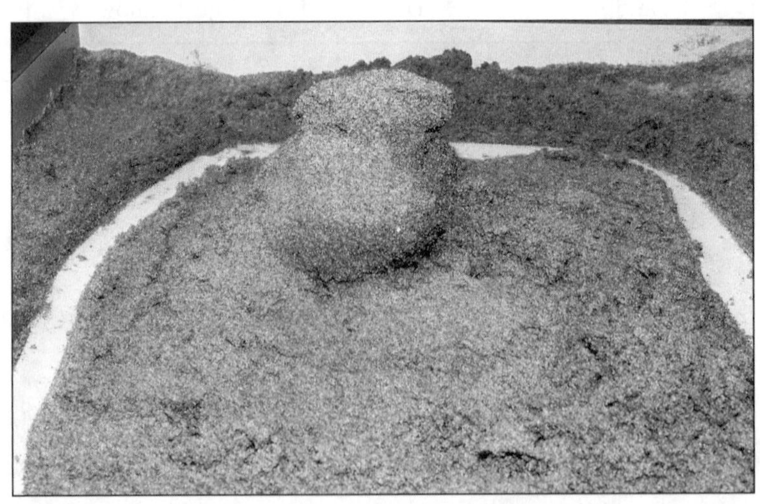

Maizie
Tray 1b ~ Detail

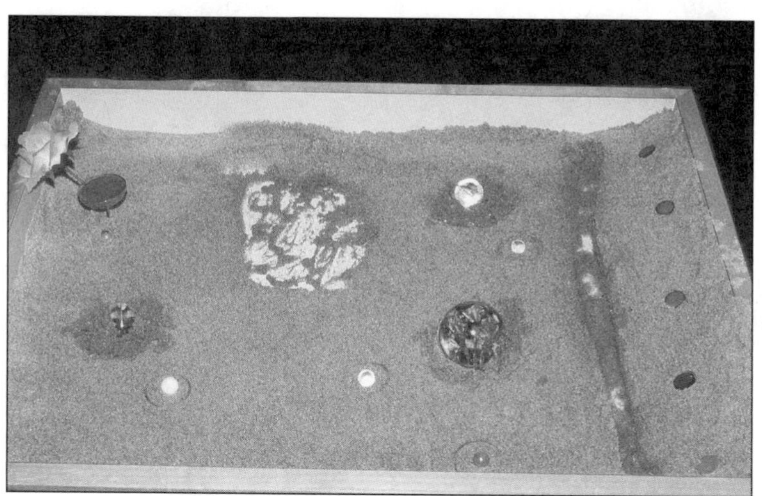

Maizie Tray 9a ~ 7 Months 2 Weeks Later

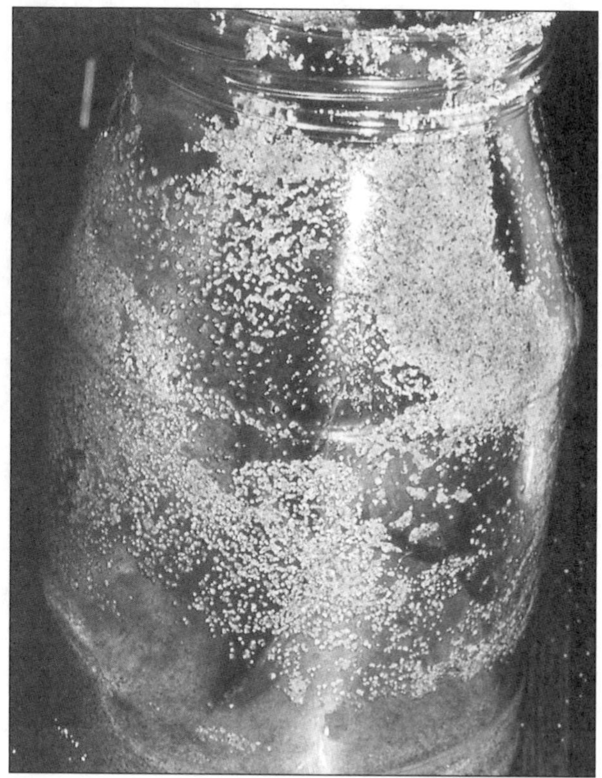

Maizie
Tray 9b
Detail

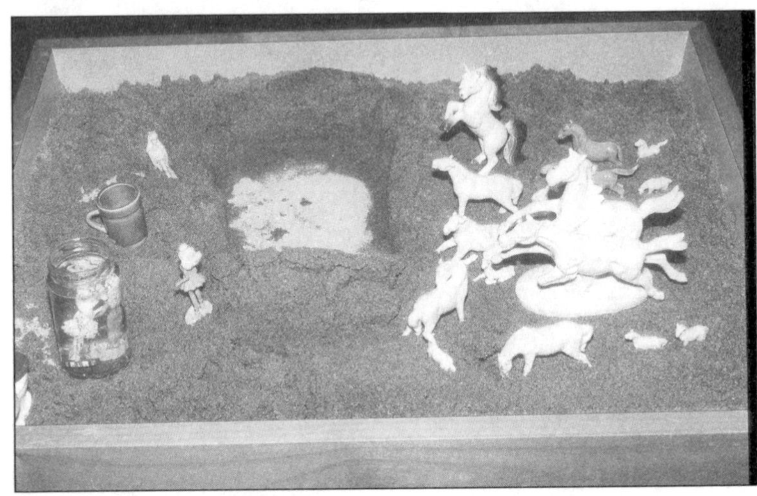

Maizie Tray 10a ~ Final 3 Months 2 Weeks Later

1 Year Since Tray 1

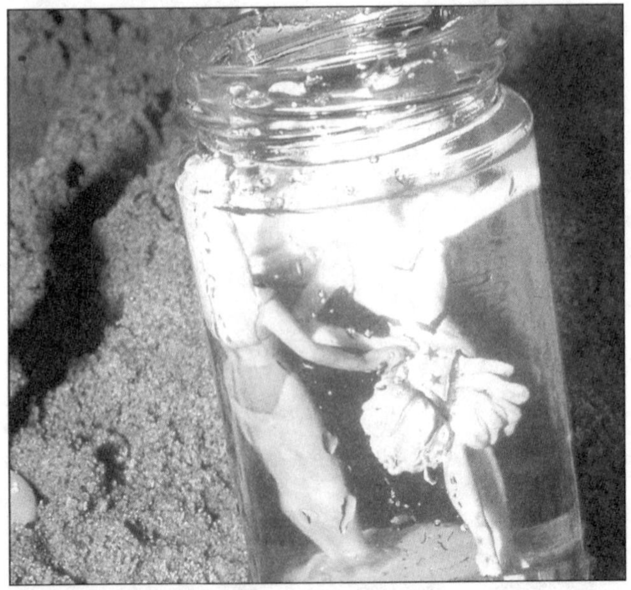

Maizie Tray 10b ~ Detail

Client Profile
MALCOLM

Boy, eight years old
Brought to treatment by Father
Parents divorced, lives with Father
Mother severely depressed, many hospitalizations and suicide attempts
Visits Mother when she is well enough
Father concerned about child's depression and expressions that he does not feel like living

Sandplay	Discussed on Page Number
Tray 1	241
Tray 2	241
Tray 8	240-1
Tray 9	240-1
Tray 27	241

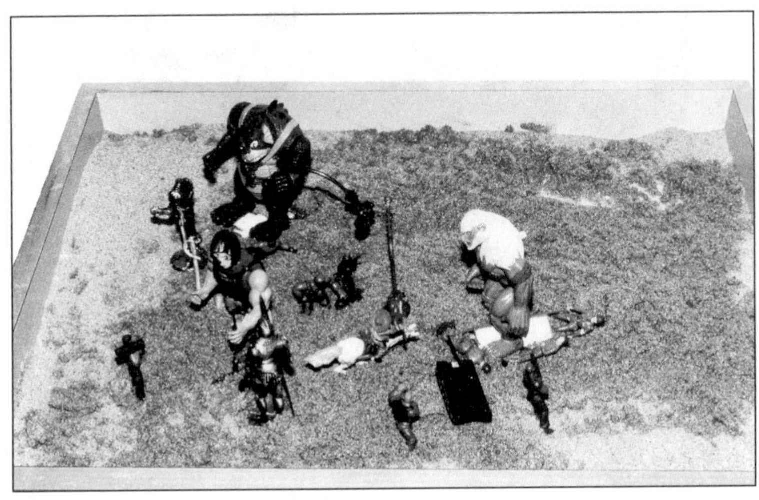

Malcolm
Tray 1~ Session 1

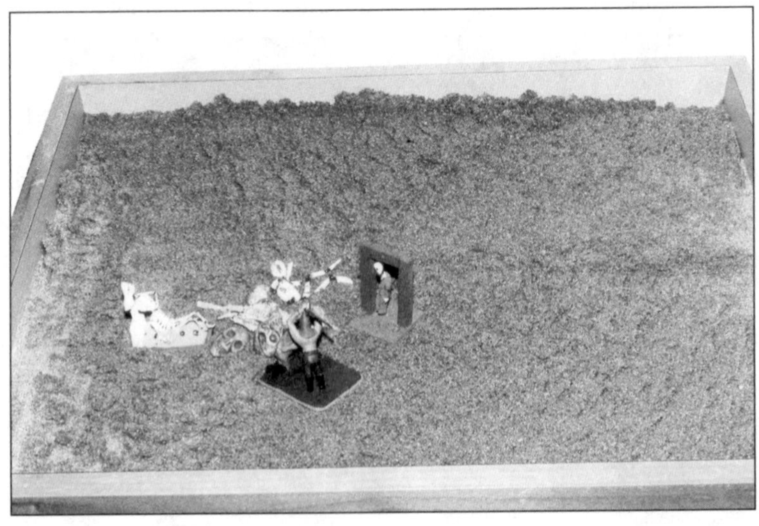

Malcolm
Tray 2 ~ 1 Week Later

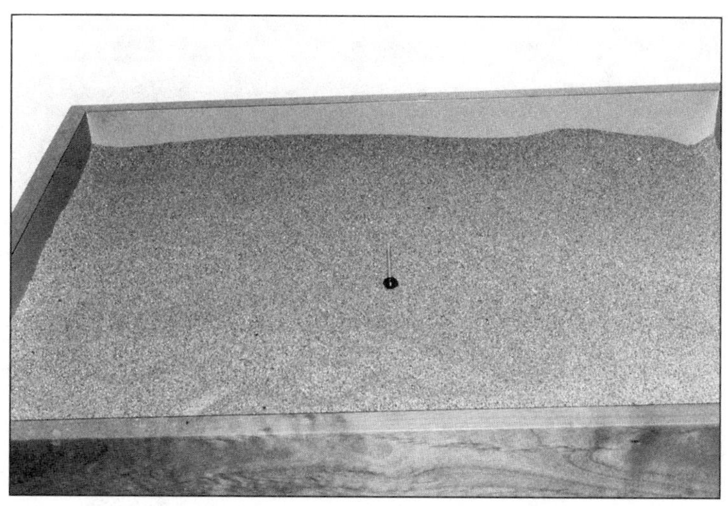

Malcolm Tray 8a ~ 3 Months 2 Weeks Later

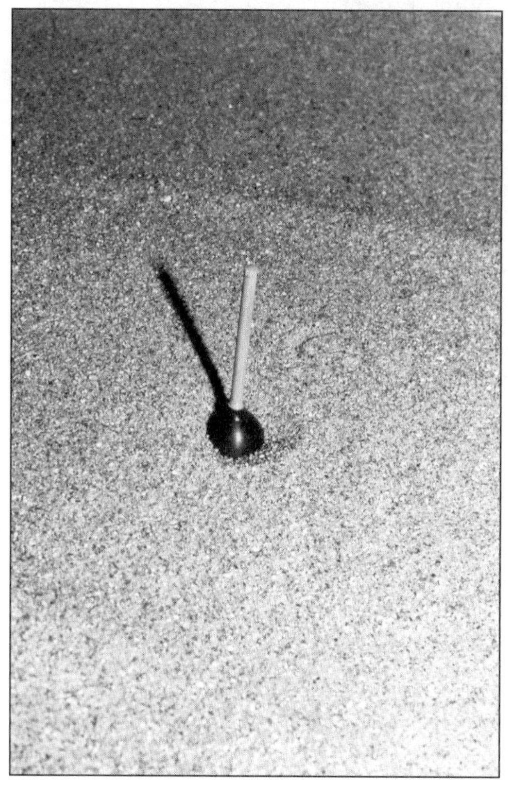

Malcolm
Tray 8b ~ Detail

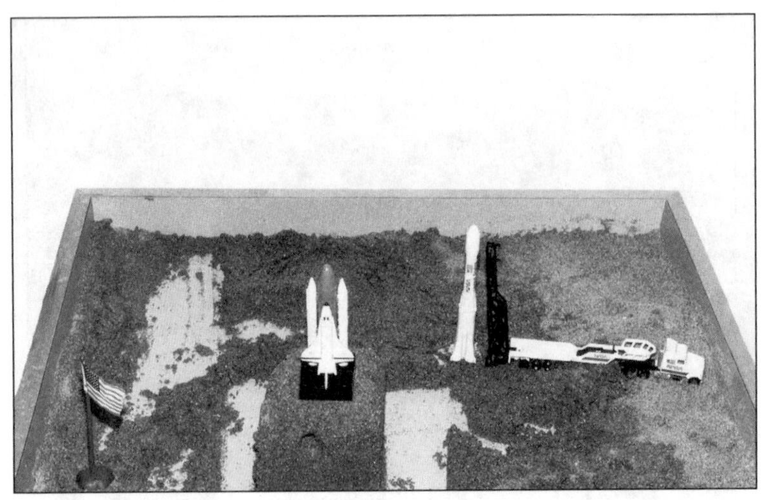

Malcolm
Tray 9 ~ 1 Month 1 Week Later

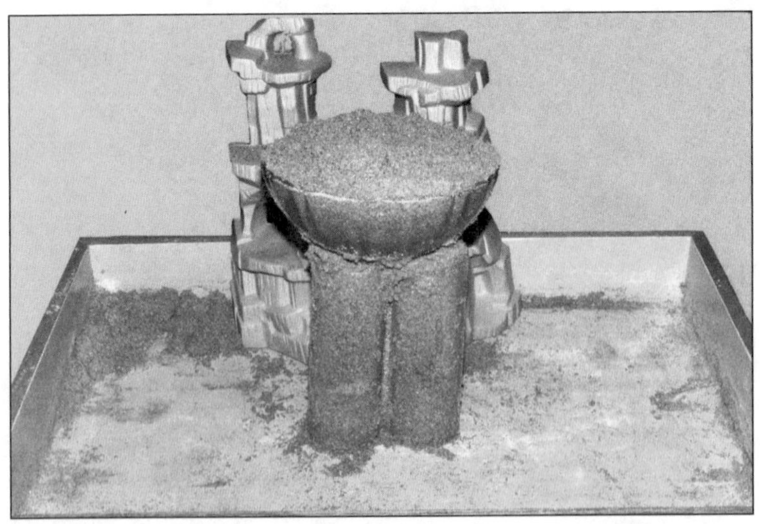

Malcolm
Tray 27 ~ Final ~ 1 Year 10 Months Later
2 Years 3 Months Since Tray 1

Client Profile
MARK

Boy, age 4
Parents separated and recently divorced
Brought to therapy by Mother
Shared custody
Father recently re-married
Two new step sisters
Nightmares, difficulty getting to sleep
Low frustration tolerance
Regressive behavior

Sandplay	Discussed on Page Number
Tray 1	
Tray 4	394
Tray 5	391-2
Tray 20	394
Tray 25	

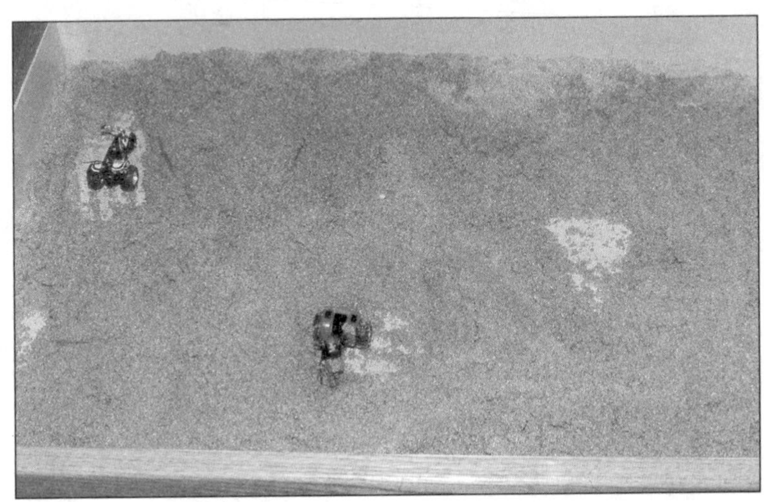

Mark
Tray 1a ~ Session 1

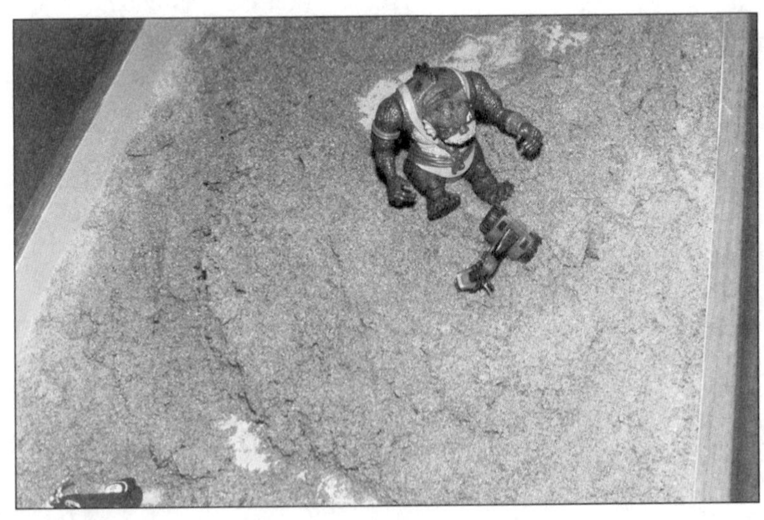

Mark
Tray 1b ~ Detail

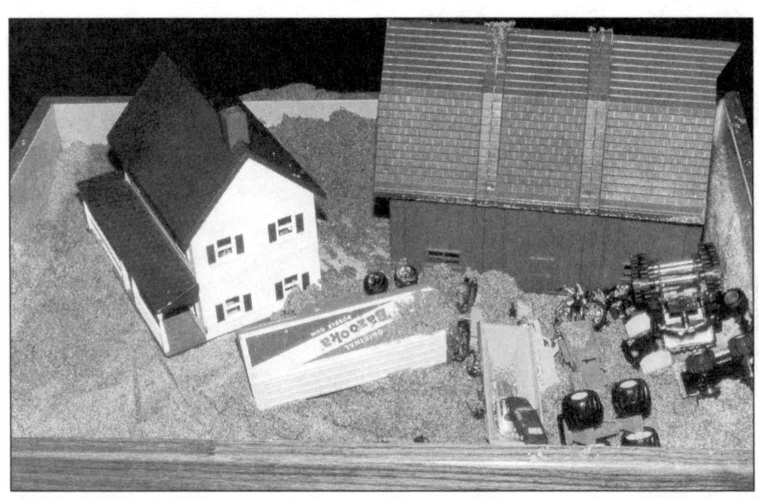

Mark
Tray 4a ~ 5 Weeks Later

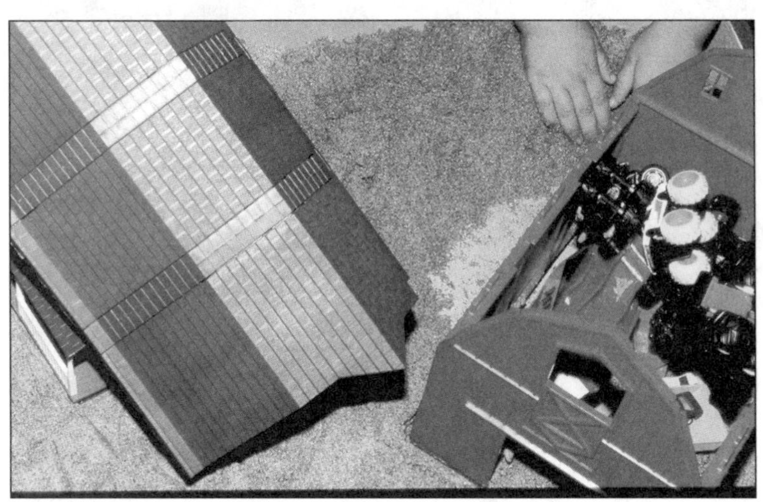

Mark
Tray 4b ~ Detail

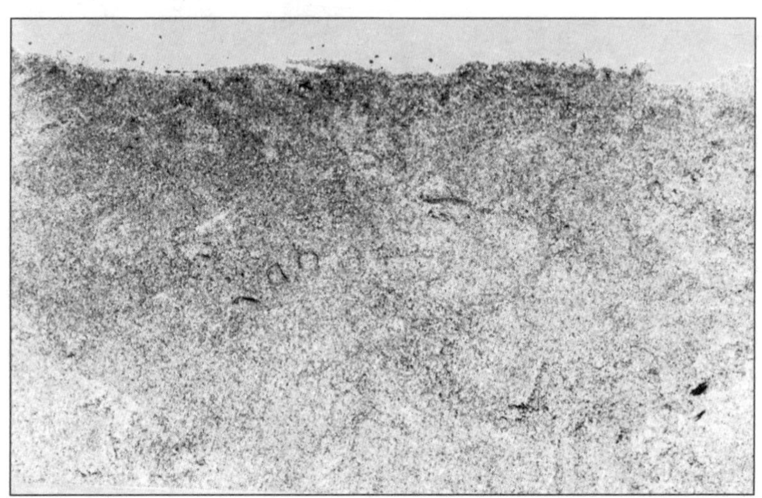

Mark
Tray 5 ~ 1 Month Later

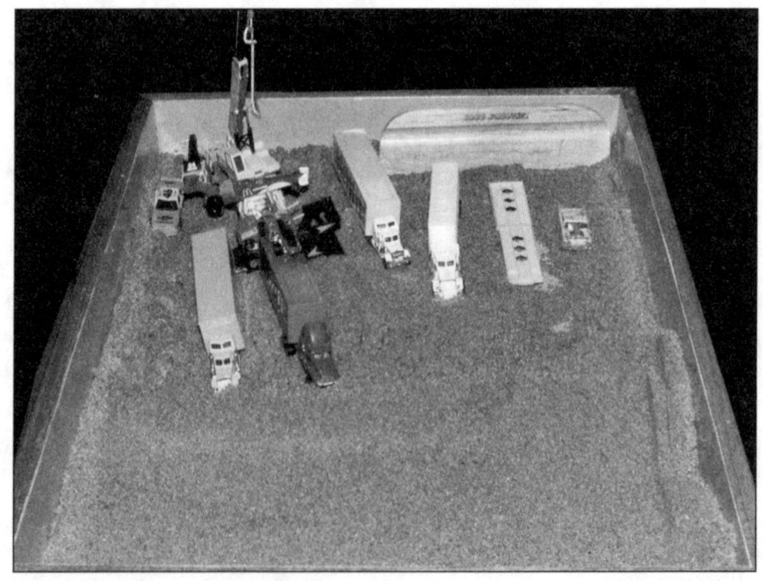

Mark
Tray 20 ~ 1 Year 3 Months Later

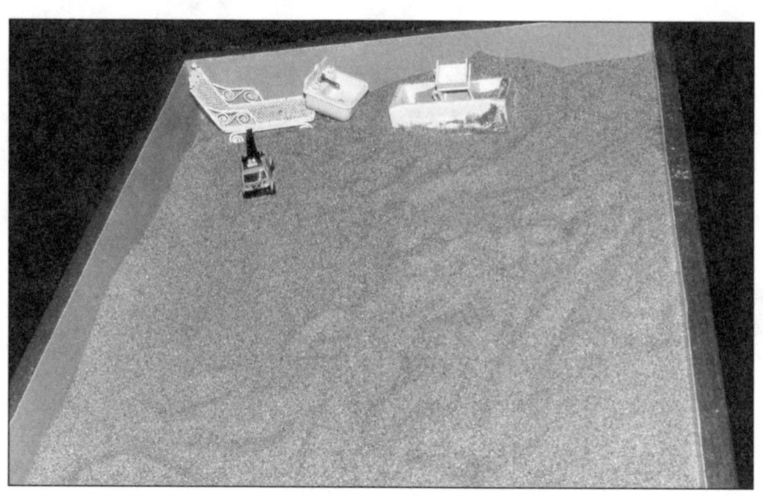

Mark
Tray 24~ 3 Months Later

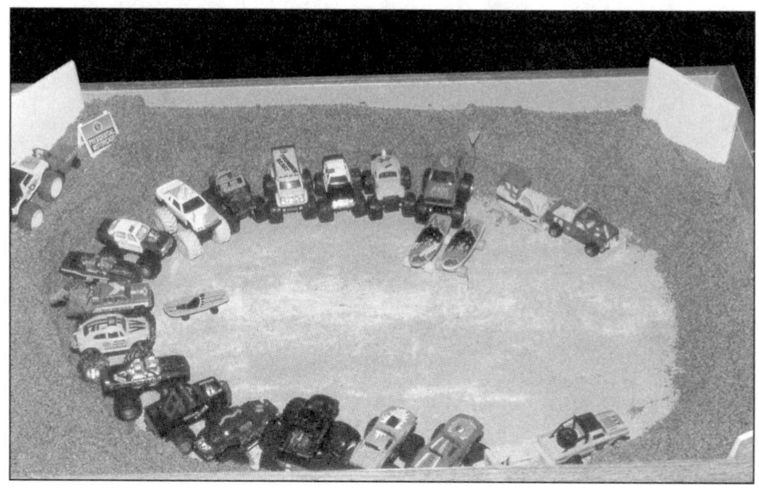

Mark
Tray 25 ~ Final ~ Same Session
1 Year 8 Months Since Tray 1

Client Profile
MARTINA

Girl, age five
One older brother
Father alcoholic, in and out of home
Parents currently separated
Brought to therapy by Mother, concerned about effects of parental conflict
Originally treated for 5 sessions
At age 6, Martina was sexually molested by a male babysitter, age 13, and returned to therapy
Following that treatment period, she was seen periodically through age 18
Martina completed her final sandplay at age 15

Sandplay	Discussed on Page Number	Sandplay	Discussed on Page Number
Tray 1	101	Tray 29	
Tray 5		Tray 32	
Tray 10		Tray 34	
Tray 11		Tray 36	
Tray 15		Tray 38	
Tray 19		Tray 40	
Tray 22		Tray 41	
Tray 25		Tray 42	
Tray 26		Tray 44	
Tray 28		Tray 45	

Note: Martina's sandplay work is specifically mentioned on page 101. A selection of her work, spanning age 5 through age 15, is included to illustrate developmental changes through childhood.

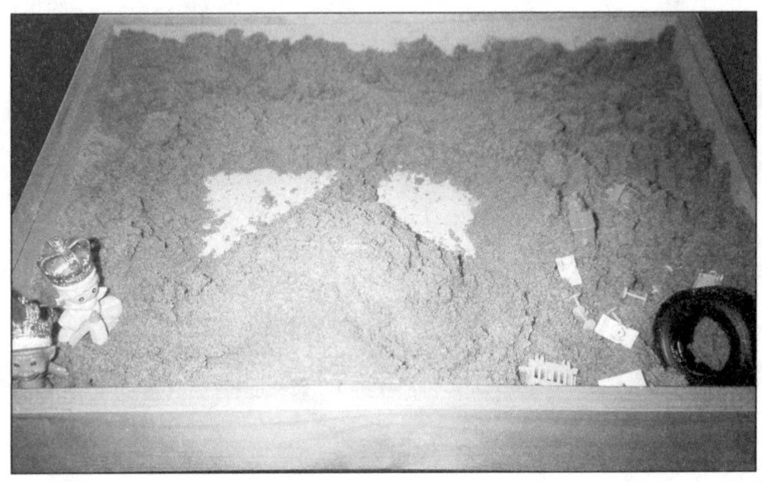

Martina
Tray 1 ~ Session 1

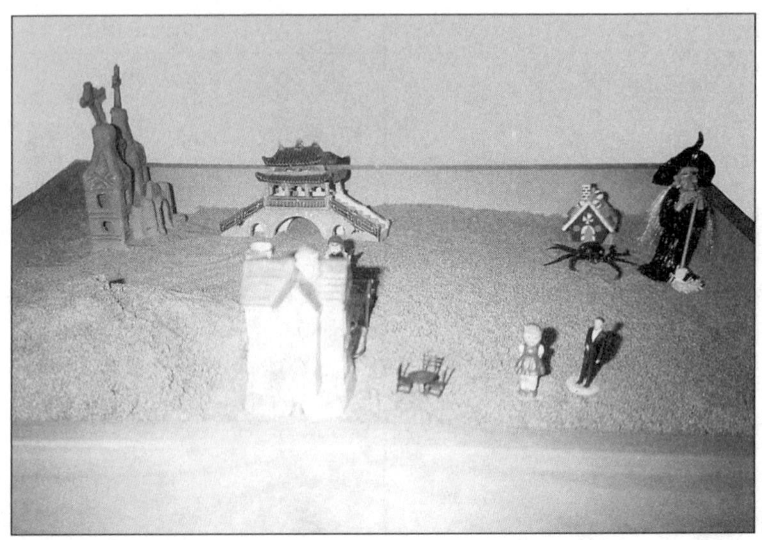

Martina
Tray 5a ~ 1 Year Later

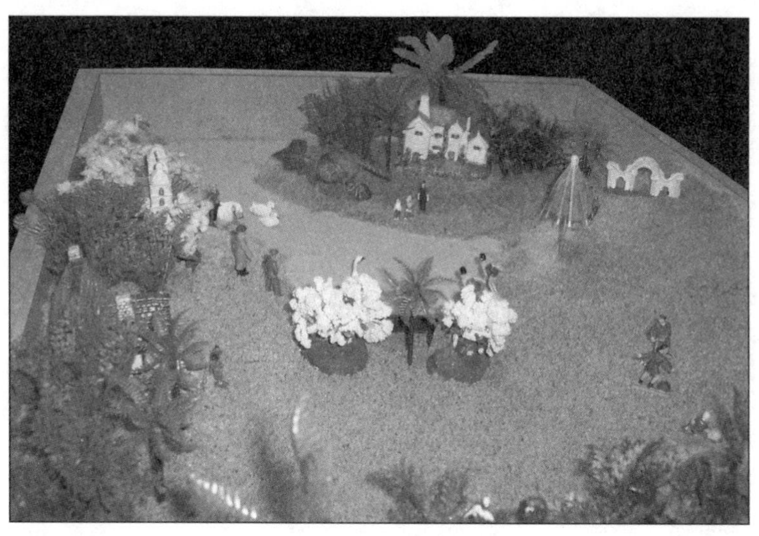

Martina
Tray 5b ~ Detail

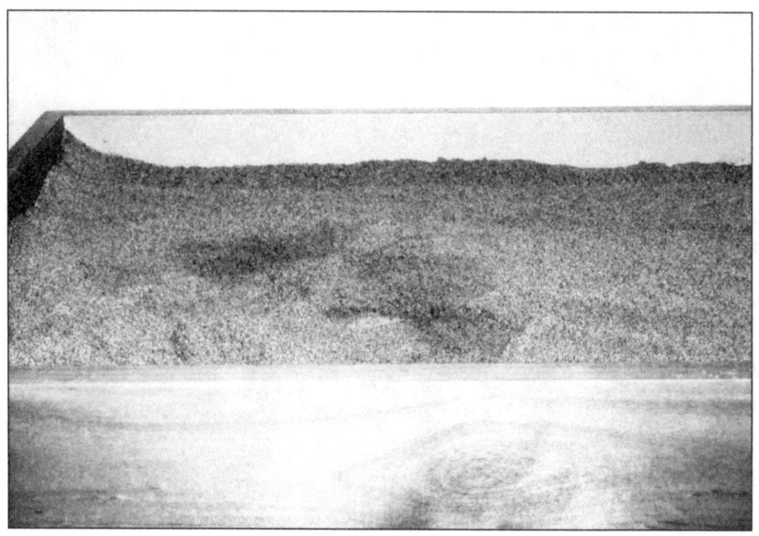

Martina
Tray 10a ~ 5 Months Later

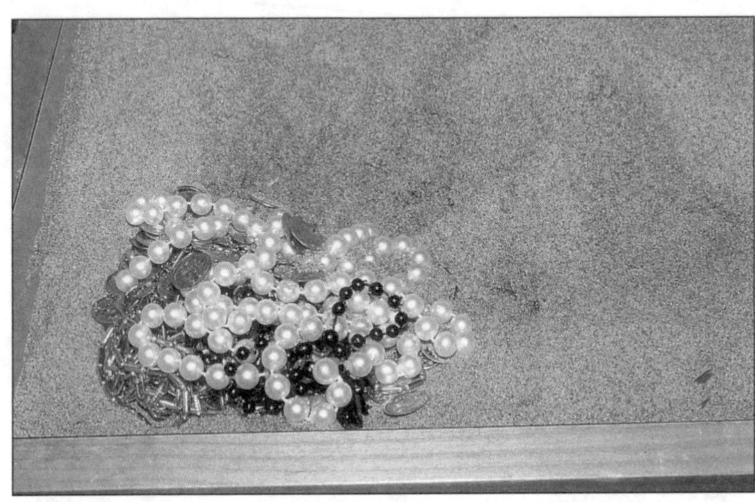

Martina
Tray 10b ~ Detail

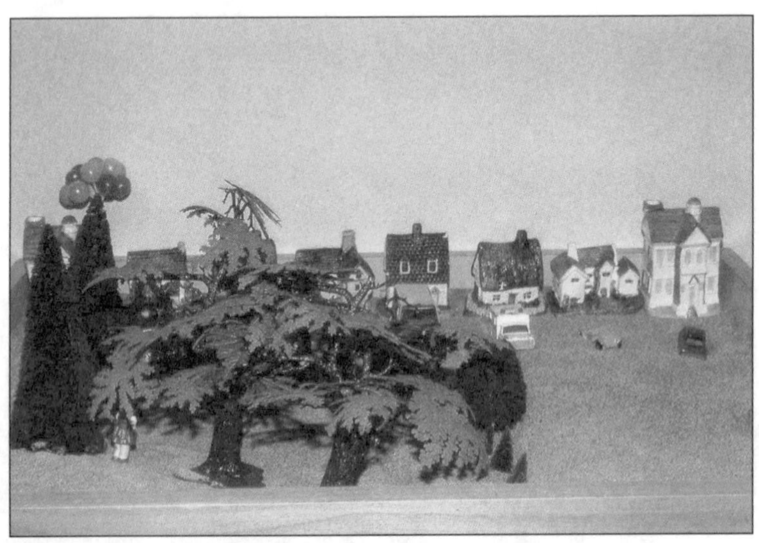

Martina
Tray 11a ~ 1 Week Later

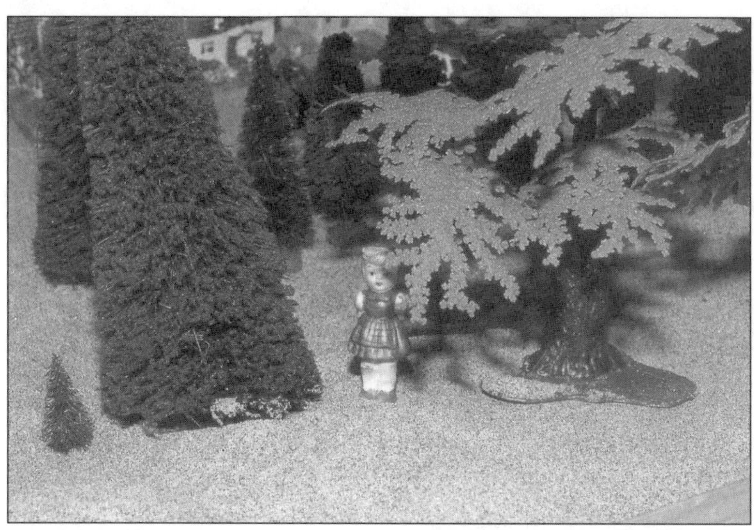

Martina
Tray 11b ~ Detail

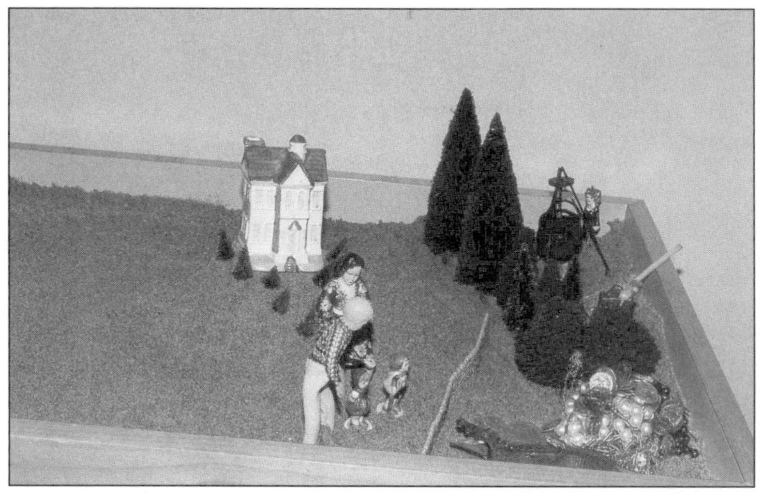

Martina
Tray 15 ~ 6 Months Later

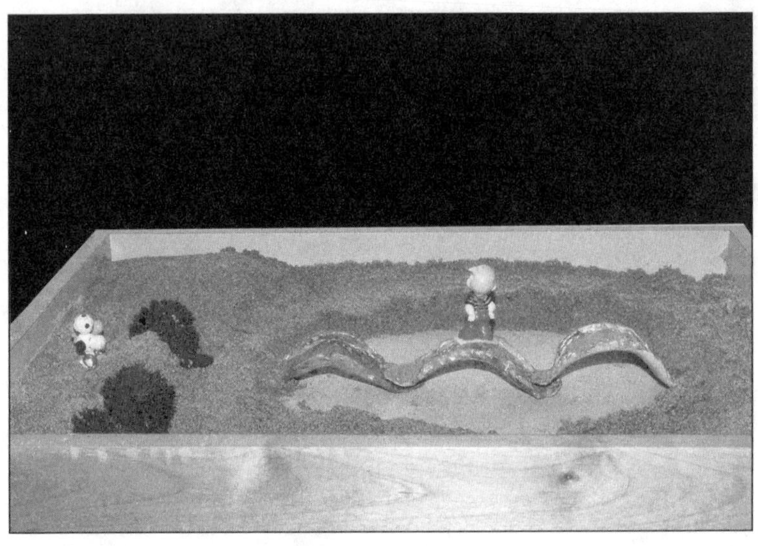

Martina
Tray 19 ~ 3 Months Later

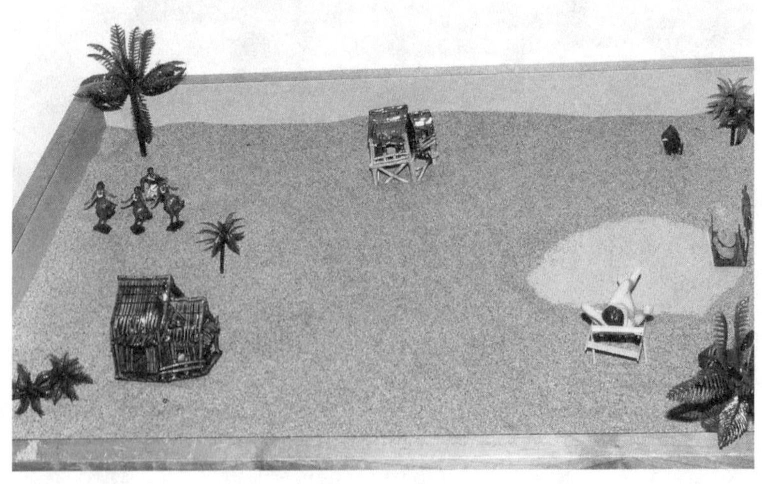

Martina
Tray 22a ~ 5 Months Later

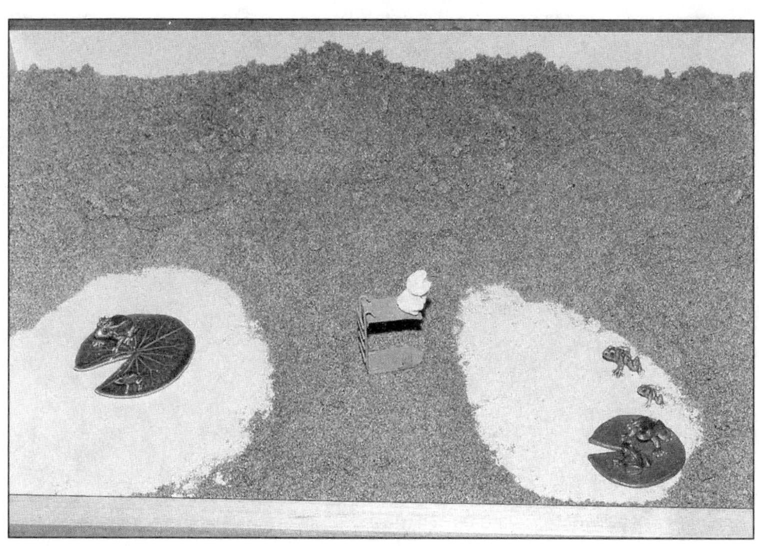

Martina
Tray 22b ~ Uses Wet and Dry Trays Simultaneously

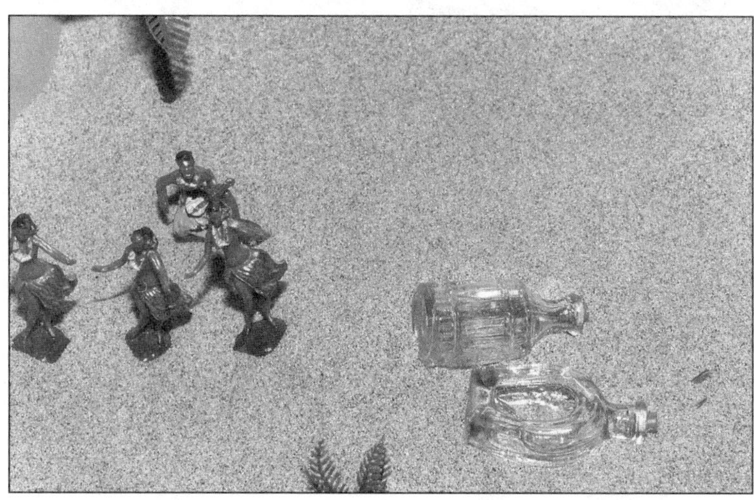

Martina
Tray 22c ~ Detail

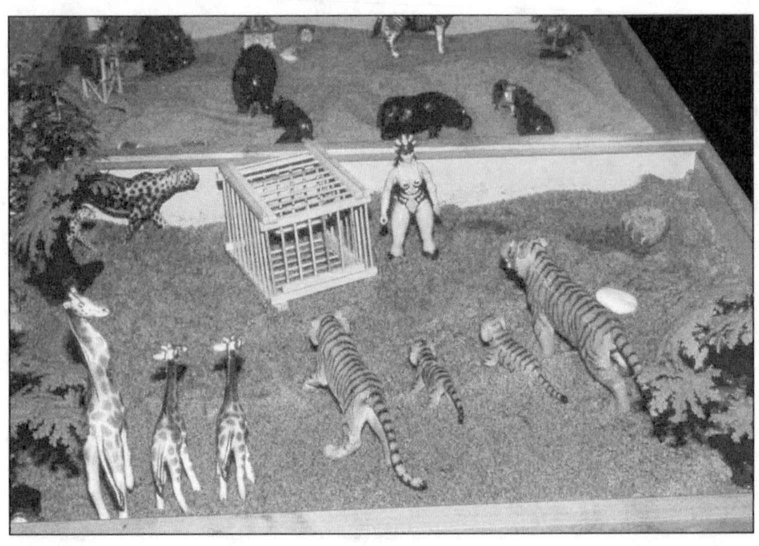

Martina
Tray 25a ~ 6 Months Later
Uses Wet and Dry Trays Simultaneously

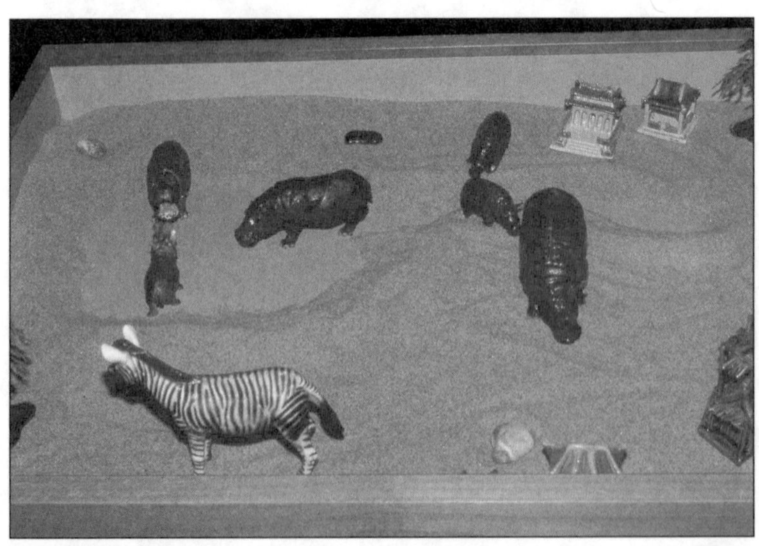

Martina
Tray 25b ~ Detail

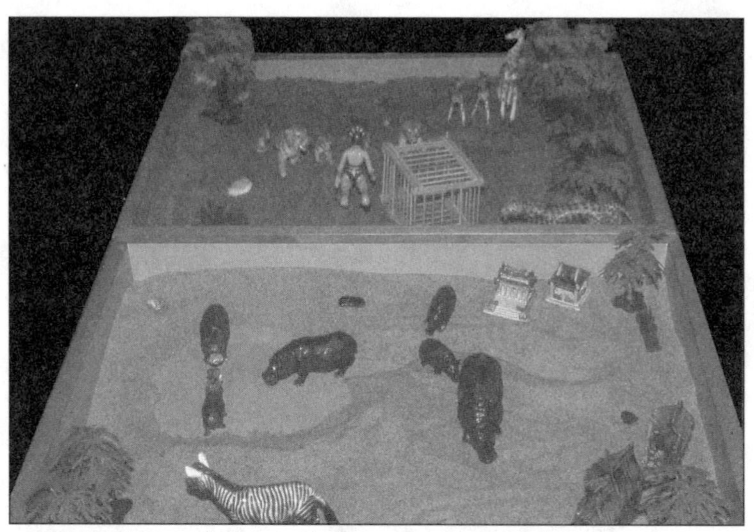

Martina
Tray 25c ~ Detail

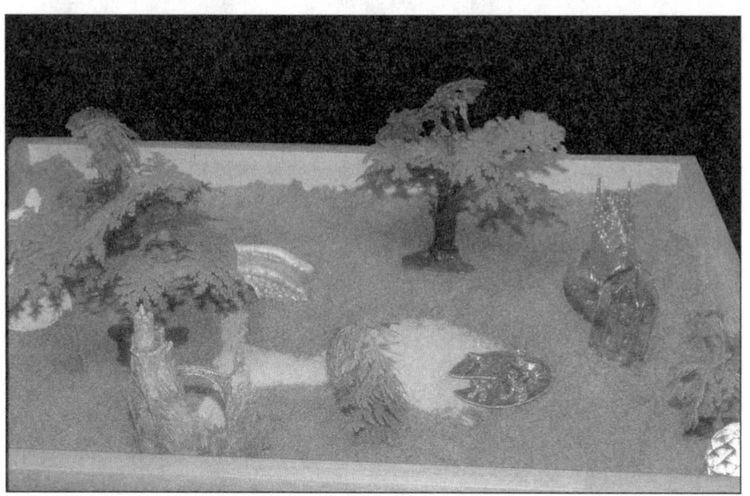

Martina
Tray 26 ~ 5 Months Later

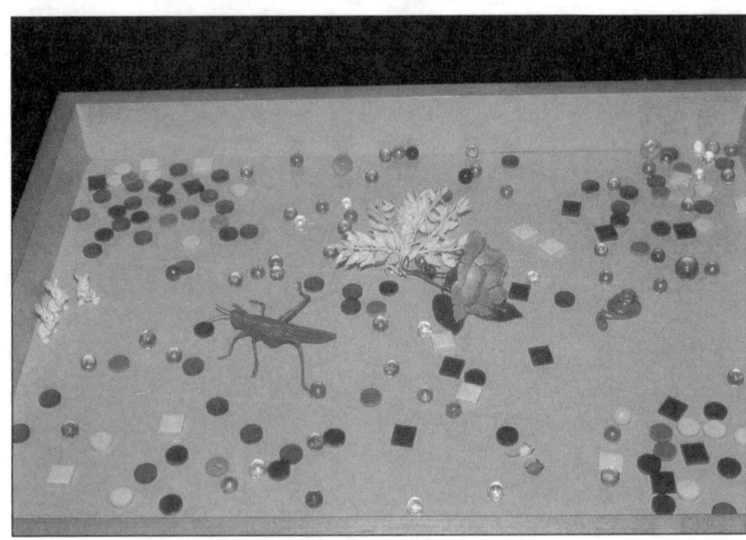

Martina
Tray 28 ~ 3 Months Later

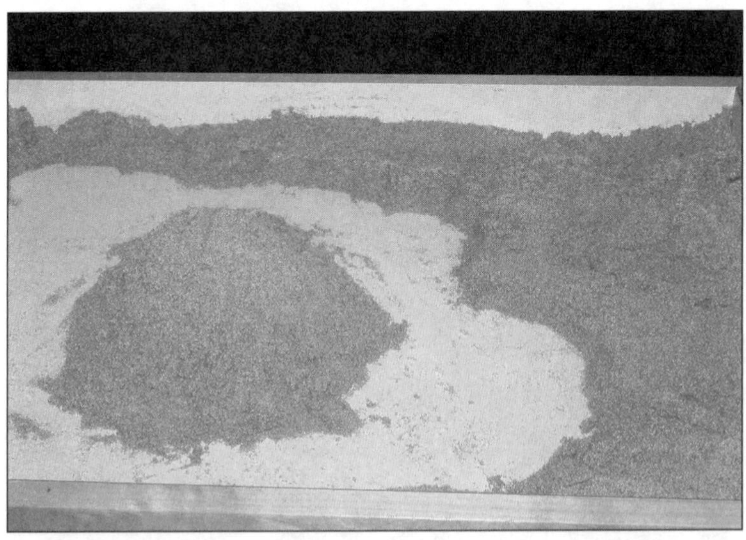

Martina
Tray 29a ~ 3 Weeks Later

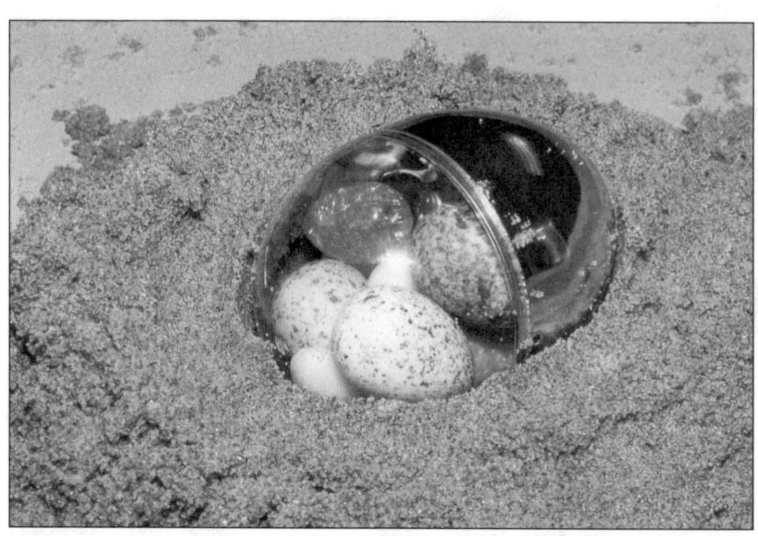

Martina
Tray 29b ~ Detail

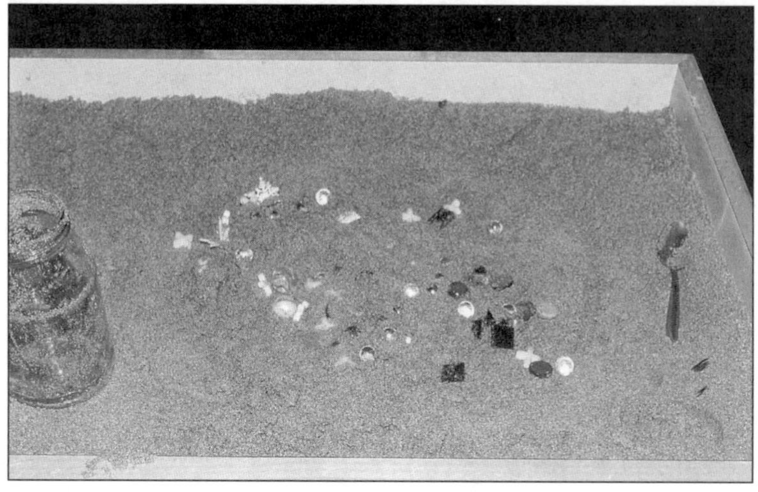

Martina
Tray 32 ~ 2 Months Later

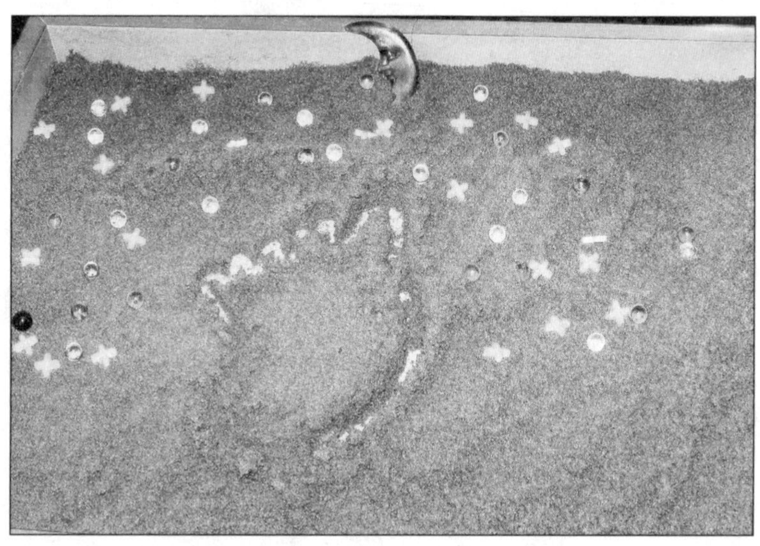

Martina
Tray 34 ~ 4 Months Later

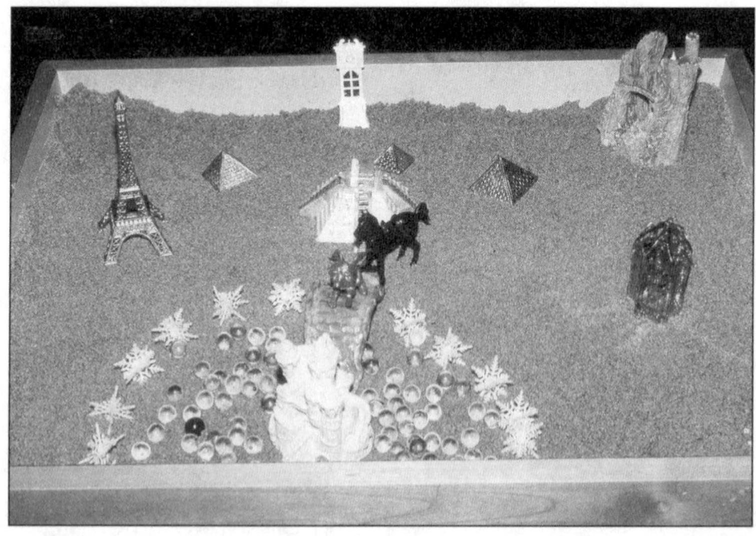

Martina
Tray 36 ~ 6 Months Later

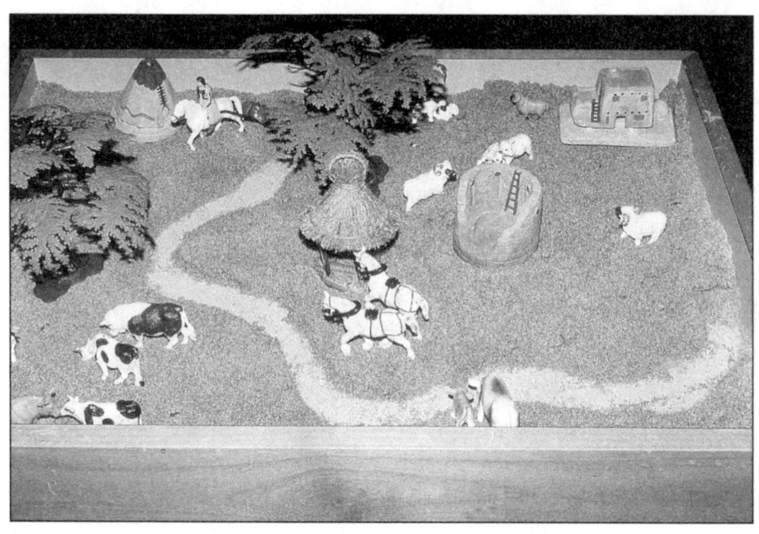

Martina
Tray 38a ~ 4 Months Later

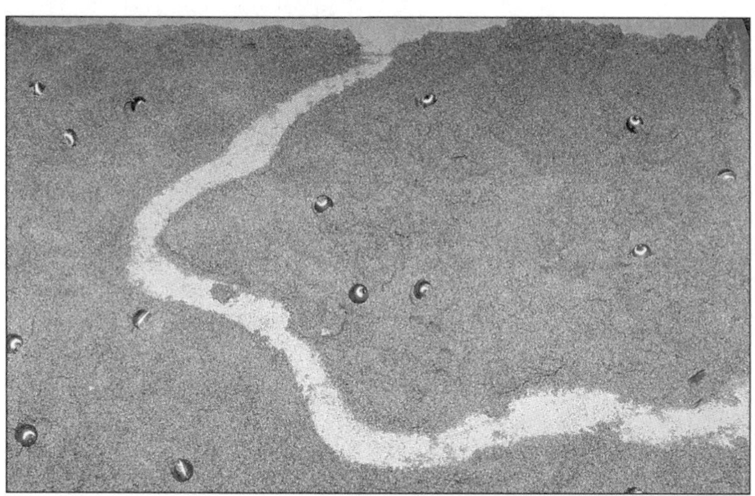

Martina
Tray 38b ~ Detail

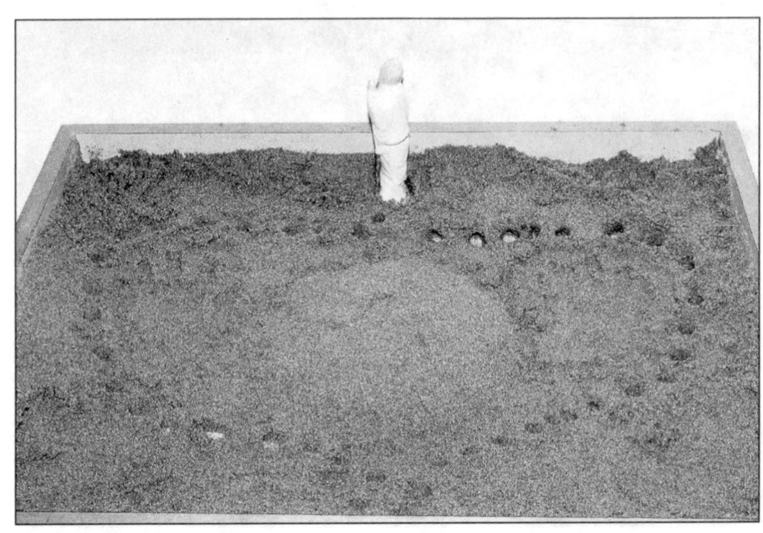

Martina
Tray 40 ~ 6 Months Later

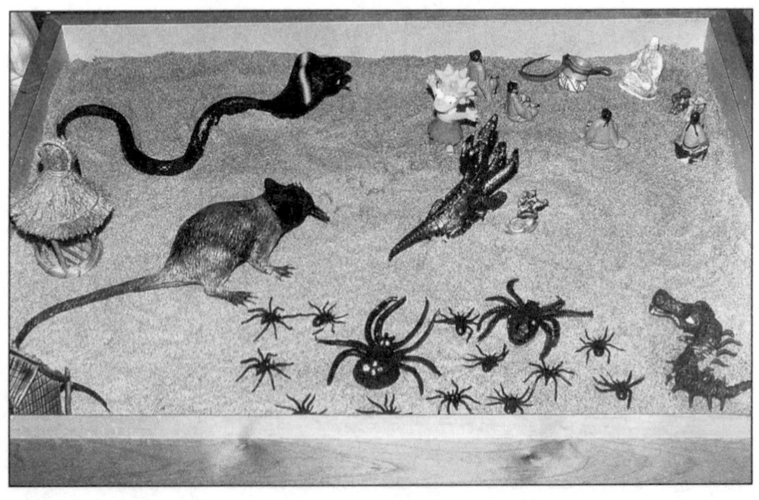

Martina
Tray 41 ~ 1 Month Later

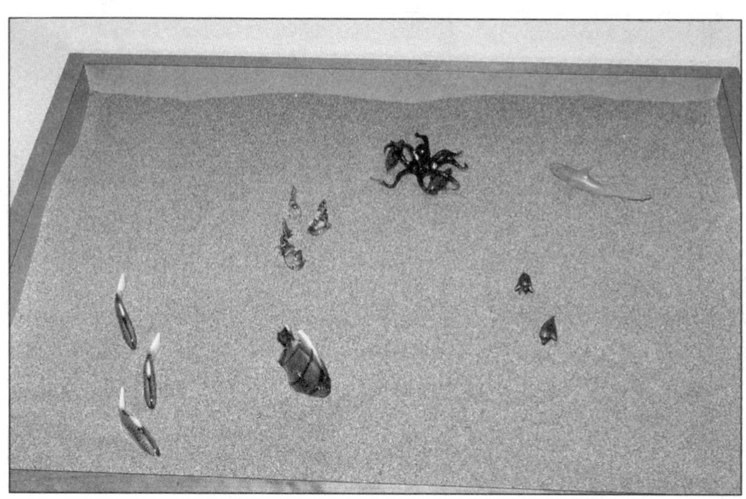

Martina
Tray 42 ~ 1 Month Later

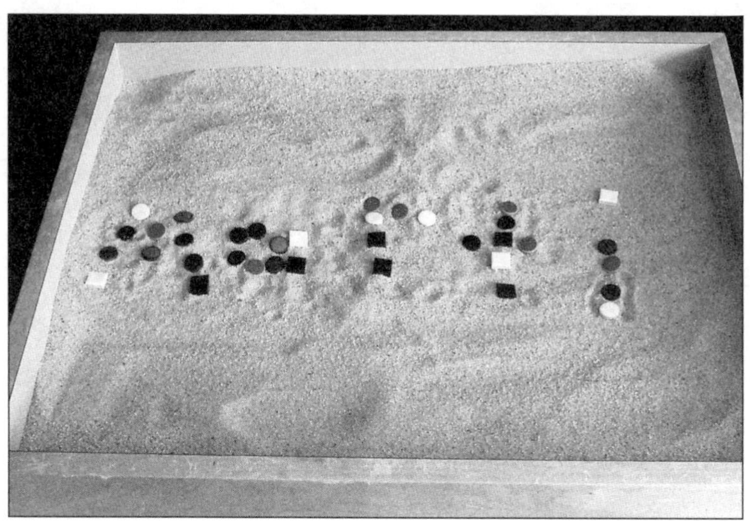

Martina
Tray 44 ~ Final ~ 4 Months Later
6 Years Since Tray 1

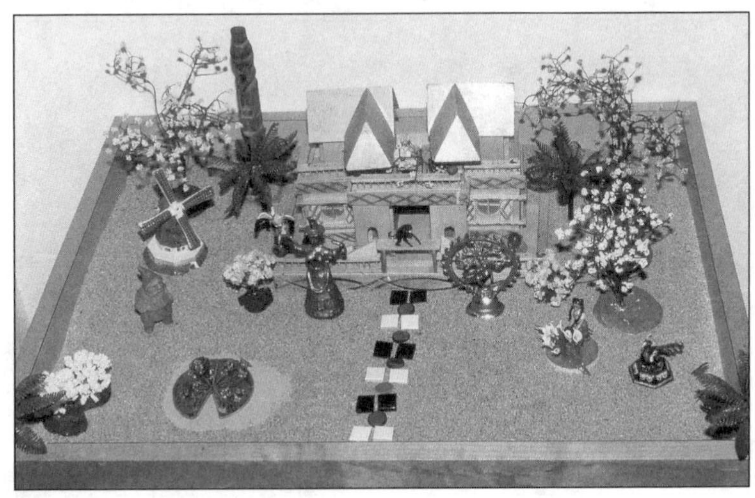

Martina
Tray 45 ~ 3 Years 6 Months Later
Returns For One Visit

Client Profile
NORMAN

Male, mid 40's
Divorced
Two older children living with their mother
Entered therapy to deal with erectile dysfunction and relationship difficulties

Sandplay	Discussed on Page Number
Tray 1	24-5, 301-2
Tray 5	25
Tray 11	
Tray 12	
Tray 13	
Tray 14	

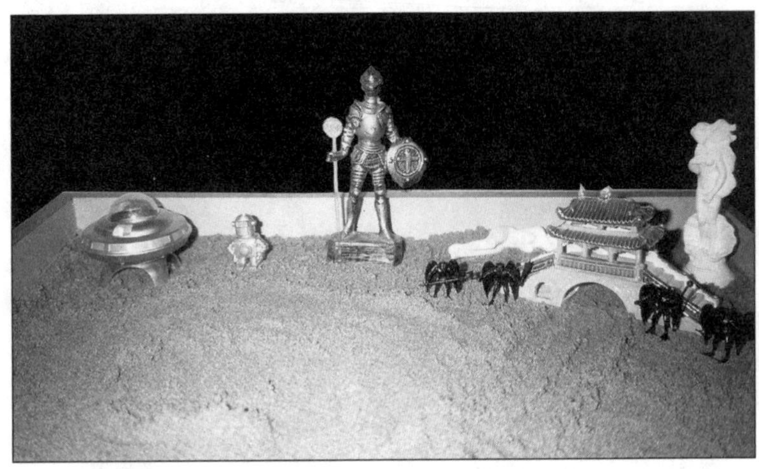

Norman
Tray 1a ~ Several Weeks into Treatment

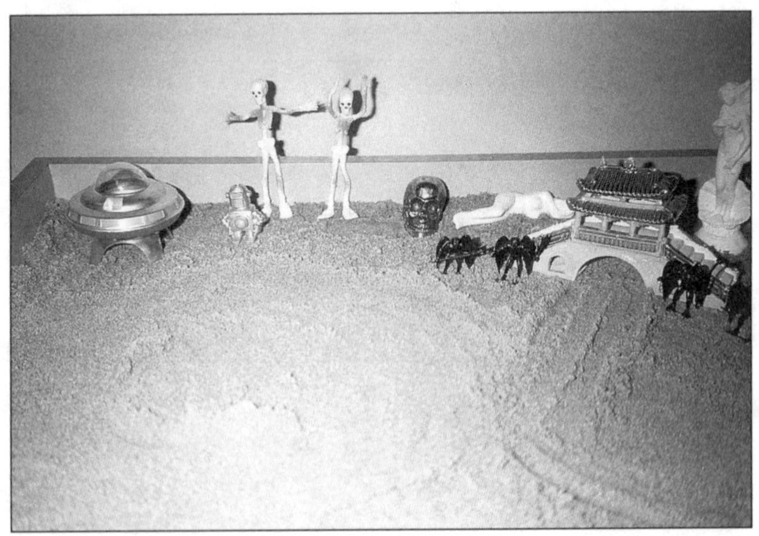

Norman
Tray 1b ~ Detail

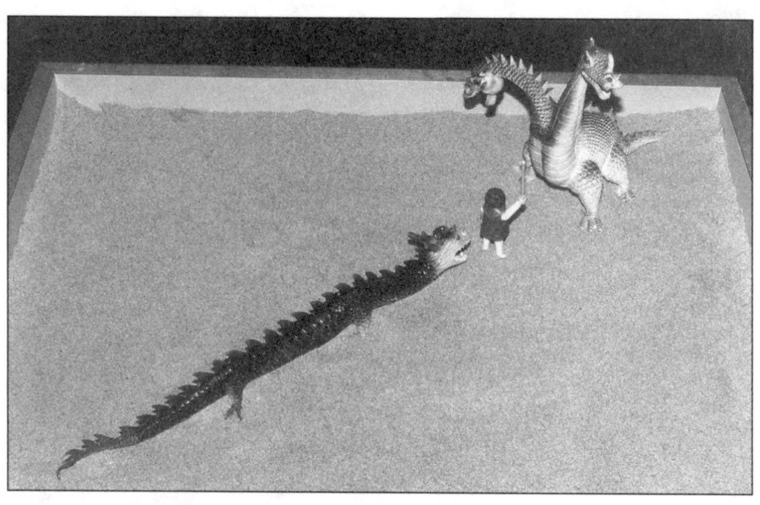

Norman
Tray 5a ~ 1 Year 10 Months Later

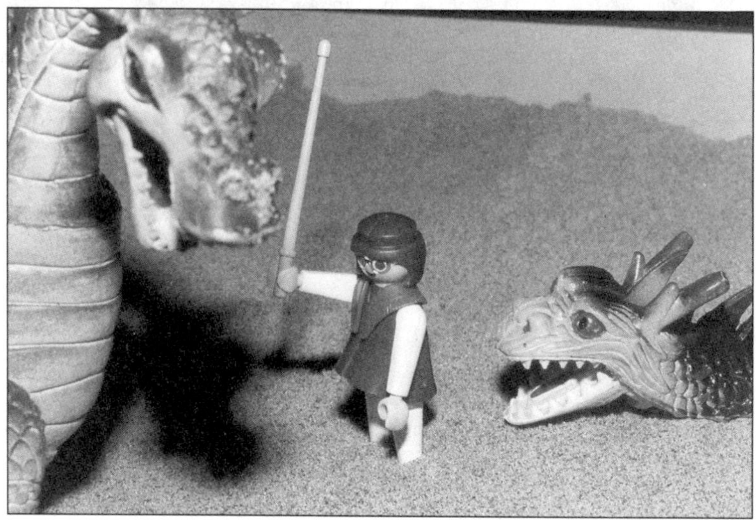

Norman
Tray 5b ~ Detail

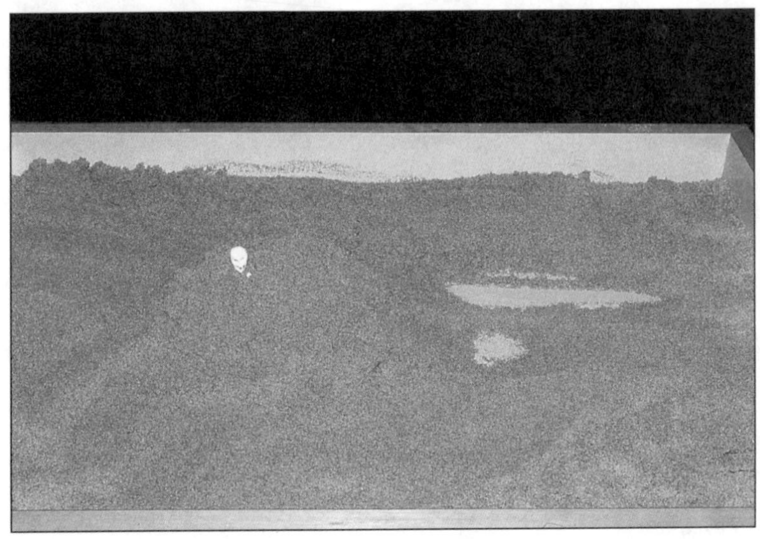

Norman
Tray 11 ~ 6 Months Later

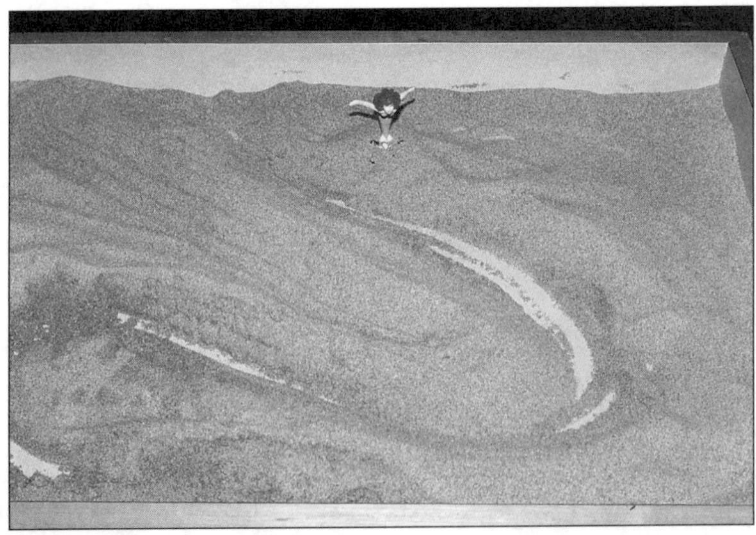

Norman
Tray 12 ~ 1 Week Later

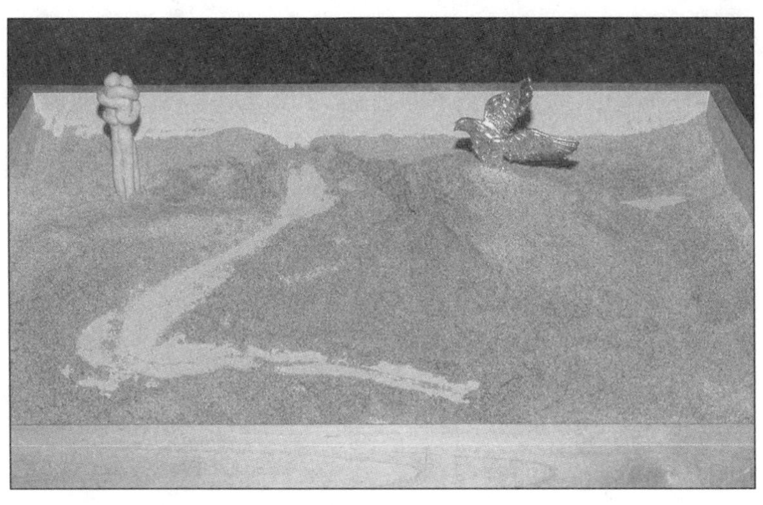

Norman
Tray 13 ~ 6 Weeks Later

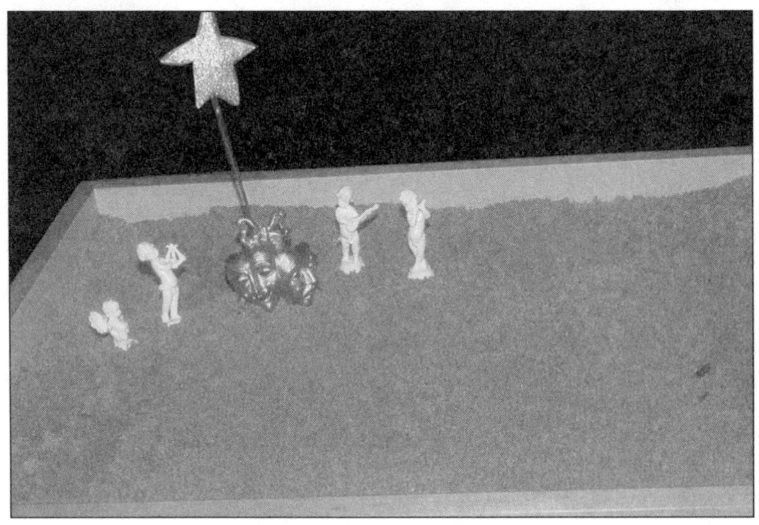

Norman
Tray 14 ~ Final ~ 3 Weeks Later
2 Years 6 Months Since Tray 1

Client Profile

RACHEL

Girl, age fifteen
Extensive history of neglect, physical and sexual abuse, violence
Likely fetal alcohol and/or drug involvement
Both birth parents suffer serious mental illness
Removed from family of origin with 7 siblings, all in foster placements
Mood swings
Academic and social difficulties
Brought to therapy by foster-adopt parents

Sandplay	Discussed on Page Number
Tray 1	216
Tray 5	216
Tray 9	216

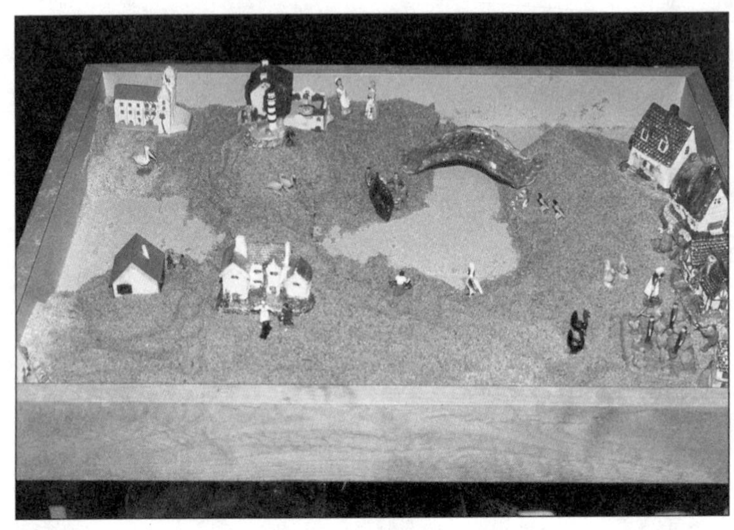

Rachel
Tray 1 ~ Session 1

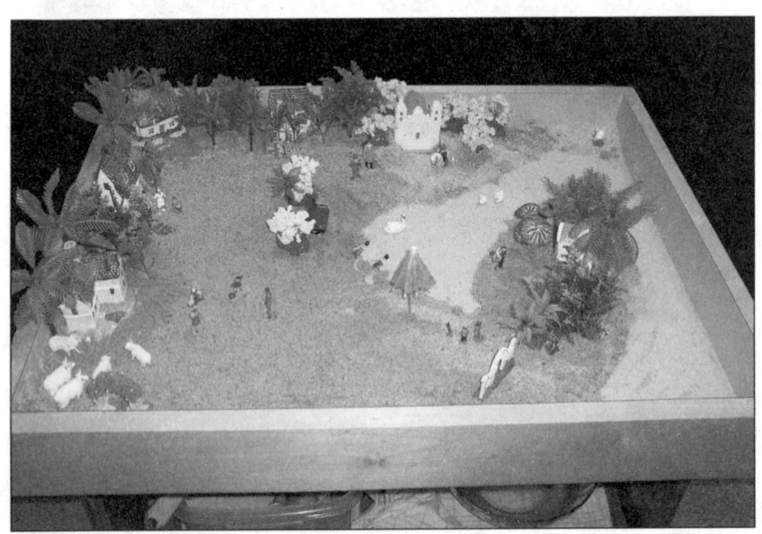

Rachel
Tray 5a ~ 1 Year 10 Months Later

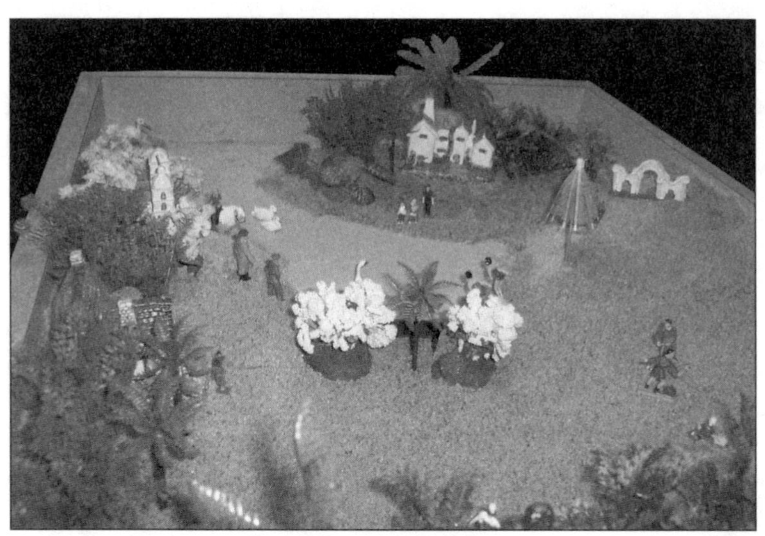

Rachel
Tray 5b ~ Detail

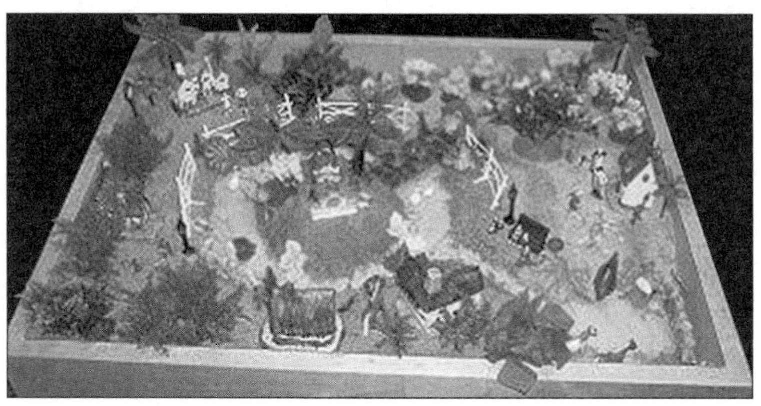

Rachel
Tray 9a ~ Final ~ 8 Months Later
1 Year 9 Months Since Tray 1

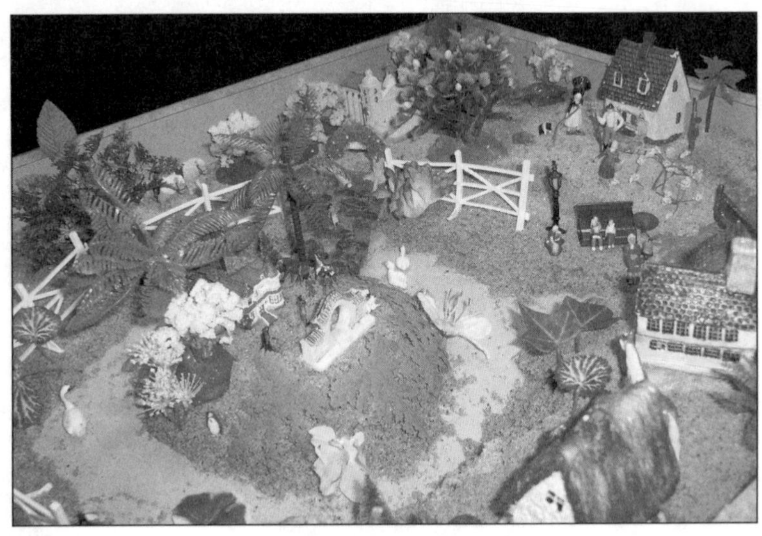

Rachel
Tray 9b ~ Detail

Client Profile

REGINA

Girl, age 7
Mother and Father drug and alcohol addicted
Born positive for amphetamines
Unstable, street life with Mother
Father not involved with child
Removed from Mother's care following Mother's arrest for attempted murder
Child witnessed crime
Recently moved into stable home with paternal grandparents
Academic and social developmental delays

Sandplay	Discussed on Page Number
Tray 1	172-3
Tray 2	172-3
Tray 3	173
Tray 7	173
Tray 12	

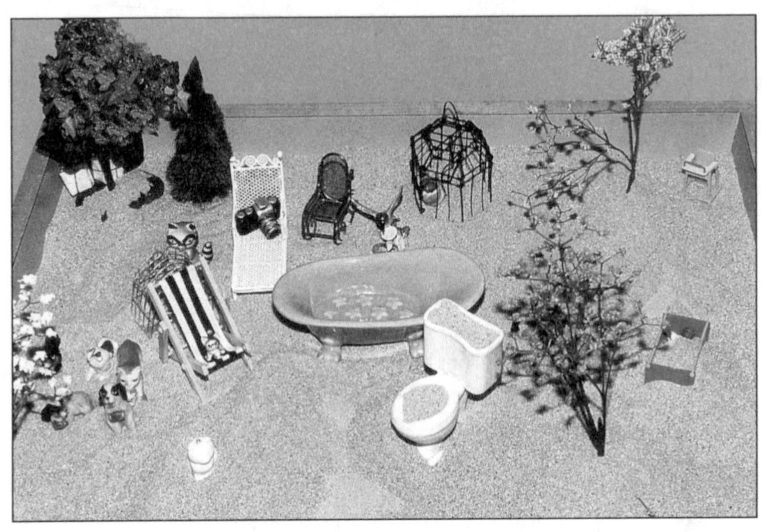

Regina
Tray 1 ~ Session 1

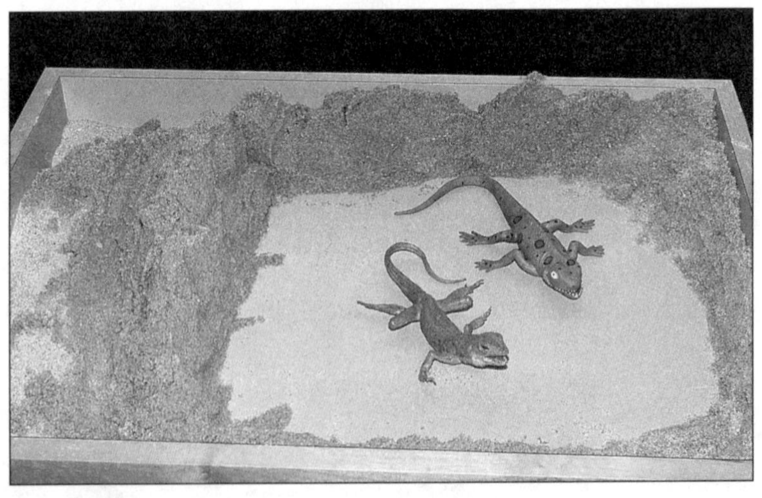

Regina
Tray 2 ~ Same Session

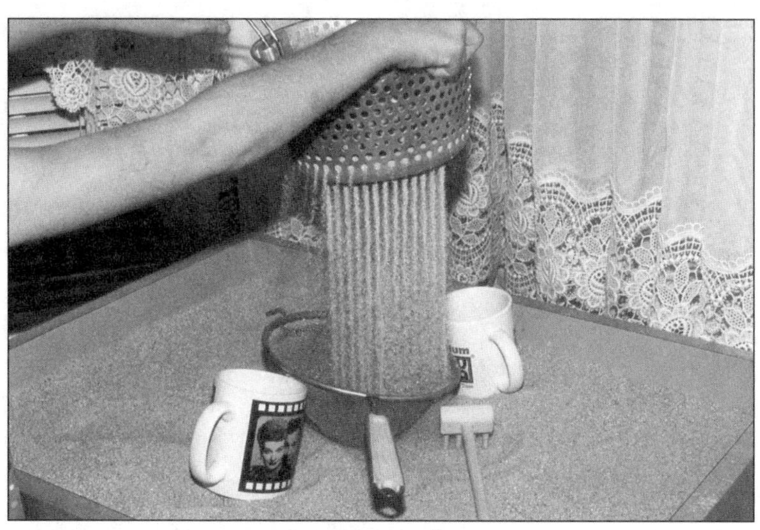

Regina
Tray 3 ~ 1 Week Later

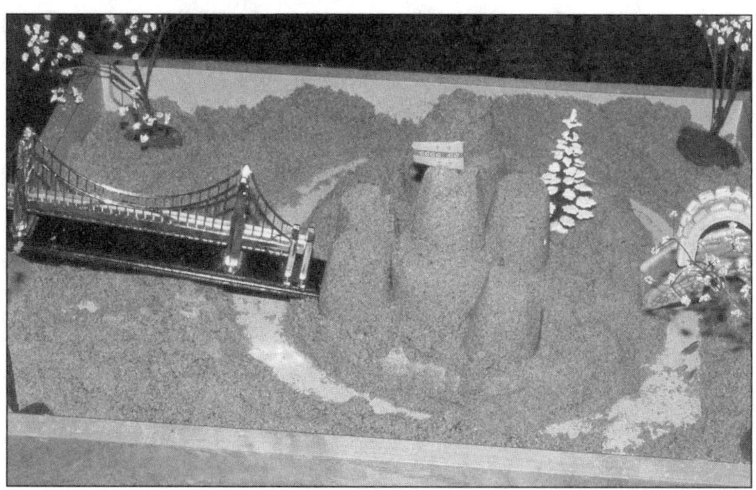

Regina
Tray 7 ~ 4 Months Later

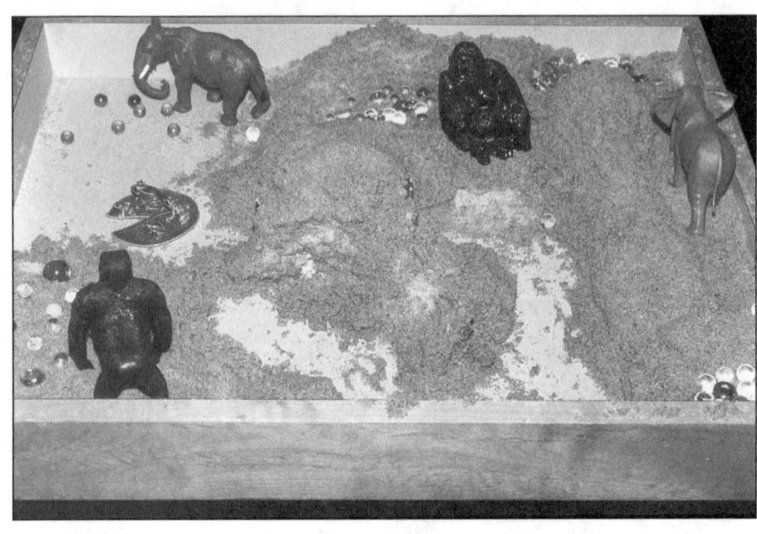

Regina
Tray 12a ~ Final ~ 1 Year Later
1 Year 5 Months Since Tray 1

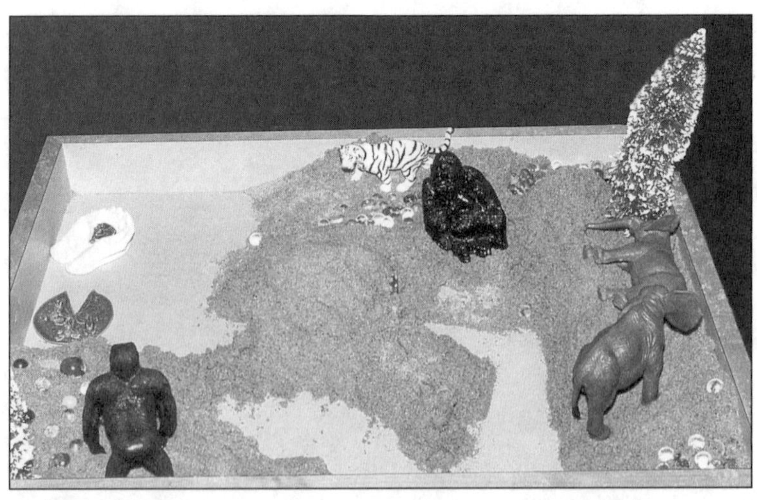

Regina
Tray 12b ~ Detail

Client Profile
ROSA

Girl, age 12
Oldest of three siblings, one sister, one brother
Fundamentalist religious sect
Mother and Father have some high school education
Mother reports child has been moody since age 9 and began over eating heavily at age 10.5
Born 6 weeks prematurely
Pregnancy was healthy - 70 hour labor
No friends
Does poorly in school

Sandplay	Discussed on Page Number
Tray 1	18, 278-80
Tray 2	278-80
Tray 3	278-80

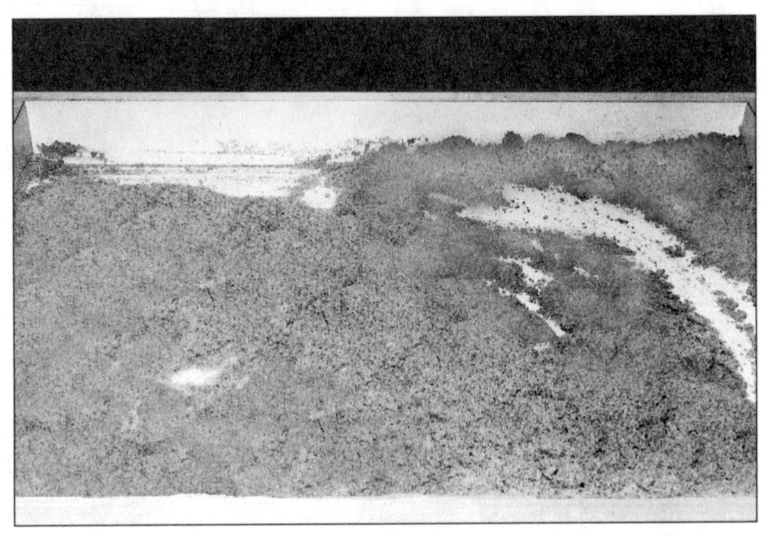

Rosa
Tray 1 ~ Session 1

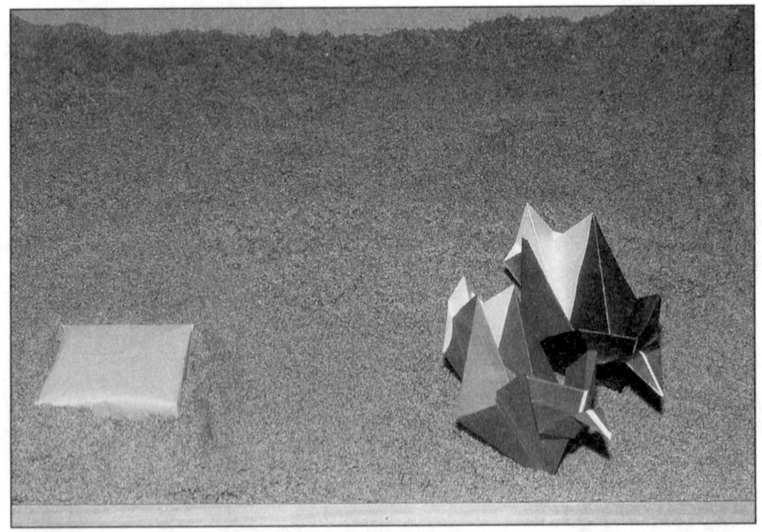

Rosa
Tray 2 ~ 1 Month Later

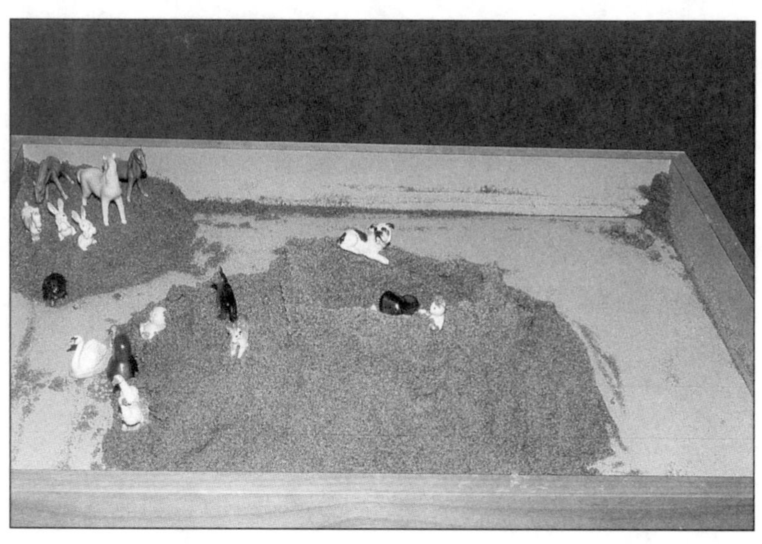

Rosa
Tray 3a ~ Final ~ 1 Week Later
6 Weeks Since Tray 1

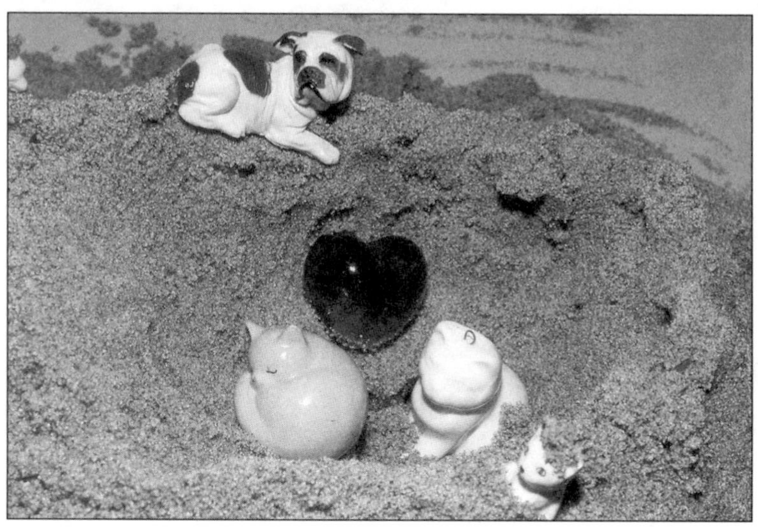

Rosa
Tray 3b ~ Detail

Client Profile
SANDER

Boy, age 7
Middle child of three
Chronic parental conflict
Serious emotional distress during pregnancy
Brought to therapy by Mother, who is concerned about child's disturbed sleep, nightmares and fears of being alone

Sandplay	Discussed on Page Number
Tray 1	
Tray 9	230
Tray 22	
Tray 23	

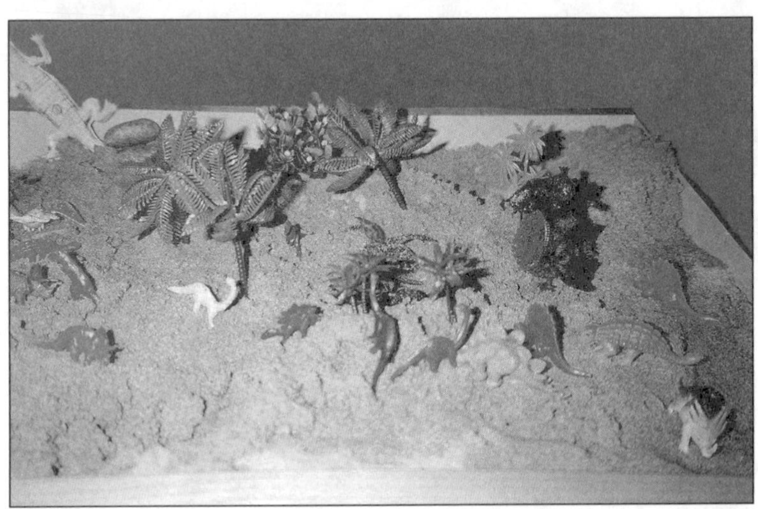

Sander Tray 1 ~ Session 1

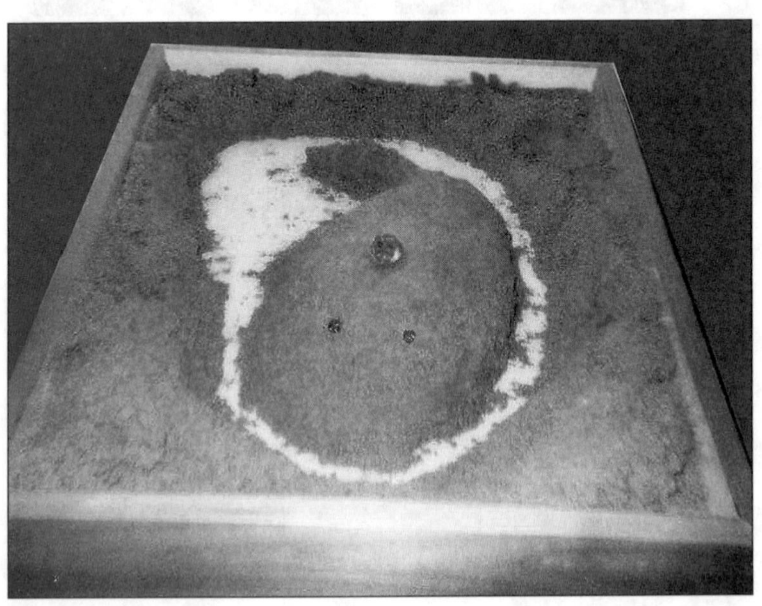

Sander
Tray 9 ~ 4 Months Later

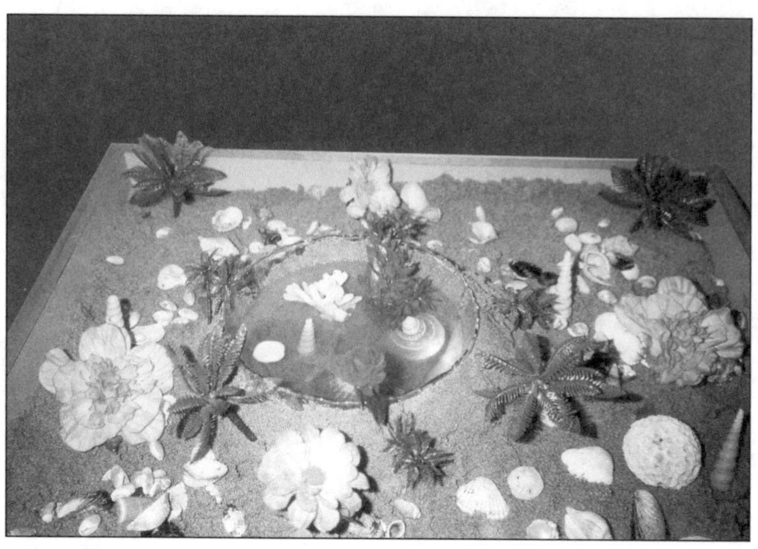

Sander
Tray 22 ~ 11 Months Later

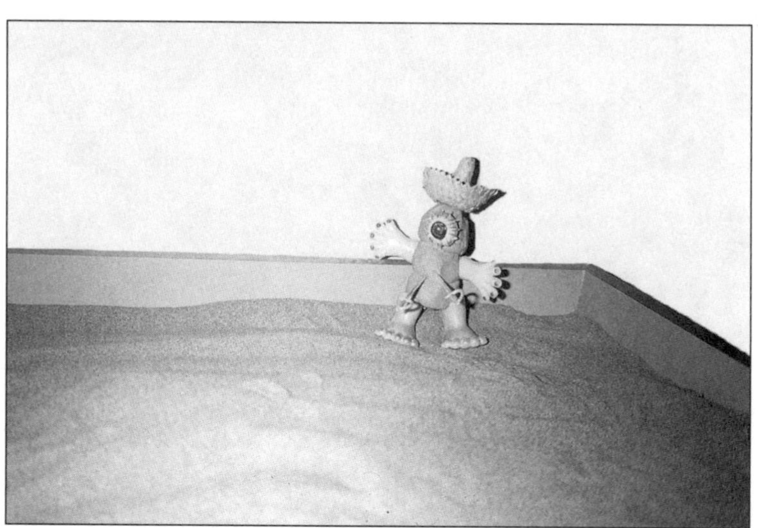

Sander Tray 23 ~ Final ~ 1 Week Later
1 Year 4 Months Since Tray 1

Client Profile

SHANNON

Woman, mid forties
Divorced
Self-educated
Two older sisters - oldest suffers serious developmental delays, close to middle sister
Alcoholic parents, neglectful
Childhood sexual abuse
Describes herself as always unhappy
Entered therapy to gain a "*...new perspective on life*"

Sandplay	Discussed on Page Number
Tray 1	266, 375
Tray 6	266
Tray 8	232, 266
Tray 10	232
Tray 15	266
Tray 17	266
Tray 39	373, 375

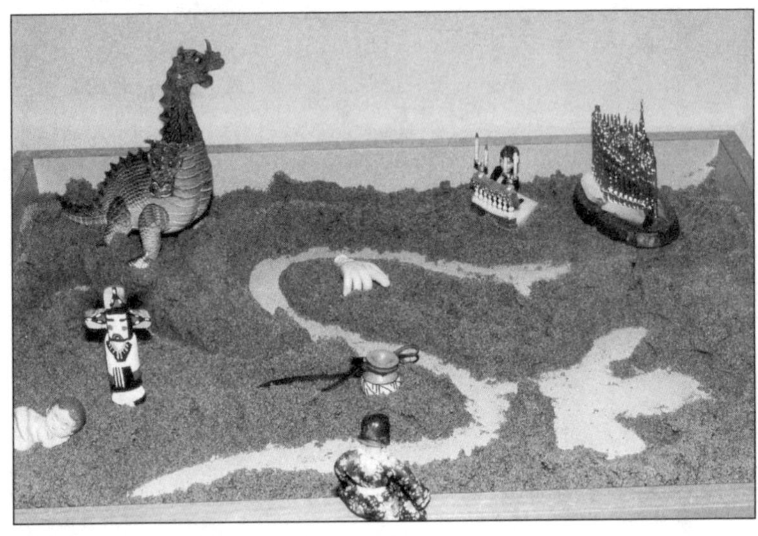

Shannon
Tray 1 ~ 1 Year 4 Months into Treatment

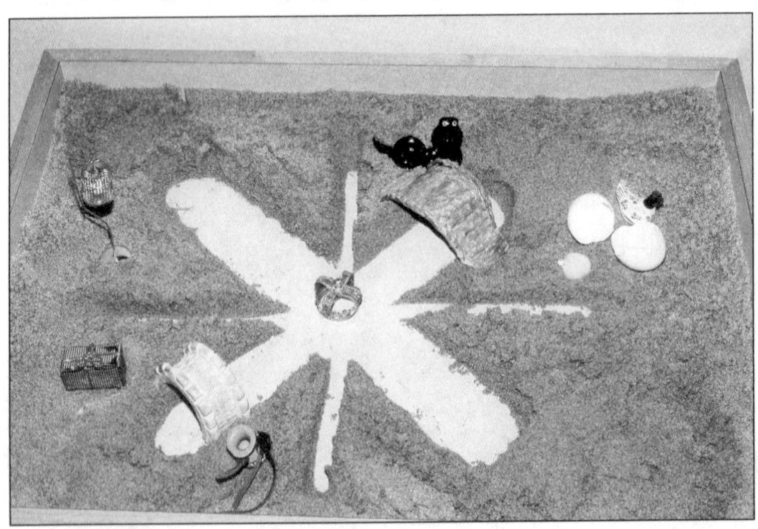

Shannon
Tray 6 ~ 6 Weeks Later

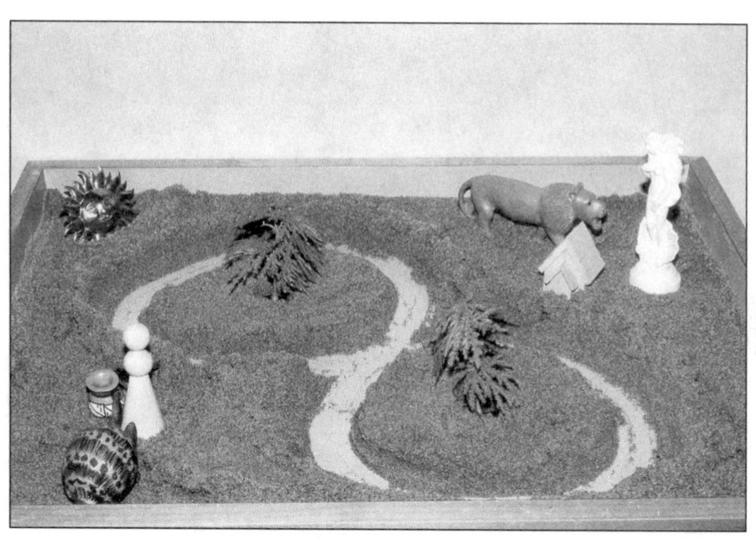

Shannon
Tray 8 ~ 6 Weeks Later

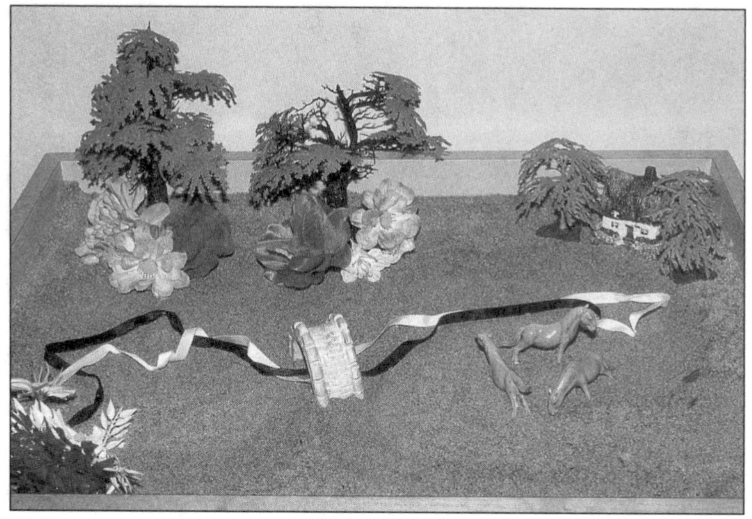

Shannon
Tray 10 ~ 5 Weeks Later

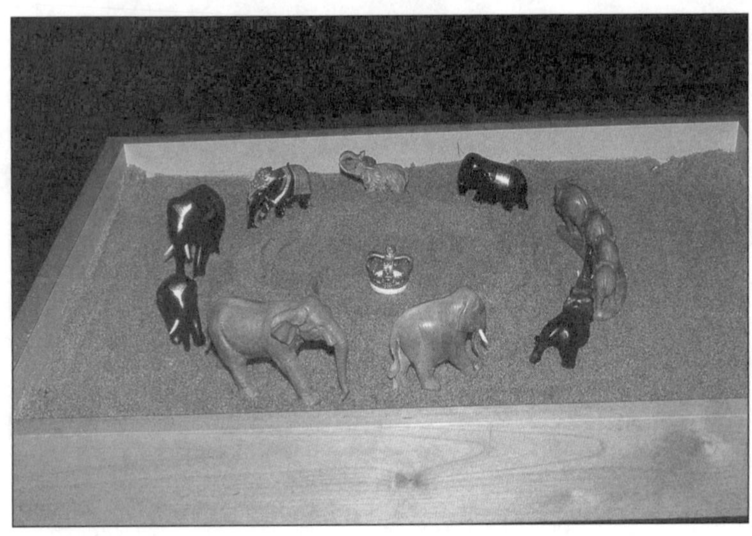

Shannon
Tray 15 ~ 3 Months Later

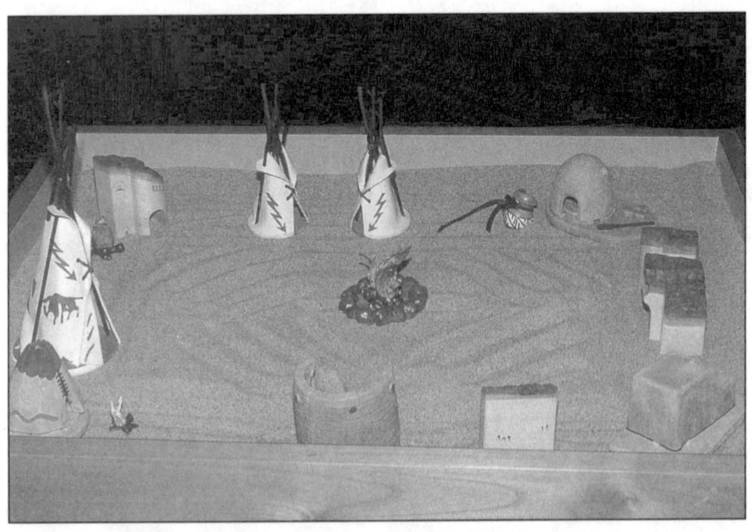

Shannon
Tray 17 ~ 3 Weeks Later

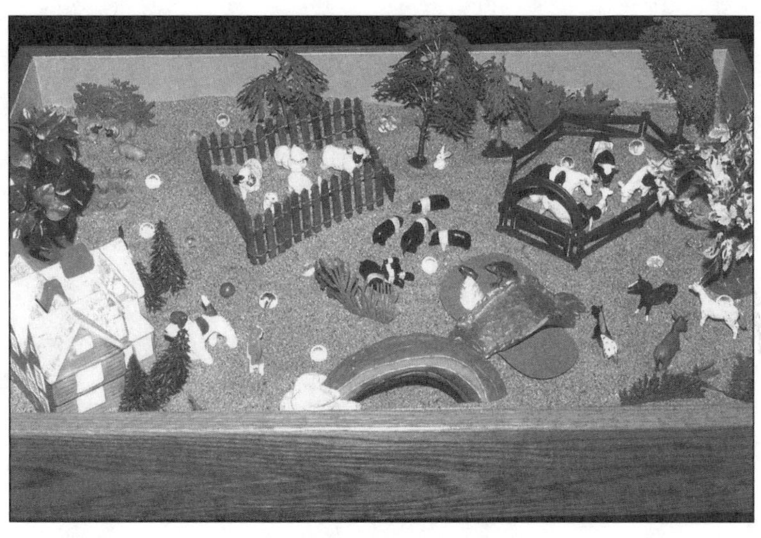

Shannon
Tray 39 ~ Final ~ 10 Years 9 Months Later
11 Years 4 Months Since Tray 1

Client Profile
TARA

Woman, age 32
Entered therapy to address relationship issues
History of childhood sexual abuse

Sandplay	Discussed on Page Number
Tray 1	18, 233
Tray 19	
Tray 20	19

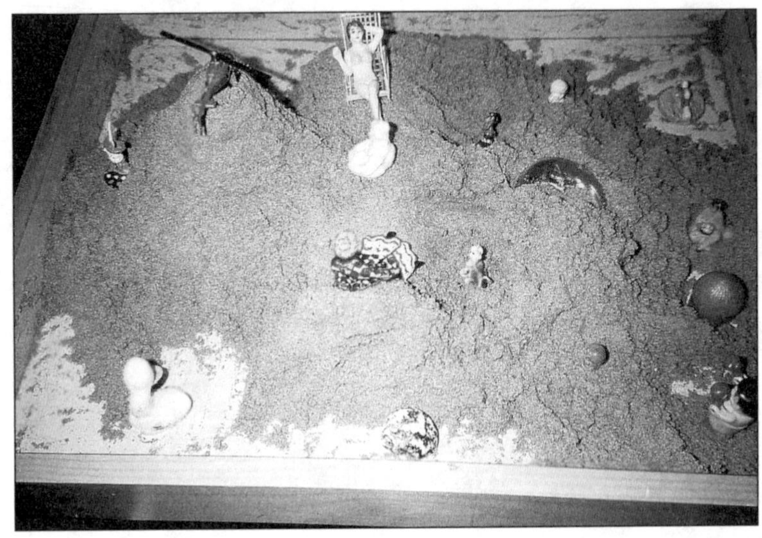

Tara
Tray 1 ~ 1 Month into Treatment

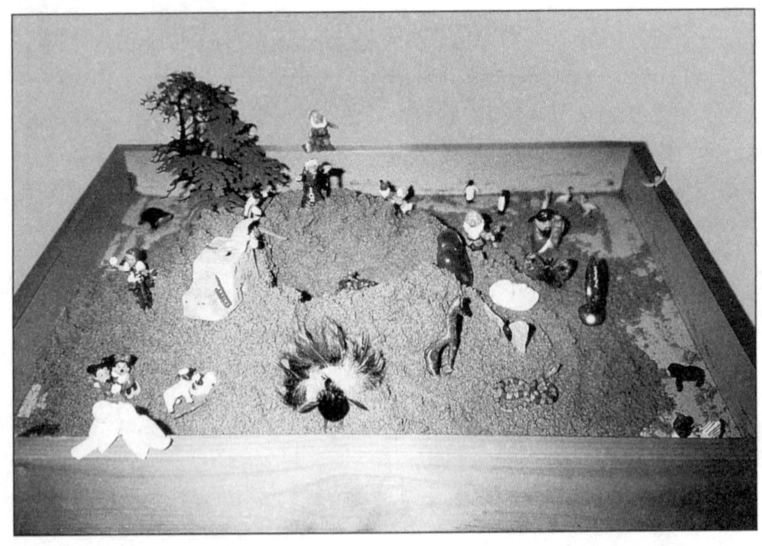

Tara
Tray 19 ~ 11 Months Later

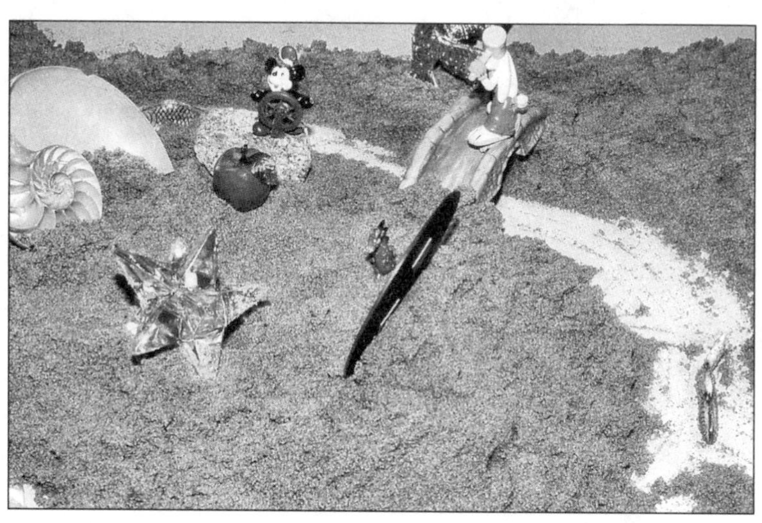

Tara
Tray 20a ~ Final ~ 6 Months Later
1 Year 5 Months Since Tray 1

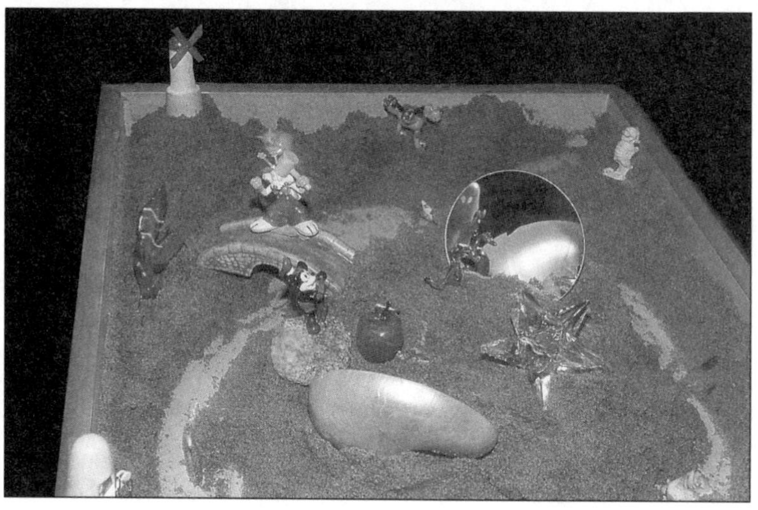

Tara
Tray 20b ~ Detail

The Sandplay Case of Aaron

A Nine-year-old Boy Defines His Masculinity

What follows is an example of a written account of a completed sandplay case. Sandplay cases are generally analyzed and written up in this manner when they are used as learning and teaching tools. I have chosen Aaron's work in order to complete the documentation of his case material, which includes the photographs of each tray, the Sandplay Record Forms, and the Subjective Immersion Analysis log.

We know that there is no complete or right way to fully account for the complexities of symbolic process. What we hope to achieve in a written case is a penetrating account of the work that adequately encompasses the scope of the transformational process. At the same time the written account must demonstrate a deep respect for the sandplay process and its proper containment.

Note: For pictures of the trays described in the case, please refer to Aaron's sandplay pictures in the previous section

Introduction

This is the sandplay case of a nine-year-old boy who elected to have himself referred to by the pseudonym, "Aaron Smith." Aaron was brought into therapy by his mother in February of 1990, as he experienced frequent outbursts of rage. His mother explained that Aaron, an otherwise quiet and highly responsible boy, had been having trouble with these angry outbursts since her separation and subsequent divorce from Aaron's father two years prior to treatment. Aaron was the middle child of three. His older sister was an energetic teenager who was involved in numerous activities outside the home. In keeping with his serious and responsible nature, it fell to Aaron to look after his younger seven-year-old brother on their visits with their father on alternating weekends.

Aaron's mother explained that Aaron's father was actively alcoholic and drug dependent, that he had used methamphetamines, and that he had a violent temper. Mrs. Smith recounted that Aaron's father screamed at him, and that Aaron had witnessed his father pounding his fist through walls during violent fits of rage. Aaron's mother appeared to have a sincere and earnest concern for the protection and wellbeing of her sons. She said that although she truly hoped the boys would be able to develop a good relationship with their father, she feared for their safety. Mrs. Smith commented that her former husband had recently become interested in guns. She had secured a restraining order to prohibit the boys' visits if the father were drinking or using drugs. Regarding Aaron's explosive outbursts, she confided that she was "beginning to see his father in him and was frightened."

Mrs. Smith, a refined, articulate woman of Jewish heritage, explained that Aaron had admitted to discomfort and embarrassment at some of his father's life style choices, particularly his interest in motorcycles. Although his father was Italian Catholic by heritage, Aaron was active in the synagogue, and he was currently in Hebrew school preparing for his bar mitzvah. It soon became apparent that, in addition to having to address the impact of the divorce and the attendant financial hardship on his family, Aaron would have a considerable challenge reconciling and integrating the temperamental life style and religious disparities between his very different parents. Furthermore, the discovery and definition of his own sense of masculinity in the context of this family that modeled two substantially different ways of being in the world would prove a demanding obstacle to Aaron's development.

The discovery and definition of his own uniqueness in this tumultuous family context of violence, divorce, and very different cultural and religious backgrounds was no small task for this nine-year-old, yet the sublime and wondrous drive of the psyche to reorder and heal was manifest in the protective container of his sandplay work. Aaron completed a total of 15 sand trays in his 30 sessions, which encompassed his 18 months of treatment. In October 1995, over five years subsequent to the end of treatment, Aaron returned with his mother to review his sandplay process. Now fifteen, a football player, doing well in school and deeply religious, it was a moving experience to look back together at this difficult, yet profoundly healing work undergone so many years before.

Sand Tray Number 1
Description

This tray was done in wet sand. It has an island formed in the middle of the tray by a waterway that approximates the number nine reversed if regarded from the left side of the tray. A tall silver knight stands on a hill in the center of the island. Three black clothed ninja warriors stand toward the front center of the island. A bridge connects the island with a peninsula on the left. A racecar approaches the island on the bridge, followed by a police squad car. Toward the near left of the tray, two Oriental men gaze into a crystal ball. In the far left corner, a wild animal tamer faces a large tiger. Behind the tiger stands a large oak tree in the center back of the tray. A small deciduous tree grows on the small island on the left. In the far right corner of the tray two skiers race down a steep hill behind Batman, Robin, the Riddler and the Penguin, who encounter one another on the right side of the tray by a bright red raft.

Sand Tray Number 1
Analysis

Prominent in this tray is the large, central figure of the knight, who stands facing the left side of the tray. His back is to the right. Perhaps he looks in the direction of the unconscious for something new to come as he turns his back on the ways of the battles of the super heroes, Batman and Robin, who now appear comedic and absurd. Standing higher and larger than all else save the lone oak on his right hand, the knight appears stiff and cold. Removed from the other figures because of his height and the heavy metal encasement, perhaps the tall knight speaks to Aaron's subjective experience of object relatedness, painfully holding his aloofness, his guardedness, and perhaps a certain lack of grounding. Disconnected and unable to make contact with the other figures in this tray, the knight's metal encasement works not only to protect him from what transpires around him, but to hold him captive. Upon completion of the tray, Aaron reflected that, "This is a statue of a guy who fought."

The knight shares his central island with three Asian ninja warriors. Poised in a threatening stance, they impose a fearsome face in the front, central portion of the tray. This fierce persona stands in dramatic contrast to the knight, all locked up, cut off and cold in his steel prison behind. With a profound sense of sadness, I wondered what aspects of Aaron's character, personality, and deeper self had to retreat to this encasement, as if his survival depended upon it.

Speeding across the bridge to the central island comes a hot racecar, followed closely by a squad car. Perhaps there is a sense that justice will be brought to this speeding, unlawful way of being in the world. Perhaps there is a reference here to justice and rectitude being brought to Aaron's relationship with his father, who used speed and was somewhat of an outlaw. Notably, both cars are headed in the direction of the central knight. Perhaps they allude to help being on its way, or to a sense of life and vitality that might help free the central figure from his metal prison.

Two Asian men sit meditating contemplatively on the little island by the police car. They gaze into a crystal ball, as if looking toward the future. One wonders what they see. Do they see the way out? Upon completing the tray, Aaron commented that, "The Chinese guys are doing magic." In contrast with many of the other elements of this tray, the Oriental figures seem calm and still. Older wise men from the East, perhaps this portion of Aaron's first sand tray holds a wise, spiritual part of himself far off in his own psyche. Perhaps the two wise men, as rudimentary poles of duality, refer to an aspect of this boy that begs to manifest. Perhaps it is the wholeness of the Self that they contemplate between them as the crystal orb. Perhaps they, along with the graceful and well-balanced male and female skiers on the diagonal to the upper right, allude to the direction of Aaron's healing as a balanced integration of masculine and feminine elements oriented toward a spiritual wholeness. This ordering toward wholeness is mirrored by the backdrop of the tall oak tree. Known for its strength, longevity, and immortality, it is related to the Sun king as masculine, and is sacred to the Great Goddess as feminine. (De Vries, 1984, pp.347-348)

These two Oriental men are very different from their warring counterparts on the central island, who are all dressed in black, brandishing weapons and posturing for attack. The serenity of the two Asian wise men gives the sense that Aaron was very tired of having to posture angrily as they do. In contemplating this first tray, I wondered if Aaron was not very tired of feeling he had to fight all of the time, pretending to be a ninja, or a super hero like Batman or Robin. I wondered if he did not long to be free, like the two skiers, gliding so joyfully down the slope behind Robin in the upper right corner. It was painfully apparent though, that he would be unable to ski while undeveloped or suppressed aspects of his psyche remained confined to this steel cage. It was also clear that the fuller expression of himself would not be able to emerge until he had developed the psychological and circumstantial tools he required to be safe. The small green tree in the left of the tray is a hopeful reference to the potential for growth and development.

Significantly, there is a bridge connecting the central island of the knight with the Eastern wise men and the police. The bridge was the first figure Aaron placed in the tray. As the initial gesture in his first sand tray (after shaping the sand in the shape of a figure "nine," his age at the time,) Aaron's sandplay process functioned to form a connection between these hitherto disassociated aspects of his psyche. Immediately subsequent to making his "signature number nine," Aaron set about re-ordering his sense of who he was to the Self. As he placed this bridge, these aspects of himself formed a connection, setting in motion a formidable process of healing and development. In the free and protected space of the sand tray and the watchful containment of the therapist, Aaron launched immediately into the process of establishing a way he could be safe in the combative and difficult circumstances of his world, remaining rooted in the spiritual, and perhaps gentler, aspects of himself as a male.

Across the water to the right of the metal knight, a wild animal tamer faces a huge tiger. Standing directly in front of the tiger, unprotected, it appears that the animal trainer has a lot of work to do to tame this beast. Yet with his left hand raised to this fierce presence, he appears confident of his position. He knows what he is doing. Perhaps the tiger wants his raging ways tamed and is glad there is an able trainer here. The tiger's apparent respect for the tamer's gesture might function as a transference allusion to Aaron's unconscious sense of the healing containment that is possible in his sandplay process.

It is not difficult to imagine how that part of Aaron's psyche that feels constrained to living behind the steel armor of the knight might manifest itself as the rage of this tiger. The devastation of the divorce and the shameful financial hardship resulting from his father's drug and alcohol use hurt Aaron deeply. Additionally, Aaron's father's modeling of what it means to be a man disappointed him deeply. It demonstrated that to be a man, he must fight and be tough, leaving no room for Aaron's real and gentle strength. Aaron's father left the family in a painful and hurtful way. It is easy to understand the sources of Aaron's pain. After a while, that hurt becomes hard and turns to rage.

Sand Tray Number 2
Description

Tray two was done in wet sand. There is a square enclosure molded from sand in the upper left corner within which a small boxer defeats a larger enemy. A rutabaga vegetable man and a banana lady look on from the upper left corner. A small boxer stands on a mound on the left center of the tray. Mickey Mouse videotapes the boxing match while Minnie acts as a cheerleader. Behind the small deciduous tree in the front left corner stands a small duck figure holding a golden spyglass to its eye pointed in the direction of Scrooge McDuck in the center who holds a gold coin in his hand. Behind another small green tree, Mickey, Minnie and Pluto convene in a circle in the upper right hand corner, while Dorothy, the Tin Man, the Cowardly Lion and the Scarecrow from the *Wizard of Oz* (Hearn, 1973) encounter the witch who stands to the right of the old oak tree in the back center of the tray. Glenda the good witch looks on from the upper right corner edge of the tray. A small blond Gretel from "Hansel and Gretel" (Grimm, 1972) stands face to face with a large gray wolf in the front right corner, while a Smurf with a large wooden mallet sneaks up behind another to knock him on the head.

Sand Tray Number 2
Analysis

As he began clearing the square area in the upper left corner of the sand tray, Aaron announced that he, "...was thinking of making a 'cartoon land' today." Here he fashions a fantasy world, allowing a colorful and imaginative aspect of his creative inner life to emerge as he continues his healing journey.

Standing on a mound at the left of the tray, a small boxer calmly surveys the many activities in this tray. He stands above things, as if to get a clear view of what transpires around him. Directly in front of him to the left, a duplicate of himself defeats a huge opponent with a swift blow. The square clearing has become a boxing ring, a defined and regulated arena for battle. Mickey and Minnie Mouse look on. Minnie cheers the victory as Mickey videotapes the event so that it will be recorded and preserved for all to see. They appear excited and exuberant in their celebration of the defeat of this enemy. Their red clothing and pompons are affirming in their energetic witnessing. Perhaps Aaron begins to tap the source of his own vitality and feeling in relation to this budding aspect of his own empowerment.

A very odd couple stands to the upper left on the opposite side of the boxing arena. The man is a goofy looking vegetable and the woman is a gorgeous banana lady. One wonders how it is that this fruit and vegetable are paired as they are different species and appear ludicrous as a couple. Perhaps this is Aaron's comic representation of the marriage of his mother and father. They, too, were so different as to be a different species. Perhaps Aaron begins to attempt to reconcile this aspect of his heritage as this odd couple witnesses the small fighter (a normal looking young man) defeat his opponent. It appears important that they be here. They stand very close and on the side of the opponent.

In the center of the tray, the elder Scrooge McDuck displays a gold coin in his open palm as the younger duck regards it through his golden spyglass from behind the tree in the front left corner. It is as if the crystal orb from the first tray takes even greater definition as the gold of the Self and assumes a central focus in this sand tray. It is clearly seen, perhaps held as a possibility, as the younger duck looks to his elder for wisdom and direction. Perhaps this inner treasure that presages the Self emerges as Aaron's psyche rallies to overcome his oversized opponents in his family context.

Far across the tray on the upper right another representation of Minnie and Mickey Mouse stand gaily engaged in talk with a roller skating Pluto. Aaron commented that Pluto, "...was skating in and fell over." Perhaps Aaron's instinctual animal nature is beginning to emerge and has not yet found a stable footing. They all appear happy, smiling as they talk together. Perhaps Aaron needed these fantasy friends to help him understand what life was like and to serve as a compensatory relief from his hurts and sorrows just to survive. Aaron does appear to make productive use of his rich fantasy life. For whatever comic relief it affords him, it is suffuse with the content of his inner and outer struggles and is anything but pure escapism.

Toward the front right, sweet little Gretel reaches out to the wolf. Aaron described this as "scary" saying, "He is trying to eat her." In the Grimm's (1972) fairy tale, Gretel lost her way in the woods, as she and her brother Hansel were cast out of their home by their wicked step mother and compliant father when there was not enough to feed them. Lured by a wicked witch deep in the woods, Hansel is imprisoned in a steel cage until Gretel effects his rescue by overcoming the cruel old witch. As with the encasement of Aaron's masculinity behind the cold steel armor of the knight in the first tray, it begins to appear that the assistance of this young emerging feminine figure is necessary to bring about his release. The young, healthy, and innocent feminine energy must assist by transforming the witch who embodies the dark qualities of the repressed feminine.

In the fairy tale, Gretel laments at their predicament, "If the wild beasts in the forest had but devoured us, we should at any rate have died together." (Grimm, 1972, p. 92) In the sand tray she faces the wolf who is the wild counterpart to the cartoon dog Pluto. Will he devour her? At this moment in the process they stand in dramatic tension.

Contemporary developmental research indicates that modern Western culture demands severe sacrifices of both its girls and boys (Gilligan, 1993; Levinson, 1978; Miller, 1984, 1986 & 1991). Girls in adolescence are required to surrender their voice, which is their connection to their inner feminine nature, as a consequence of wanting to maintain relationship in the culture. Boys in latency are required to push away the mother, who is their teacher and guide to their own inner feminine qualities. A boy's prolonged closeness to his mother is considered a threat to patriarchal culture's demands for autonomy in its males. Historically and symbolically, the witch carries these cast off aspects of the feminine: the relatedness that is forbidden the boy and the voice that is denied the girl (Turner, 1996a; 1996b). For the male to re-own the witch (to reintegrate these powerful disowned aspects of himself) he must establish connection with others and learn to maintain a sense of self in connection. For the female to re-own her witch, she must own her uniqueness, honor her strengths, and maintain this self in the relational context. Each gender must come to honor both the masculine and feminine qualities in themselves and each other, working cooperatively in a new paradigm of connectedness.

Reference to the witch is made three times in this sand tray. In the back central portion of the tray, Dorothy, the Cowardly Lion, the Scarecrow, and the Tin Man encounter the Wicked Witch as Glenda the Good Witch looks on from above and behind them. Although the Witch is terrifying, each of these characters has needs and is not about to give up. The Tin Man needs a heart so he can feel. The Scarecrow needs a brain so he can think clearly. The Cowardly Lion needs courage so he can live without fear. And Dorothy needs to find her way back home (Hearn, 1973). All of these missing aspects of Aaron must face the horror of this witch in order to find what has been lost. Aaron must confront this dark specter of what has been cast off or denied in his own development and integrate the missing elements. Dorothy, the Tin Man, the Cowardly Lion, and the Scarecrow here bravely confront the witch. As they do so, Glenda stands watchfully above. Dorothy and her wounded friends do not see her though. Perhaps they cannot see the presence of new light until they fully confront the abyss of the darkness.

Glenda stands above the tray overseeing it all. Her knowing and positive presence feels hopeful, as she appears to see how the all of the elements function as a whole. Perhaps Glenda holds the containment of the co-transference actively created by the mutual engagement in the symbolic process by Aaron and the therapist.

Two Smurfs stand in front of the sand tray to the far right. One is sneaking up behind the other with a huge mallet, poised to hit him over the head. He appears angry. Perhaps he wants to knock some sense into his counterpart. The Smurfs live underground. Like dwarves and the cabiri they know their way around down under, in the unconscious (Jung, 1953/1977). Perhaps the angry one with the mallet wants to wake something up or to make something conscious about this situation. No wonder he is angry. All of the elements must join forces and work together to attain the gold.

Upon closer scrutiny, the direction of Aaron's healing and development becomes clearer as we witness a duplication of the elements in parallel themes within the sand tray. The Smurfs mirror the Scarecrow's need for greater consciousness. Minnie and Mickey's family appear to mirror the Tin Man's longing for loving acceptance and connection. Gretel and the wolf reflect the soft courage required to tame the beasts sought by the Cowardly Lion. And Scrooge McDuck holds the golden treasure of Dorothy's longing to return home to the Self. It would appear that in this second sand tray, the nature of Aaron's wounding and the healing required have become more clearly defined.

Like the white ducks who carry the gold in this tray, it is on the back of a white duck that Hansel and Gretel were able to cross the water back to ordinary life in the fairy tale bringing their jewels and treasures with them (Grimm, 1972). The prognosis for Aaron's healing and resumption of healthy development is strongly evident in this sand tray as the elements of his healing are defined and manifest in the context of a powerful co-transference.

Sand Tray Number 3
Description

This tray was done in wet sand. In the upper right hand corner, Superman is face to face with a large two-headed dragon, a smaller three-headed dragon and an even smaller two-headed dragon. A lone palm tree stands behind the large dragon. To Superman's left, a white and blue unicorn rears over the skull of a cow. In the front center of the tray, two Star Wars figures and a blue Pegasus stand facing a dead man hanging from a gallows. Behind the gallows is a grave with a skeleton sitting on it. Behind the large oak tree in the front left of the tray, a golden coach heads toward the gold castle in the back left of the tray. A pathway to the castle is clearly carved in the sand. In the front right, two white suited astronauts approach a round silver space ship.

Sand Tray Number 3
Analysis

Superman, the hero from afar, boldly raises his left hand to the three dragons as if to say, "Halt. You will go no further." The three dragons recall the three witches in the prior tray, here confronted in the classic form of the hero's journey: the masculine quest to slay the negative feminine and distance himself from the mother (Neumann, 1971). Backed by a single palm tree, perhaps reflective of the primitive qualities of these dragons, the task of this hero is formidable as the dragons have seven heads among them. Superman does not raise the right hand as if to attack but raises the left. Very different from the masculinity modeled by his father, perhaps this gesture indicates the gentler form of masculinity that Aaron begins to define as his own as he separates from his identification as mother's little boy and moves into his role as a man. Perhaps the seven dragon heads allude to the numbers three and four and the deeper purpose of this work as the integration of the masculine and feminine, the spirit and the body.

As the monsters are halted, a death scene appears behind Superman. Flanked by a warrior and an alien, Pegasus regards the skeleton sitting on a grave and the hanging man. According to Greek legend, the winged horse Pegasus emerged from the blood of the slain Gorgon queen, Medusa (Leach & Fried, 1972). Like the witches in the prior tray and their reflections in the dragons of this tray, Aaron's journey requires that he confront this image of the dark feminine within himself in order to move into a mature form of his own masculinity. In keeping with the patriarchal cultural demands that its developing males disconnect from their mothers and from each other in order to become men, traditional psychodynamic theory would define this confrontation as the hero's "overcoming" or "slaying" of the dragon (Neumann, 1971). It is highly interesting that Aaron's symbolic process is not a separation by violence but rather one established by the very firm setting of boundaries between himself as male and the dark feminine energies that threaten to devour him. Rather than severing himself from the feminine with the raised left hand, Aaron establishes a way of remaining in contact with these powerful aspects of his own psyche. Rather than cutting himself off from the mother's world and eschewing his own inner feminine nature, as modern Western culture would have its sons do, Aaron finds a way of confronting these powerful inner energies. This allows him the potential to be whole as a man while remaining connected to other people and to his deep inner experience of feeling.

The power of Aaron's connectedness to the feminine is further reflected in the image of the large unicorn, which rears over a two-horned skull lying dead and dry in the back center of the sand tray. A symbol of chastity and fierceness, the unicorn symbolizes the power of love. Legend has it that the horn of a unicorn is an antidote to poisons, and if dipped into water, purifies it (Leach & Fried, 1972). Perhaps this is the loving power with which Superman raises his left hand to bring the seven dragonheads to a stop. Mythologist Robert Graves describes the unicorn's horn as "...'the upper pole' which reaches from the king directly up to the zenith, to the hottest point attained by the sun" (1994, p. 411). It would appear that as Aaron confronts and forms a relationship to the darkest feminine, he simultaneously establishes a solar connection through this pure and loving creature. The various faces of his limited ego identification die and are cast off, thus making room for the arrival of new aspects of himself.

Jung observes that the theme of the unicorn is also found in the Hindu epic *The Ramayana*, wherein Rishyashringa (the horned one) is rescued from isolation by the king's daughter Shanta. By their marriage, the horrible drought that ravaged the earth was ended (1953/1977). For Aaron, it would appear that it is not only a solar connection that is established through the unicorn but also a connection to the feminine that will water and fructify the earth itself.

In the right front corner of the sand tray, a round silvery space ship has just landed from a far off place. Two well-equipped astronauts wave their arms happily, eager to greet the newcomers. Upon completing the sand tray, Aaron commented that, "These [astronauts] will not be hurt when the aliens come out." I recall feeling excited with the anticipation of seeing how these emerging elements from Aaron's unconscious might manifest and was comforted by the knowledge that Aaron was ready to receive them.

Round and shiny, the space ship appears to be another allusion to the Self. Positioned on a dramatic diagonal is a golden castle in the upper left corner of the tray toward which moves a golden coach from behind the protection of the stately oak tree, Aaron said that the coach "...is going to a ball." With the power of his gentle masculinity, the way is clear to go home. Scrooge McDuck's gold from sand tray two now finds a place and a vehicle.

Sand Tray Number 4
Description

Tray four, done in damp sand, has a circle of male and female Native Americans around a large contained fire in the center. Four trees form a square on the periphery of this central event. Between three of the trees stand masks of Rama, Sita, and Ravana, figures from the Hindu *Ramayana* (Reyna, 1984). A kachina stands in the upper left plane of the square formed by the trees. Behind the kachina stand three teepees, the largest of which houses a baby. A snake draws toward the fire from the right. A lone brave aims an arrow at a figure of Davy Crockett who stands on the left center edge of the tray (not visible). A young Indian maiden stands on the center back edge of the tray to the left of a large silver moon.

Sand Tray Number 4
Analysis

Presaged by the prior allusions to the Self, Aaron created this tray in complete silence. Although many years have passed, I still recall the numinosity that surrounded and continues to characterize this tray in which Aaron experienced the manifestation of the Self. This tray was, and remains, an experience of the sacred.

Aaron began with the central placement of the fire. Then forming a squared circle, the archetypal symbol of wholeness spoken of by Dora

Kalff (1980/2004), Aaron placed a ring of Native Americans within the square frame of four trees and "...the gods they pray to." A perfect union of spirit (the circle) in matter (the square), Aaron's unique manifestation of centering holds within it the rectification of the very conflict, which lay threat to his being. Here he unites the warm connectedness of the Native Americans to the earth, her rhythms, the body, and instinctual nature with the profound spirituality of ancient India. Here, with a simple reverence, this child of nine contacts within himself the way he can be religious and of this world, and the way he can be strong and safe while remaining with others in loving connection.

Tapping the collective unconscious, Aaron returns to the symbolism of the ancient *Ramayana*. The masks of Rama, Sita, and Ravana from this ancient Hindu epic poem mirror the essence of Aaron's struggle and its remedy. In the Hindu tradition, Rama and Sita are considered the ideal man and woman. Rama, an incarnation of the god Vishnu, is widely revered for his gentle strength and steadfastness (Mitchell, 1993). Sita, a derivative of the goddess Lakshmi, embodies the essence of the feminine and is said to have been born from a furrow in the earth itself. The *Ramayana* recounts the tale of how Sita was stolen away from Rama by the evil king Ravana of Sri Lanka. Rama was distraught without his beloved feminine counterpart and struggled valiantly to retrieve her. Finally enlisting the aid of the monkey king Hanuman, she was wrested from the grip of Ravana and restored to Rama (Reyna, 1984). Completely unconscious to this child of nine, this ancient myth drawn from the collective defines the devastation of the masculine alienated from the feminine and the need to enlist the instincts to bring about an embodiment of the spirit with the body.

All of the earth people gather around the central ring of fire. They come together in its warm glow as the cool light of the moon shines from above. The serpent moves in for warmth. It feels as though its quiet power is welcome here. The central fire is powerful yet contained in its ring of stones. It is a great power harnessed for the use of the native peoples, who now bask in its warmth, celebrate its strength, and revere its might. Here Aaron symbolically identifies the central archetype of the psyche. While its power and energy are acknowledged, they pose no threat. They serve as a rallying point around which his various ego identifications may organize and relativize (Weinrib, 1983/2003).

A beautiful Native American princess looks on from above by the gentle light of the moon. Aaron commented that, "She was the first Indian, who is now dead. She is a spirit, who hangs above the fire [watching as] they have an Indian ceremony." As the Self is constellated, the spirit of an ancient feminine figure is released above the central fire. Ancient and archetypal, this spirit is at the same time young, for she makes her appearance here as a child. It would appear that as the Self is constellated, the anima emerges in potential to be developed more fully when Aaron reaches adolescence and young adulthood.

It is a sacred ceremony that takes place below the spirit. Like this "first Indian," the kachina is also a supernatural being. Representing the mythical ancestors of the present humans, the Hopi and other Pueblo Indians believe the kachinas return to the earth half of every year during the winter months to fructify the earth (Leach & Fried, 1972, pp.566-567). This kachina is the "butterfly," which perhaps alludes to the deep order of transformation Aaron undergoes as the spirit re-enters the earth in this sacred centering. Mirroring the germinal manifestation of the anima in the spirit of the first Indian, the butterfly is thought to represent the soul's release from unconscious matter (Woodman & Dickson, 1996). Aaron, at only age nine, has a great deal of development to undergo in the years ahead of him but his work in sandplay has afforded him access to all of the necessary elements of a full and rounded masculinity with an abiding connection to the deepest reaches of his soul.

The inner feminine soul is now aligned in relationship to the central masculine fire. Aaron's fire is tempered and guided by this gentle earthy spirit. Now anchored to his soul his masculinity has shape and direction. No longer will it blaze out of control. His empowerment as male is now connected to his deepest inner truth, to the truth of his very being. This fire can now be harnessed for Aaron's productive growth and creativity. Aaron's artistic creativity burgeoned at this point in treatment. Giving productive and safe vent to the anger he had held onto for so long, he did a series of luscious paintings of volcanoes in various states of eruption, and sculpted an exploding volcano.
The energy and creative fluidity he directed into these projects delighted both of us during this phase of his work.

Three native homes stand in the upper left corner. One contains a baby. Perhaps the ceremony is a celebration of the birth of this new child, the new potentials opened in Aaron, and the promise he now has to move forward in wisdom from this place. Davy Crockett stands on the far left of the tray as an Indian brave directs an arrow his way. It would appear that there is no place for this Western invader in this holy fire circle. Perhaps Aaron releases the dictates of Western patriarchal culture as this new child is born to him.

Sand Tray Number 5
Description

In the center of this tray, done in damp sand is a baseball game taking place on a diamond with second base closest to the front center of the tray. The players, all gold in color, are poised for play. A cameraman views the game from the first base line. Eight men in tuxedoes stand in a "V" formation, watching the game from behind the catcher at the top center of the tray. Behind them at the apex of the "V" is an older man who holds a boy upon his shoulders. Three men watch the game from the upper left corner: a farmer, a man seated holding a beer, and a man holding a hammer who has just hit his thumb. In front of them is a small pond dug in the sand by which stands a sign saying, "No fishing." A large oak tree stands in the front left of the tray by which is parked a pick up truck (out of view). In the upper right corner, behind a small tree, a drunken man is passed out in a chair with an ice bag on his head. In front of him, a golden sun hangs above the tray on the right

Sand Tray Number 5
Analysis

Subsequent to the manifestation of the Self in the previous sand tray, Aaron here continues the nascent ego's task of differentiating the masculine and feminine elements of the personality. The squared circle of the last tray now becomes a baseball diamond manned by golden players. The wholeness of the Self is reflected in the undertaking as the central figures are gold and their field of play is a diamond. All of the people in the sand tray are male. The sun, which hangs above the far right corner of the sand tray, is identified with the male creator, heaven, and the hero, further defining this as a masculine enterprise (De Vries, 1984). Perhaps Aaron undertakes the task of reordering his identity as male.

The men that have come to watch the game vary widely in their countenance and demeanor. When Aaron returned to review his sandplay process at age fifteen, he commented, "These are all parts of my father." At age nine, from an ordered center now his own, Aaron examines each face of masculinity modeled by his father. Importantly, it is the "fathers" that come to witness Aaron's game. All players are in place, a game is underway, and there are rules, which govern its progress. Upon completing the sand tray, Aaron commented that, "The pickup truck had lost its way, but had finally found his way to the game." It felt that Aaron had indeed found a center from which he could sort things out.

Eight men in tuxedos stand in a "V" formation as if to anchor the game from behind home plate. Behind them at the apex, an older man lifts a young boy on his shoulders. He supports the boy with his older masculine wisdom. These men assume a rather normal looking appearance in contrast with their counterparts to the left and right who range from comedic to pathetic. Perhaps Aaron was most closely identified with these qualities of his masculinity, although he would certainly have to contend with and address the less admirable aspects on the periphery.

On the far left is a humble earthy farmer who rests his hoe long enough to watch the game. As a farmer, he tills the earth and cultivates plants so they might grow and provide nurturance. I recall feeling a sense of hopefulness that this figure was present. To the right of the farmer is a "No Fishing" sign beside a tiny pond. It seemed important for the time being to leave the fish alone, to let them be, deep in their pond. Perhaps this alludes to a deeper sense of spirit that requires time to grow and develop. Much as the farmer attends to the growing of things, perhaps the fish are being protected so that they, too, might grow. Aaron's associations to this figure, upon completion of the tray, contrast rather dramatically with the farmer's physical appearance. Aaron commented that, "This guy is fishing and is breaking the law."

On the farmer's left sits a man with a beer. Although somewhat comedic in appearance, he seems ordinary. On his left stands a man who has hit his right thumb with a hammer. He is hurting and he has done it to himself. He will need to heal. He will need to learn to use the hammer properly or he will hurt himself again. The juxtaposition of these three figures may be reflective of the various effects of Aaron's father's alcoholism, which Aaron would have to reconcile for himself. When the man drinks his beer, he seeks spirit in the wrong way, fishing where he should not and breaking the law. He also hurts himself. The fourth figure on the periphery of the baseball game in the upper right corner painfully illustrates the pathetic aspects of alcoholism as a drunken man slumps in a chair. This man is not even conscious. This aspect of the masculine sits behind a tree that would block his view even if he were awake. In his drunkenness he cannot see the golden diamond game of his son. He sits in darkness, as he is behind the sun. I wondered if the farmer-as-cultivator might somehow be contained within the farmer-as-law-breaker-and-alcoholic. I wondered if these very different associations to this figure would hold, albeit painfully, the growth and wisdom that might derive from Aaron's early experiences with this unconscious and unavailable father.

Sand Tray Number 6
Description

Two armies square off for battle with soldiers facing each other lined up along the right and left sides of the tray. In the center of this damp tray, Adolph Hitler and a bugler face a Confederate and a Union soldier who prepare to fight. In the front center of the tray, two medics carry a wounded soldier on a stretcher. One large oak stands in the upper left of the tray diagonally across from another large oak in the front right.

Sand Tray Number 6
Analysis

Aaron begins this sand tray by announcing, "I'm going to make a war going on." In a serious and sober fashion he proceeds to arrange two opposing armies, aligned facing each other. Aaron commented, "They are getting ready to start the war. When [the bugler] blows the horn, it will start. This guy [behind the bunker] will be disqualified, because he already shot a guy. He is a bad guy. The good guys are on the left and the bad guys are on the right. This guy [Hitler] is the commissioner of the bad team; this [the bugler] is the commissioner of the good team."

Here the opposite poles of the symbolic process face each other in dramatic tension. Jung observed that a condition of such parity is intolerable to the ego. An opposition of such equal and powerful psychic forces creates a condition of tremendous pressure, and with appropriate and stable containment results in the descent of psychic energy into the unconscious activating new content around the issue at hand (Jung, 1960/1981). Aaron completed the tray with the placement of the two oak trees, as if to punctuate the balance of pressure between the two warring armies. The dynamic tension in this sand tray was tremendous, yet the firmness of the two solid oak trees appeared to underscore the strength of the containment that obtained between therapist and client in a powerful co-transference.

The central metal figure has now become the bugler's horn, poised and ready to sound the commencement of the transformation. The horn is thought to be androgynous in shape. As long and penetrating, it is considered active and masculine. At the same time, its bell is a container and is thought to be feminine (De Vries, 1984). As it sounds, it hails the spirit to fight the holy battle (Cirlot, 1971). Drawing from the Hindu themes that run through Aaron's case, I am reminded of the field of battle upon which Arjuna fought in the *Bhagavad Gita* (Edgerton, 1944). Arjuna's battlefield was, as is Aaron's, the transformative possibility of this moment. As for Arjuna in the ancient Indian scripture, this battlefield was for Aaron the point at which the temporal meets the eternal; the crossing point of will and destiny through which the Self gains liberation.

Perhaps Aaron continues the process of differentiating the masculine aspects of himself, here battling the opposite qualities of his own gender as he attempts to arrive at his own sense of masculinity. It is interesting that the "good guys" are on the left side of the tray. Perhaps, as was evident in the first sand tray, the healing energies required for Aaron's growth and development come from the direction of the feminine. Aaron acknowledges the wounding that has already taken place by noting that one man has been shot. At the same time, there is evidence of a taming of his aggressions as we note the animals are now all domestic. Additionally, the two central swordsmen who battle with their metal weapons appear evenly matched. Swordsmanship requires a keen sense of balance, order, and poise. It demands a quiet strength. Although the dynamic tensions of this impending battle are great, there is order to it. Aaron is clear that someone who broke a rule, "...has been disqualified." Although there is tremendous transformation to be undergone, there will be no more uncontrolled fighting and raging.

Sand Tray Number 7
Description

This tray, done on wet sand, is the layout of a room. The bathroom with tub, sink and toilet is in the upper left. There is a small bath sponge in the tub. A white iron bed sits in the center of the tray. A table holding a computer stands in the upper right with a chair facing the computer. On the right side of the tray is a dresser with a large mirror above it. Upon the dresser sit four small army tanks. To the right of the dresser, toward the front right of the tray is a folded pink parasol and a cabinet upon which sits a small sailboat. An empty ping-pong table sits to the front left of the tray and a small red stepladder in the left corner. In the front center of the tray stands another small cabinet, which holds a large silver loving cup. In the center of the tray, to the left of the bed, stands a golden birdcage, which holds a small white bird.

Sand Tray Number 7
Analysis

The shiny bugle of the previous tray now becomes a golden cage, which holds a single white bird. Located in the center of the sand tray, it appears that the spirit is now manifest and is housed in a safe and beautiful container. The masculine spirit is here emerging in Aaron, with the balanced acknowledgment of the containing presence of the feminine. This room, which has emerged out of the dramatic opposition of the last sand tray, has a quiet sense of order to it. Here Aaron returns to ordinary life, to every day consciousness, bringing with him the transformed qualities of the masculine resulting from his transcendent experience.

This room is open and welcoming to those who live here. There is a nice bathroom for washing up, beautiful furniture, a computer area for creative work, a red stepladder for reaching up to high places, and a ping-pong table for games. The clear surface of the ping-pong table with its two sides so clearly marked is reminiscent of the battlefield of the previous tray. Here it is cleared and a place for new life has emerged around it.

On the dresser four small tanks sit before a mirror. It is important that they be seen. They are small now, like memories of past battles. Recalling the size and dominance of the suit of armor in the first tray, perhaps these miniature tanks speak to the burdensome constraints of the past. Although the spirit is present here as the bird, it remains confined in a metal encasement. Now behind golden bars and no longer the dark heavy cold steel of the armor of the first sand tray, the bird is not yet free to fly. A model sailboat sits atop a small end table. It looks so light and breezy with its sail open to the wind. Perhaps this boat suggests a freer way to catch the wind of the spirit. The presence of the folded parasol also feels hopeful, as it appears ready to provide shade and protection.

A glimmering silver loving cup sits in the front center of the tray in the position of the wounded man in the prior tray. Trophies are awarded to victors. Its presence here is hopeful and assuring. It speaks to the success of Aaron's undergoing to date, as well as his potential to see the process through. This trophy is silver, the color of the moon. Sometimes referred to as a "loving cup," it recalls the moon spirit in sand tray four and is, perhaps, a testament to her triumphant yet nurturing presence in the center of Aaron's life. The place where the bird is caged is gold, the color of the sun. Perhaps Aaron is in some way still captive of a solar force. Although the encasement is much more open and radiant, he is not yet free. I recall hoping he would be able to fly out and claim the silver loving cup.

Sand Tray Number 8
Description

A small river running from left to right divides this tray. On the front side of the riverbank stands a lone fisherman who looks at a small fish he has caught. A stone bridge connects the two banks and is directly to the fisherman's right. A yellow rubber raft sits on the far side of the riverbank to the left of the bridge. Two white geese stand to the right of the bridge. Three blue fish swim from left to right, approaching the bridge from the left. Behind them is a Venetian gondola, covered with a parasol and steered by a gondolier. A dog sits on a bench in the back left corner of the tray, shaded by a large oak. A small white bird sits on the ground to the right of the bench. Another small white bird flies from a hook overhead on the left. Flanked by two large oaks, a large house occupies the back right corner. A blue car is parked to its left.

Sand Tray Number 8
Analysis

The prohibitions against fishing from tray five have been lifted, and the fisherman is here free to probe the depths. He holds high the fish he has brought up. The act of fishing speaks to inquisitiveness about the deeper elements, the elusive treasures of the unconscious that are available to the seeker (De Vries, 1984). Aaron is now able to tap these resources in him. Three large beautiful blue fish swim in from the left. The fish, as a multivalent symbol encompasses life, abundance, sexuality, and fertility. It also suggests the soul, immortality and the Self (De Vries, 1984). As three, the dynamic number of change, these fish allude to the transformation of Aaron's masculinity and an abundant, fertile possibility for its growth and development. They approach from the left, bringing a healing, softer energy, and are followed by a beautiful Venetian gondola. An elegant vehicle from far off Italy, perhaps the fish usher in a resolution to Aaron's conflict with the form of masculinity modeled by his Italian father. Perhaps the troublesome and out of control racecar in the first tray is here replaced by this quiet water vehicle. Unlike the driver of the racecar, who sped himself into trouble and danger, the gondolier guides his boat quietly yet powerfully with his oar that reaches to the bottom of the water. The man who guides this vehicle is in touch with and secure in the depths of him. The parasol from the previous sand tray reappears to protect the rider from the burning rays of the sun. While the presence of the masculine sun is acknowledged, it sheds a softer, gentler light on the passengers of this boat.

The bridge leads to the inviting domestic scene ahead. To the left a dog sits peacefully on a park bench and a tiny sea gull sits quietly on the ground as the gondola passes by. Two geese walk to the right of the fisherman. Usually watchful and vigilant, this pair appears quiet and unthreatened. All of the animals appear natural and comfortable. They are at home and unthreatened. Perhaps the animal, instinctual parts of Aaron are beginning to find their home. Forming a connection between the world of the fisherman and that of the house and garden, this bridge appears to connect ordinary life with the contemplative life. As his sense of masculinity is reordered to the Self, it appears that Aaron is simultaneously able to bridge this very important connection to his own reflective and spiritual nature.

High overhead on the left flies a single white bird. The little bird in the cage from the previous tray is here set free, allowing this serene world to emerge. I will never forget Aaron's utter delight as he gleefully suspended the bird on a string above the sand tray, nor how my heart soared when I recognized that this little bird was now free of its cage. As the bird flies above, the spirits are drawn up from the depths. Here Aaron achieves a profound partnership between the masculine and the feminine, the heavens and the earth, as his new potentials arrive from the left.

Sand Tray Number 9
Description

Tray nine, also transversed from left to right by a river, is dotted with Oriental buildings. A large pagoda-like Oriental bridge joins both sides of the river in the center of the tray. To the right of the bridge swims a large blue dolphin. A wooden Chinese junk floats on the river to the left of the bridge. Three trees mark the upper right, upper left, and front center of the tray. A single silver pine tree stands to the back right side of the central bridge.

Sand Tray Number 9
Analysis

Aaron noted that, "This is China. Everyone is in his or her house. This boat is leaving. It is early in the morning, because it just dropped off food and stuff. This is a dolphin. It is swimming to the ocean. The fishers [men] tried to get it, but it got away." In this sand tray surrounded with a sacred quietude, Aaron travels so far that he comes to the most remote place possible within himself. It is as if he travels to the inner side of being. Having bridged his inner and outer lives in the previous tray, Aaron goes deep within his unconscious to a very special and holy place.

As in the previous tray, this boat also follows fish. This boat is a junk, upon which people live and work, conducting all of their lives on the water. Having resolved the primary conflicts with his father, Aaron is able to find deep within himself the vehicle that allows him the on-going lived connection with the unconscious that he so yearned for, yet was previously denied by a masculinity that demanded an exclusively outward focus. Aaron tells us that this boat has brought food and supplies to feed and nurture these remote regions of his psyche. The boat and the fish, having escaped the grasp of the "fishers" (the men who would have stopped him) now make passage through the archway pagoda that appears to mark the border between the inner and the outer worlds. As they make their exit from this sacred place, it is apparent that Aaron now has access to these deeper regions of himself and that his own sense of masculinity which affords a profound connection to the spiritual and inner life, is firmly in place.

Sand Tray Number 10
Description

Made entirely of colorful plastic toys, this tray done in damp sand depicts a classroom with the teacher seated at her desk by the blackboard in the front and students at their desks. A lone child sits facing the corner in the front left. To the right is the playground with swings, slide, and merry go round. Children climb and play on the equipment, while a woman sits on a bench looking on from the upper right. Her child, in a stroller, sits to her left.

Sand Tray Number 10
Analysis

In this sand tray, Aaron returns to ordinary life, creating a colorful and well-equipped school. Upon completing the tray, Aaron reported that, "They are watching a film about dinosaurs." It would appear that Aaron has gone from facing monsters directly to looking at them from a distance as remnants of the past. As he does so, a lively learning environment manifests around him. Aaron commented that, "The teacher is trying to get them to be quiet, but they are not, [so full of energy is this colorful place.]" However, even in this highly active environment, a sense of order obtains. Aaron notes that the little boy had to sit in the front left corner as, "He is a dunce who was playing with his pencil." This teacher has things well in hand, for highly energized creative play and learning are now free to take place within the safe containment of her clear structure. It was deeply moving to recognize that Aaron had found that place within himself where he was free to playfully create and explore while remaining safe.

A playground with children gaily romping on swings and merry-go-rounds extends the classroom, as if they are all of a piece. Perhaps Aaron realizes that play is very much a part of his life and learning, as it appears he is finally able to surrender his guarded, serious, overly responsible demeanor and unleash his playful spirit.

A mother sits with her young child in the upper right hand corner. Although her baby is too young to send to school, this mother, like the teacher, gives the impression of being nurturing and supportive of her child's growth as she watches the children. I wondered if this guardian mother in the upper right corner might not also be an allusion to the containment of Aaron's work in the co-transference, as this was the corner in which I sat during Aaron's work in the sand.

Sand Tray Number 11
Description

Done in wet sand, tray 11 has a small waterway across the front along which four blue fish swim from right to left. The front edge of the tray (not visible in photograph) is lined with a rock wall. A snow pine and a bench sit on the right side near the bridge, which connects both banks of the tray. There is a water well on the left front. Set off with green pines and flanked by two large stones, a large black train moves from left to right toward the top center of the tray. A large golden sun hangs overhead at the point of the front of the train. An ornate gazebo sits in the center of the tray. It houses a table and chairs. There is a large house in the upper right corner and a smaller house in the right center. The small house has a silver pine to its right, the large house a snow pine to its right. Another snow pine stands between the train and the gazebo and a solitary tall green pine sits directly in the front center of the gazebo.

Sand Tray Number 11
Analysis

Creating this tray with a penetrating intensity, Aaron announced that, "It is Christmas time. Everybody decorated everything and went to see their families. That is where the train is going -- to the families, and that is why no one is around." The train, of dark and heavy cast iron, is reminiscent of the armored metal encasement in tray one. Here, as it passes under the sun, it returns people to their families. Perhaps the shadowy rage contained beneath his armored encasement moves toward further integration as this train passes from the land of the sun to the snowy land ahead. A stone wall defines the front boundary of the sand tray, as if to solidly underscore what transpires here. I recall feeling that it said, "Take notice," and firmly so.

The large golden sun hangs above the train at the very point of the head of the train. To the left, in the area of the train, are green trees. To the right, the trees are covered with snow, as if at the interstices of summer and winter, Aaron tells us that this is Christmas. This is the darkest time of the year into which appears the first new light. As the train leaves, it passes a heavy fossil rock. As Aaron's train heads for the land of winter, it leaves the remnants of the past behind, perhaps opening to him the possibility of connecting with others, with the family, in a way that allows him the security of his wholeness and uniqueness with genuine closeness and feeling.

A single silver tree stands to the far right of the house. Recalling the silver moon to the right of the native princess in sand tray four, perhaps Aaron's train moves from the land of the golden solar form of being masculine, to a more silver lunar way of being a man, as he continues the process of differentiating the masculine and feminine aspects of his personality.

A well stands on the front left. It recalls the small pond in tray five in which fishing was forbidden. Now four fish swim up the stream from right to left, moving in the opposite direction from which they swam in prior trays. Perhaps they swim in the direction of the well and toward the source of the water. As four, perhaps, the fish allude to the material manifestation of Aaron's "fish-ness," his sexuality and spirit, now firmly in form. As his outer masculinity moves into new territory, refining its manner of manifestation, he remains inwardly aware of its eternal source in the depths of the headwaters. From the well, water is drawn up from the depths of the earth. Ahead of the train in the land of winter, the water is transformed into beautiful crystal ice and snow. With its source deep in the wellspring of his being, Aaron is now able to artfully and exquisitely manifest his own way of being male in this world.

Sand Tray Number 12
Description

Tray 12, done in damp sand, has a small waterway angling diagonally across the front right corner of the tray. Two ice cubes stand in the river and two polar bears stand nearby. A large white igloo occupies the upper right corner. Ensconced by two snow pines, it is topped with a crystal ring. Two skiers race down a slope in the upper left corner, as two galloping white horses approach from the front left. The landscape is dotted with large snowflakes and a large crystal star hangs over the tray.

Sand Tray Number 12
Analysis

All is crystalline and snowy white in this exquisite sand tray Aaron called, *Winter Land*. In a rarefied, muffled quiet, as if it had actually snowed, Aaron paired two horses, two bears, two cubes of ice, two snow pines, and two skiers. As if newly emerging from primal wholeness, these dualities call to be seen in their pristine purity in this archetypal land.

The black iron train of the previous tray has moved fully into the land of winter and has transformed into a magnificent pair of charging white horses. It is as if Aaron's spirit has been set free in a powerful and glorious way.

To the right, a pair of pure white polar bears approaches the icy stream. Large and powerful, they are very much at home in this environment. Perhaps they are a male and female, a balanced whole. The larger of the pair approaches two cubes of ice in the stream. The water has been transformed, freezing and assuming the form of a cube. Like a square, the cube alludes to all dimensions of spatial reality (Smith, 1992). There are two cubes here and the bear appears to point them out. Perhaps this pairing of wholeness in material manifestation calls out to be seen.

Behind the bears is an igloo. Beautiful and round, it is made of cubes of ice. It is as if the wholeness of the ice cubes comes together to form a round home. In three-dimensional reality, Aaron now integrates the circle and the square, creating a place to reside in his new wonderland. A pair of crystalline snow pines flanks the igloo, ensconcing it, and planting it firmly in this snowy habitat. His last gesture in the creation of this sand tray, Aaron crowned the igloo with a crystal ring, as if to emphasize its sacredness and its wholeness. I was certain that Aaron would never again feel the sense of displacement with which he began his work, knowing that he carried deep within his psyche this pure, whole, simple home that belonged solely to him. Although he may have struggles with his sensitivities and his quiet strength, he now belonged to himself in the fullest and truest way.

The skiers from the first tray have returned, here moving to the far left corner. A matched pair, male and female, they are skillfully able to negotiate their way through this snowy land. It would appear that Aaron has found a beautiful balance between his masculine and feminine energies.

Above the tray now hangs a many-pointed crystal star. Perhaps the sun of the previous tray has set as the train moves into darkest winter. Perhaps it is nighttime and this is the rising of a glorious new star. The light of this star is gentler than the light of the sun and seems fitting in this sublime new land.

Sand Tray Number 13
Description

Done on damp sand, Tray 13 contains a variety of soldiers and military implements encircle the tray, facing inward. The medics carry a wounded soldier on a stretcher in the upper right corner, while a jet plane hangs above the tray.

Sand Tray Number 13
Analysis

Walking around the tray as he quickly placed the figures, Aaron created this sand tray with a disgusted air of resignation. This was the day that war broke out in the Middle East in early 1991. Aaron announced, "This is the war in the Persian Gulf. It stinks and they are acting like kids." It is as if international events reflected the warring, oppositional way Aaron used to be in the world. Stimulated by external circumstances, Aaron returns to this familiar way of being with others and with himself in his sand tray, but brings with him a reordered relationship to the Self. No longer acceptable, he finds it despicable and immature. He no longer sees himself in relationship to others in this way, but painfully recognizes that many others, adults and world leaders, continue this oppositional struggle. He is repulsed, yet wisely aware.

Sand Tray Number 14
Description

In this tray, done in dry sand, a skier followed by a large polar bear heads up a hill dotted with snowflakes in the upper left corner. A large black train sits in the upper central section of the tray, headed from left to right along a pathway dug into the surface of the sand. Dick Tracy and Inspector Clouseau face a golfer in the left front of the tray. A well sits near the center of the tray. To its right are two gasoline pumps and two cars. A cow moves from left to right toward a golf green. Behind this on the right, the space shuttle points toward the sky. In the front right a bridge spans a small waterway that crosses the front of the tray. A scuba diver lays prone on top of the bridge while five bicyclists pedal along the river. A large fish bone sits at the left end of the river (not visible in photo).

Sand Tray Number 14
Analysis

Done in a playful, teasing mood, Aaron called this sand tray, *Crazy Land.* Saying that it takes place on a golf course, he laughingly described how, "...the cyclists are riding in a river. The space shuttle is taking off. People are inspecting the golf ball because they think there is a bomb in it and the skier is going uphill." He added that this place, "...is not very safe. You can't get hurt, but you can't count on things." It was very interesting to note that five months subsequent to completing this sand tray, Aaron spontaneously referred back to it, likening it to his life, saying, "Like my life, I can't always count on things to be the way I think they should." After his deep, inward explorations, Aaron returns to his ordinary life able to see it in a completely new way. From the vantage of a new ego state, his vision of what obtains is humorously reordered. Everything appears to be "stood on its head," and nothing is as it should be.

What transpires here in "Crazy Land" is very like the humorous antics of the clowns in the kachina ceremonies alluded to in tray four. In the Hopi and Zuni traditions, the clown kachinas frequently invert themselves and climb down ladders head first to illustrate the human tendency to do things in the most difficult way. These native peoples believe that the clowns prevent them from taking themselves too seriously. Like the trickster, these clowns hold the compensatory balance in life, often doing the opposite of what is expected (Griffin-Pierce, 1995). Anthropologist Geoffrey Turner refers to this behavior of the kachina clowns as a, "...Licensed inversion of the rules of good behavior," (Turner, 1979, pp.89-90) which serves as a safety valve for the tensions that build up under the native societies' insistence on self-discipline. Here Aaron, with renewed vision and a playful spirit regards the ironies of his life. His overly serious persona is tempered now with humor and wisdom.

Even with all of the distractions on this comic strip golf course, the golfer is focused and has his shot clearly lined up. Aaron, like this golfer, now appears to know exactly where he is headed. Witnessing this tray, I recall feeling a profound sense of confidence in Aaron's ability to handle not only the immediate challenges of his family, but anything that life might hand him. At the same time I delighted in the intelligence and humor with which he set about the task.

Poised to take off, the space shuttle was the last figure Aaron placed in this sand tray. I recall wondering if he might be nearing the end of his process and preparing to leave. As it would come to pass, he would complete just one more tray.

Sand Tray Number 15
Description

In this tray, done in wet sand, a curvilinear water way divides the tray left from right. The two sides of the tray are connected with a bridge, atop which sits a small blue car headed from left to right along a road traced in the sand. On the left side of the tray, Superman faces the two-headed dragon, the three headed dragon, the Penguin, Davy Crockett, Hulk Hogan, and Hitler. A tall silver statue of an early nineteenth century French soldier stands in the front left corner, encircled with a small train track and small black train engine headed toward the left. A small boxer stands in the center of the left section beside a silver loving cup. In the far right upper corner, a woman sits on a bench. The Rocket Man hangs above the tray in the region of the river. The landscape is dotted with trees.

Sand Tray Number 15
Analysis

Ending his process as it began, Aaron's first gesture in this last sand tray was the placement of the bridge. Unlike the troubled racecar chased by the police in tray one, here the little blue car from the peaceful domestic scene in sand tray eight makes its passage from the left to the right. Identifying himself as the triumphant boxer who returns from tray two, Aaron said, "This is me and these are all of the bad guys that I killed or that are about to die." Referring to the soldier in the front left corner he said, "This is a statue of me and this is a train with me leaving the battle. This is the Rocket Man, who helps me kill all of the bad guys, and this is a lady watching the fight. This is my Mom. Superman is helping me, too." Then, with a final gesture, he added the silver trophy, placing it to the left of the boxer, saying, "This is the trophy I get. It's as tall as me!"

The tall, silver loving cup reappears from tray seven and stands to the boxer's left, his feminine side. Now liberated from the metal encasement of the first sand tray, he rejoices in his far-reaching personal triumph. The burdensome armor that was once his defense and his prison is now transformed and stands as a gleaming testament to the victories and capabilities of his emerging self.

As Aaron leaves the battle behind, and prepares to cross the bridge to the other side where all is peaceful, he ceremoniously gathers his antagonists and stands triumphantly before them. Well prepared now with able helpers, they no longer threaten him. The Rocket Man flies along the path of the river, marking the division between the old world and the new. No longer at the mercy of his explosive rage, his fiery aggressive energy has been transformed and channeled into his service as rocket fuel. Powerful and exercising great alacrity in the skies, the Rocket Man has command of the reaches of the heavens, as does Superman. Acknowledging a remarkable integration of body and spirit, Aaron honors his capacity to move between the earth and the heavens in himself. Now at home and safe in both dimensions, this young man has found peace with the beginnings of his own unique balance between masculine and feminine energies.

Although it was anticipated that Aaron would have more work ahead of him in terms of further discovery and differentiation of masculine and feminine energies as he continued to grow and develop, his sandplay work provided him a clear reordering and a firm foundation upon which to build. Aaron commented that the woman sitting in the upper right corner was his mother. The loving support of Aaron's mother was clearly present throughout his work. I recall feeling deeply touched by his reverent respect for her presence. Given the multi-dimensional quality of symbolic process, I wondered if this woman might also hold the further differentiation and integration of the anima that lay ahead for Aaron. Additionally, as this was the corner of the sand tray at which I sat, I wondered if this figure might serve as a reference to the presence of the therapist and the strength of the co-transference throughout this profound healing process.

The Sandplay Case of Aaron
Postscript

Follow-up with the client and his mother in the fall of 1995 indicated that Aaron had made an excellent social adjustment. He was popular with the girls and doing very well in school. Both Mrs. Smith and Aaron affirmed Aaron's deeply religious nature and his continued involvement in the synagogue. Mrs. Smith, rightfully proud of her son, noted he had a clear career direction and planned to go to the university to study engineering. Both mother and son gratefully acknowledged that Aaron's relationship with his father had been healed. His father was able to be present for Aaron and they saw each other frequently.

APPENDIX A

Subjective Immersion Analysis
The Sandplay Case of Aaron —
Transcript of SIA Inquiry

Following is the original transcript of the Subjective Immersion Analysis of Aaron's sandplay. Only minor spelling and language corrections have been made to the original log. Reading it through with frequent reference to the photos of Aaron's trays demonstrates my experience of the SIA inquiry into the symbolic context of this case.

This SIA was done over the course of several days. It was undertaken many years after Aaron completed his work. It was done prior to the written case analysis and before Aaron's later review of his work..

After completing the SIA of some of the sandplays, thoughts and understanding continued to occur to me. It appears that the SIA continued even after I had consciously dis-identified with the focus figures. These are included as *Post SIA Reflections.*

Although each therapist's SIA examination of any sandplay work will be different, reviewing my SIA experience of this case is a good way to develop familiarity with this tool.

Intent of Inquiry

I propose to study the sandplay process of Aaron from the vantage point of a central, or prominent figure within the sand tray. The objective of the study will be to gain greater and deeper understanding of the sandplay process through the subjective experience of witnessing the tray from the perspective of an element of the tray itself.

An orienting question for this study is,
What is it like to be here in this tray now?

Tray 1
Focus Figure — Central Knight in Armor

As the knight in this tray, I am covered with metal. I think ahead to the tray with the little bird in the metal cage in the center of the tray and later, in the last tray, to the victorious boxer with the metal loving cup next to him. The flesh has come out of the metal and stands strong on its own.

I stand here facing left. My back is to the right. Perhaps I look in the direction of the feminine for what is to come. Behind me are the battles of superheroes. Batman and Robin defeat the Joker and the Penguin.

I stand on an island and am larger and higher than everything else save the lone oak to my right hand. I'm stiff and cold and isolated. I'm disconnected and unable to connect with anyone or anything else. I'm too far removed, because of my height and this heavy metal encasement.

I share this island with three Asian ninja warriors. They are scary and fierce and put on a fearsome face, but how I really feel is this way. All locked up, cut off, cold in this steel prison. Why have I had to retreat to this encasement? It is as though my survival depended upon it. I feel profoundly sad.

Here comes a hot racecar, speeding across the bridge to my island. There is a squad car after him. That will fix him. That will bring justice. He won't be able to get away with this speeding, this unlawful behavior, any more. You are coming my way. Well, I can use the help. Maybe someone can help, so I can get out of this metal prison and be safe, and be myself.

Two Asian men sit meditating contemplatively on the little island by the police car. They gaze into a crystal ball, as if looking toward the future. I wonder what they see? Do they see the way out? They seem very calm and still. It looks as if it is very warm over there. They are very different than their warring counterparts on my island, all dressed in black, brandishing weapons, and posturing for attack. I'm so tired of having to be like that. No wonder I've hidden my real Self in steel armor. At least I will preserve it and be safe.

I'm tired of fighting these cartoon battles, too. I'm not really a superhero, like Batman. I'm just me. Oh, but I tire of fighting all of the time. How I long to be free, like the two skiers gliding so joyfully down the slope behind Robin. I can't ski in this steel cage. I can hardly even move. At least, though, I'm protected from the inevitable blows that come my way.

I'm glad there is a bridge between my island and that of the Eastern men and the police. Maybe I'm more connected to this than I think. Perhaps I have a way of accessing these helpers and this peaceful, contemplative way of life. Ah, that feels hopeful.

Across the water on my right, a lion tamer faces a huge tiger. He has a lot of work to do to tame that beast, but seems confident of his position. He is there directly in front of the tiger, unprotected. I think he really knows what he is doing. I know that tiger. He is mean and full of rage. He doesn't want to be, but he is. Sometimes he just viciously attacks. I think he wants to be tamed and is glad that there is an able trainer here. (Transference to the therapeutic containment) When you have to live locked up in one of these steel suits long enough, you get very angry. When you are told that, to be a man, you have to fight and be tough, like the ninjas, but your real, gentle strength isn't even seen, you get really hurt. After a while, that hurt gets hard and turns to rage. Yes, that tiger really wants to be tamed.

I don't want to have to pretend I'm Batman, slaying enemies any more.

Post SIA Reflections

The moment I identified with the knight, I felt and understood the role that metal encasement had played throughout Aaron's sandplay case. Regarding the transference, the client felt safe enough in this first tray to reveal his inner struggle between the fierce qualities of the masculine, modeled and valued by his father and his own gentler strength that found no place in his outer world. That he was able to reveal his quieter masculine qualities in the figures of the older Asian men, suggests that, at least, he felt safe enough to risk this part of himself being seen in the therapeutic setting. The very able lion tamer, face to face with the huge beast, suggests great possibility for the taming of his raging inner beast in his work. It is a powerful statement of his positive transference to the potential for transformation within this therapeutic setting.

Tray 2
Focus Figure — The Small Boxer

I stand here with gloves on, poised, ready to fight. I'm small, though. I feel calm and centered as I look around me. There is a lot going on here. I stand on a mound, so I can see over things, so I can see what's going on around me.

Right in front of me, in the boxing ring, I defeat the huge enemy with grace and power. I overcome what seems an impossible battle. My cartoon friends, Mickey and Minnie Mouse look on. Minnie cheers my victory and Mickey videotapes the defeat, so it will be recorded and preserved for all to see. They seem excited and exuberant in their celebration of my overcoming. Their red clothing and pompoms are very affirming in their energetic witnessing of my victory.

To the far left stands an odd couple. They are fruit and vegetable people. The man is a goofy, stupid looking vegetable. The woman is a gorgeous banana lady. How is it that they are together? Their pairing does not make sense. They are different species. I wonder if this is Mom and Dad? They watch, also, as I defeat the huge opponent. It is important that they see this. They stand very close and on the side of the opponent. I make it though. I knock him out and they see it. Maybe the marriage of a vegetable and a luscious fruit creates a monster. This is my legacy.

There is Scrooge the Duck in the center of the tray showing his gold. He must want me to see it. He doesn't make any effort to hide. His little nephew duck stands behind the willow tree in the front to my right, with a golden spyglass aimed directly at him. This wealth, this gold, must be seen. Maybe this is my inner treasure that emerges as I overcome this oversized opponent.

Far across the tray, opposite me, stand Minnie and Mickey and Pluto, gaily engaged together in talk. They all smile, as they lovingly visit together. These are my cartoon friends. They are fantasy figures. Maybe I need my fantasy friends to help me understand what things are about, what life is like. Maybe I need them just to get by. They live a very nice life in my imagination.

It is not all so easy, though. Across the tray, sweet little Gretel reaches out to the wolf. Gretel lost her way in the woods, because her wicked stepmother didn't have food for her and Hansel. Will she be eaten by the wolf, or will she tame him, like the lion tamer in the first tray? She isn't a trained lion tamer, though. She is a tiny, gentle little girl, innocently extending her left hand to the wolf. It is as if this very gentle energy seeks to make contact, to make peace with the wildness of the animal. Can she do it? Will her arm be torn off?

Two Smurfs stand in front of the tray to the far right. One is sneaking up behind the other with a huge mallet, poised to hit him over the head. He looks angry. Does he want to knock some sense into his counterpart? The Smurfs live underground. They know their way around down under, in the unconscious. Does this angry one want to wake something up, make something conscious about this situation? He means business. The other one seems hapless and dopey. No wonder he is mad. We all need to work together.

Up to my far left, Dorothy, Cowardly Lion, Scarecrow and Tin Man encounter the wicked witch, as Glenda, the good witch looks on from above and behind them. The witch is terrifying, but they all have needs and are not about to give up. Even though they are very scared, they stand and face her horrific presence. The Tin Man needs a heart, so he can feel. Scarecrow needs a brain, so he can think. Cowardly Lion needs courage, so he can live without fear. Dorothy needs to find her way back home. These are all parts of me. The Smurfs mirror the Scarecrow's need for greater consciousness. Minnie and Mickey's family mirrors the Tin Man's longing for loving acceptance. Gretel and the wolf mirror the soft courage to tame the beasts. Scrooge the Duck reflects the golden treasure of Dorothy's longing for her home in the Self.

All of the missing parts must face the horror of this witch, the darkest of the dark. It is as if it is the turning point in the journey back home. In order to find what has been lost, in order to conquer the beast, they must bravely confront this darkest specter of horror of the unknown. Yet, as they do so, Glenda stands watchfully above. I feel comforted in seeing that. I see that she is there. Dorothy and her wounded friends don't see her, though. They cannot see the presence of new light until they fully confront the abyss of the darkness.

Glenda oversees it all. She stands above things, as I do. Her knowing, positive presence is very hopeful. Somehow she acts to hold it all together. All that she surveys are parts of the whole. She stands above it all and is able to see how it all fits together.

Post SIA Reflections

Hansel and Gretel encounter the child-eating witch, who burns in her own fire. The children then take her jewels and return home to live well, where they find that their wicked stepmother has died. The essential elements of the fairy tale are the child eating witch, the abandoned children, the wicked stepmother and the disappearing trail.

Tray 3
Focus Figure — Superman

I am Superman and I am strong. I come from a foreign place and have super powers. I have much work to do here, though, as I must do battle with three multi-headed dragons. There are seven heads, altogether. I face them head on and raise my left hand as if to say, "Halt. No further. Enough. You will go no further." Maybe it is my left hand, because it is the side of the feminine, gentler part of my nature. I don't raise my right hand as if to attack. Maybe the fighting is over and I can use this quieter masculinity to curb the ravages of these fearsome monsters. Behind the monsters stands a single palm tree, perhaps a primitive remnant of these ancient demons.

As I halt the monsters, something interesting appears behind me. It is a scene of death. Pegasus, flanked by a warrior and an alien watch a skeleton on a grave and a hanging man. Pegasus emerged when the Gorgon Medusa was slain. He sprang from her blood. Medusa is the mortal Gorgon queen, living in the farthest west, near night.

It appears that the Witch of Tray 2 was successfully faced, because the Pegasus has arisen. I halt the monsters and behind me is death. Perhaps it is time for something new to arise.

To my right, two well-equipped astronauts greet a ship from outer space. They wave their arms happily, eager to greet the newcomers. I wonder what will emerge from this round, silvery space ship? I feel excited with anticipation.

On my left, a large white unicorn rears over the skull of a dead head of cattle, vertical and reaching to the heavens. Has he slain it? Why a unicorn?

The unicorn, the gentle power of love, is also the antidote to poisons. This is the power with which I raise my left hand to the seven heads and bring them to a stop.

Beside the unicorn, and behind the protection of a beautiful old oak tree, is a golden castle toward which moves a golden coach. With the power of this gentle masculinity, the way is clear to go home. Scrooge the Duck's gold from tray two now finds a place and a vehicle. I want to go there. That is my true home.

Tray 4
Focus Figure — Indian Princess

I am here, dark, beautiful and ancient. Up by the moon, I oversee all. My arms are extended outwardly, palms up, as I bestow blessings on all below. This is a very sacred place. I am here in the light of the silvery crescent moon. It is a gentle light that illuminates from above.

I am the Princess of the Moon.

A sacred ceremony takes place below, where all of the earth people gather around the central ring of fire. They come together in its warm glow, as the cool light of the moon shines from above. The serpents move in for warmth. Their quiet power is welcome here. The fire is the center of all that is. It is great and powerful, yet contained in its ring of stones. It is a great power, now harnessed for the use of the native peoples. They bask in its warmth, celebrate is strength, and revere its might.

Three native homes stand by. One contains a baby. Perhaps they celebrate the birth of this new child and the potential he has to move forward in wisdom from this place.

Ancient masks, the faces of spirits from far off India, attend. What transpires here is ancient indeed. The spirits gather to witness this centering. A native kachina squares the central circle, as the fourth witness from the spirit world. These spirits come because they understand what transpires in this center. They also come to contain it with their four corners. The spirits stand between four trees, also marking this sacred grove.

Davy Crockett stands to my far right, leaving now, as a brave directs an arrow his way. There is no place for this Western invader in this holy fire circle. He may depart now, as this new child is born.

Tray 5
Focus Figure — The Pitcher

I am pitching now, from the center. I have great skill and aim. I am in the center of the game. The batter is poised to strike and all of the other players are ready. We are golden and we assemble around our diamond. I stand in the center of the diamond. The camera man records my every move for all to see.

Many men have gathered to watch the game. Eight men stand and watch from behind the catcher. They have come now to see it all, to see how this works. They are here to witness the intricacies and the perfection of this game. They stand in a "V" formation, anchoring the point of the diamond. Behind them at the apex, an older man lifts a young boy on his shoulders. He supports the boy with his older, masculine wisdom, in order that the boy might come to see how this game is played. The boy seems safe and well supported, well cared for.

From a greater distance, four other men look on, also. They, too, have come to witness. On my far left is a humble, earthy farmer, who rests his hoe long enough to watch the game. He tills the earth and cultivates plants so they might grow and provide us nurture. I feel glad and honored that he has come to witness. On his right is a "No Fishing" sign beside a tiny pond. I wonder why they don't want us to bring up the fish? For some reason they want us to leave the fish alone, let them just be, deep in their pond. Maybe that is so they might have a chance to grow and develop. Much as the farmer attends to the growing of things, maybe the fish are being protected so that they, too, might grow.

On the farmer's left sits a man with a beer. He looks like the most normal, regular guy I could imagine watching a game. It feels good to have him watch, also. On his left stands a man who has hit his right thumb with a hammer. He is hurting and he has done it to himself. He hurts now and will need to heal. He will have to learn to use that hammer properly, or he will hurt himself again.

In the far upper corner to my right, slumps a drunk man in a chair. His beer can has slipped down and he has an ice pack on his head. He isn't even conscious. He is drunk and cannot see this golden diamond game. I feel very sad about that. He sits behind a tree that flanks the spectators. The tree would block his view also, if he were conscious.

It feels good having the tree there. It seems to anchor and punctuate the attendance of the spectators. Another tree and small shrub are to the far left, sheltering the little fishing hole. The green and the growth feel good. A pick up truck has parked behind me on the left. It is nice to have a vehicle to move about with and one that can carry a lot.

High above the game in the upper right, hangs a beautiful golden sun. It casts its golden light down on all of us, save the drunk, who sits behind the sun. I feel wonderful and whole, pitching in the golden radiance of the full sun.

Tray 6
Focus Figure — The Bugler

I hold my bugle and survey the field. All are poised for war, weapons are raised. The war is about to begin. The two swordsmen in the center, directly in front of me have swords raised and ready. They represent their sides of the conflict. With the sound of the bugle, it will begin. The opposing sides will face off, do battle to the very end, and conflict will be decided.

Adolph Hitler stands directly across from me on the other side of the two swordsmen. His right hand is raised in salute. He, too, is ready to start the battle. It's good versus bad, us versus them. My team against Hitler's. The air is brittle and tense with the power of these opposing forces.

Even though this battle hasn't begun yet, there has already been a casualty. The medics are carrying the wounded man away, directly behind me.

The war field is clearly demarcated by two solid, old oak trees. One stands behind me and one behind Hitler. They stand opposite each other, defining the field of battle, as if to say, "Here we are. Here is where all is." I am reminded of the field of battle upon which Arjuna fought in the Bhagavad-Gita. His battlefield was, as is this, the transformative possibility of this moment, now. It was for Arjuna, and is now for me, the point at which the temporal meets the eternal, the crossing point of will and destiny through which the Self gains liberation.

Tray 7
Focus Figure — The Bird In the Cage

I am very special. I live in a golden cage in the center of this room. This is a very nice room. As I look around, I see it is orderly and calm. There is a sense of quiet about it, even though there are many things to do here. There is a very nice bathroom for washing up, beautiful furniture, a computer area for creative work, a red stepladder for reaching up to high places, and a ping pong table for games. The clear surface of the ping pong table, with its two sides so clearly marked, reminds me of the battle field of the last tray. Here it is cleared, and a place for new life has emerged around it.

On the dresser sit three small tanks in front of the mirror. It is important that they are seen. They are small now, remembrances of past battles. Perhaps they are remembrances of the need for heavy armor. They no longer pose a threat, but they remind me of a very constrained past. I recall the suit of armor in the first tray, of its size and dominance. Perhaps the little tanks are an artifact of that once heavily guarded past.

Now this room is open and welcoming to those who live here. A model sailboat sits on a small end table. It looks so free and breezy, its sail open to the wind. Maybe it is a reminder of a freer way to catch the wind, or the spirit, that was not possible from within the steel walls of the armored tank.

I can see this all around me, but through the bars of my golden cage. I am still encased in metal, here in the center. Although my encasement is now behind golden bars and no longer dark, heavy, cold steel, like the armor in Tray 1, I remain confined. I can see out much better now than I could in Tray 1. You can see me, too. I am a white bird. I yearn to fly and sing.

Directly in front of me sits a glimmering silver loving cup on top of another end table. Trophies are awarded to victors, to those who make it. It sits there very proudly in the front and center. It is silver, the color of the moon. I am reminded of the Moon Spirit in Tray 4. Perhaps this is a testament to her victory. The place where I am caged is gold, the color of the sun. Perhaps I am in some way still captive of a solar force. Although my encasement is much more open and radiant now, I am still not free. I want to fly out and claim the silver loving cup.

Tray 8
Focus Figure — The Fisherman

I'm a fisherman, all outfitted with my creel, hat and gear. I've caught a small fish from the stream, which I am raising up to admire. I love being here. It is very peaceful and beautiful. As a fisherman, I am a quiet man. I am attuned to nature and understand her rhythms. I am patient and quiet, as I wait for the fish. I can fish now. There are no more prohibitions against fishing, as there used to be. I can now fish deep in the stream and freely bring things up from the depths. The fish are abundant here. I can see three beautiful fish coming my way.

The fish are followed up by a beautiful Venetian gondola. This is an elegant, beautiful vehicle from far off Italy. Maybe this has something to do with rectification of this part of my heritage. My father's family is Italian. Now there comes a quiet boat, in lieu of the troublesome racecar in the first tray. The racecar has been replaced by this comfortably outfitted gondola, which is now in the same place of the car in Tray 1. The gondolier guides his boat quietly, yet powerfully with his oar. He often sings as he navigates the waters. He is a master at navigating the tiny channels in Venice. This gondola has a parasol to protect the rider from the burning rays of the sun. The sun was burning too hot. Its light is quieter and gentler here.

There is a bridge in front of me, leading to the beautiful domestic scene ahead of me. Nestled between three sturdy oaks is a commodious house with a car parked beside. It looks inviting to me. To my left a dog sits peacefully on a park bench, looking on as the gondola passes by. A tiny sea gull sits quietly on the ground to the right of the bench. These animal visitors appear so natural and comfortable. They are at home and unthreatened. Maybe the animal parts of myself have found their home, too. Down to my right stand two geese. Usually watchful and vigilant, this pair is quiet and unthreatening. They seem comfortable with me fishing in their home.

High overhead on my left flies a single white bird. Perhaps the little bird in the cage has been set free. As she flies, it feels like this serene world is free and safe to emerge. My heart soars as I watch this little bird fly so freely above. No longer held in her metal cage, she is free now to ascend to the heavens. As she flies above, I draw the spirit up from the depths. This is a beautiful crossing point.

Tray 9
Focus Figure — Blue Dolphin

I have been swimming a long way up this stream and have crossed to the other side of the bridge. I have traveled so far, I have come to the other side of being, to the most remote place possible. This is China. There is no place farther away than this.

Behind me follows a boat. As in the last tray, the boat followed the fish. This is a junk. People live and work on this boat, conducting all of their lives on the water.

Ensconced in three trees, this is a pristinely beautiful and ancient place. It is sacred. Six holy pagodas surround the central bridge. Around this sit several small temples and shrines. It is a blessing to make passage through this holy arch.

Tray 10
Focus Figure — The Teacher

I am the teacher, seated at the front of my very well equipped school. There is a large black board to my left. Beyond that a chart showing dinosaurs, remnants of a time past. There is a radio on my desk to bring music into the classroom. A television sits on the central work table, as four seated students look on from behind their desks. One child sits behind me in the corner to my right. He must have misbehaved.

I can see beyond the classroom to the playground of our school. Children are gaily playing on the swings and merry-go-round. Their play is very much a part of this school. It is all of a piece, the classroom and the play yard. Children must be free to play in order to learn and grow.

It is very colorful here. Everything is bright, alive and full of energy.

In the far corner ahead of me to my left a mother sits on a bench with her young child in a stroller. Perhaps she is thinking that one day her child will be ready to go to school and learn. Now they sit and look on, almost with longing or admiration. It is interesting to me that they are directly opposite this little malfeasant behind me in the corner. It is as if the young child of this mother wants to be here, yet this one behind me misbehaved in a way such that he is not able to participate. I wonder what he did to exclude himself so? This mother across on the bench seems supportive of helping her little one grow and develop so she might one day send her little one here to school. I care for these children and help them grow, just as this Mother does in the far corner.

Tray 11
Focus Figure — The Train

I am very dark and heavy. I pass to the right and the sun is directly overhead. I am sturdy and strong. No one can see into me. I am made of very heavy metal. Perhaps my heavy metal encasement can leave now, as the sun lights the way.

It appears to be winter. Some of the trees have snow on them. Some, however, do not. There is a large, heavy fossil rock on my right. Maybe I'm leaving the old fossils of the past behind, also. The wintery trees lie ahead of me, the green ones behind. It is as though I am at the interstices of summer and winter. In the center there is a beautiful gazebo with an inviting table and chairs. It is empty, though. No one sits there.

The village, ahead to my right is lovely and peaceful. It is very quiet and there are no people about.

Behind me, behind the tall green pine, is a well. We can reach deep places with this well. It stands at the head of the stream. Four fish swim along the stream, heading in the opposite direction from the way they were going in the past trays. They swim in the direction of the well. Perhaps they swim to the source of the water.

From the well, we draw the water up from the depths of the earth. Ahead of me in the land of winter, the water is transformed into beautiful crystal ice and snow. It undergoes a radical transformation and becomes something exquisitely beautiful.

The sun above lights the way for my passage to the land of the snow. Am I leaving the land of the sun and moving into a new place? Am I leaving this solar masculinity behind and moving on now to something very different, something transformed?

A stone wall defines the front boundary of the tray on the other side of the stream, as if to solidly underscore what transpires here. It says, "Take notice," and firmly so.

A single silver tree stands to the far right of the house beyond the gazebo. Perhaps we are moving from the land of the golden sun into the land of silver, from the golden, solar form of being masculine, to the silver, lunar way of being a man.

Tray 12
Focus Figure — The Charging Horses

Here we come now. Powerfully charging in from the near left, our thundering hooves are quietly muffled by this snowy wonderland. Nothing can hold us back now. We are here, we are strong, and we are magnificently beautiful! We are pure and glorious. This is a very special place. Exquisite snowflakes dot the landscape. All is crystalline and snowy white.

To our right a pair of pure white polar bears approaches the icy stream. They are large and powerful. Perhaps it is a pair, a male and a female. They are very much at home here. This is the place where they are completely comfortable. The larger of the pair approaches two cubes of ice in the stream. The water has been transformed, frozen, and it has assumed the form of a cube. Like a square, the cube is representative of all dimensions of spatial reality. There are two cubes here. The polar bear seems to point them out. Perhaps this pairing of wholeness calls out to be seen. There is a pair of cubes, the water has been transformed, and it is right in front. It is as if the bear wants us to know that things have dramatically changed. There is now wholeness. It is pure, beautiful and powerful.

Behind the bears is an igloo. It is beautiful and round, almost spherical. Made of cubes of ice, it becomes very rounded in shape. It is as if the wholeness of the ice cubes comes together to form a round home. It is a place of respite in this wonderland. Atop, it is crowned with a ring of crystal, as if to emphasize its sacredness and its wholeness.

A pair of crystalline snow pines flanks the igloo, ensconcing it and planting it firmly in this snowy habitat.

Directly ahead of us is a pair of skiers, artfully making their way down the snowy slope. This pair, this couple, is also very much at home here. They are skillfully able to navigate and negotiate their way through this snowy land.

There are two of us (horses) two bears, two cubes of ice, two snow pines and two skiers. Things are paired here, as they are newly emerging and call to be seen.

Above us all hangs a many pointed crystal star. Perhaps it is nighttime. Perhaps this is the rising of a glorious new star. The light of a star is gentler than the light of the sun.

Tray 13
Focus Figure — The Wounded Soldier

I am hurt. This war has wounded me badly. Help has come to carry me off the battlefield. It all seems so pointless now, all of this strife and warring.

The sides are clearly defined, lined up one against the other. Funny how they look the same now. The battle is over for me, as I now make my exit.

Tray 14
Focus Figure — The Golfer

I am concentrated and have my shot clearly lined up. I know right where I am going. It is directly ahead of me, but there are many things in the way.

Dick Tracy and Inspector Clouseau, two fictional detectives, are confronting me. They are amusing and not threatening. Clouseau examines the region of my golf ball with his looking glass. Dick Tracy's gun is raised toward the sky and isn't threatening. I wonder what they are looking for. This place is like a comic strip. My shot will not be easy with all of these obstacles. Nonetheless, I am focused. There is a well in the way. I must cross a road, which has two race cars and a gas pump on it. Not a very likely golf course, this one. There is a cow headed toward my hole, also. What is a cow doing on a golf course?

Directly behind the hole, the space shuttle is ready to take off. To my right, several bicyclists ride up a riverbed, while a diver rests prone on top of the bridge. Everything is mixed up here.

To my left, the large black train moves in the direction of the shuttle. What is a train doing on the golf course?

In the upper left corner a polar bear is chasing a skier up a snow-covered hill.

This is a very funny place where everything is mixed up, but I know exactly where I am going.

Tray 15
Focus Figure — The Boxer

I stand here glowing and triumphant next to my gleaming silver trophy. I have won. I have overcome all of my battles. I stand and face each of you, all of my antagonists, as I prepare to leave, to cross the bridge to the other side where all is peaceful. My little car stands ready on the bridge and is making the passage to the new land.

The two- and three-headed dragons—I've conquered you and can leave you behind. Penguin, Hitler, Davy Crockett and Hulk Hogan, none of you any longer poses me any threat. Even the heavy black train is much smaller and is moving away. Now it stands here among my opponents and acknowledges my victories.

Superman triumphantly backs me up, mirroring my strength and personal power. Above me, Rocket Man flies along the path of the river, marking the division between the old world and the new. He is very powerful and exercises great alacrity in the skies. He has command of the reaches of the heavens, as does Superman. We have regained the earth and the heavens as our own and move between them with ease, grace and power.

The loving cup stands to me on my left, my feminine side. I am liberated from the metal encasement of the first tray. The heavy armor that was once my defense and my prison is now transformed and stands as a gleaming testament to the victories and capabilities of my emerging self.

In the far right corner, a woman sits watching. It is as if she has always been there, knowing, believing in me, ever present as I have emerged. There is something strong and solid about her. I am glad she has been there.

— End of SIA Inquiry Log —

~ Conclusion ~

The Sandplay Case of Aaron—Transcript of SIA Inquiry

The Subjective Immersion Analysis of this sandplay case provided me a means, as the therapist, to grasp its transformative significance from within the symbolic context. By employing SIA, I was better able to understand the relationships among the figures as carriers of the psychic change process. This intimacy greatly strengthened my ability to hold the case.

I find the SIA method a helpful tool for sandplay understanding and containment. I encourage sandplay therapists to experiment with SIA to determine if it may be of help in their work.

APPENDIX B

The History and Development of Sandplay Therapy

British pediatrician and child psychiatrist, Margaret Lowenfeld (1979/1993) is generally credited with the development of the therapeutic use of miniature figures in a tray of sand at her *Clinic for Nervous and Difficult Children*, which she opened in London in 1928. Lowenfeld drew upon her memory of H.G. Wells' *Floor Games* (1911), which describes the wonders of the miniature worlds Wells and his children created on the floor with a variety of small toys and blocks (Turner, 2004). The engaging and creative nature of the *Floor Games* had impressed Lowenfeld greatly, so she set about equipping her clinic with small toys and materials in what she called the *wonder box*. It was the children that gave birth to what Lowenfeld named the *World Technique* in 1929 when they referred to the wonder box as, *—the world*, and spontaneously began fashioning miniature worlds and scenes in the sand boxes in the clinic playroom (Bowyer, 1970; Lowenfeld, 1979/1993).

Perceiving that children's thought processes were quite different from those of adults, Lowenfeld's (1939, 1946) intention was to develop a way that allowed for the direct expression of the mental and emotional experience of the child. Lowenfeld also wanted a method that would lend itself to some form of record keeping so that their creations might be studied. Lowenfeld was concerned to avoid the superimposition of any theories onto the children's productions, preferring to allow any theory to evolve directly from the children's work itself.

> My own endeavor in my work with children is to devise an instrument with which a child can demonstrate his own emotional and mental state without the necessary intervention of an adult either by transference or interpretation, and which will allow of a record being made of such a demonstration. My objective is to help children to produce something which will stand by itself and be independent of any theory as to its nature (Lowenfeld, 1979/1993, p.3).

The first professional demonstration of the World Technique was at a clinical conference in Paris in 1937. Carl Gustav Jung, who was in attendance at that conference, analyzed the world that Lowenfeld had presented (Bowyer, 1970). The therapeutic value of the World Technique was well regarded and documented in Lowenfeld's child clinic and by the mid twentieth century came to be recognized as an effective means of treatment for adults, as well (Bowyer, 1970; Lowenfeld, 1950b, 1993).

A number of clinicians were drawn to the study of the World Technique, later adapting or modifying it to suit their own particular therapeutic or diagnostic purposes. Among these was Swedish clinician Goesta Harding, who was influenced by Hanna Bratt, who had studied with Lowenfeld in 1933. Harding studied briefly with Lowenfeld in 1949, then developed what she called the Erica Method, which has since flourished in Sweden (Harding, 1969/1972). Harding credited Gudrun Seitz, who studied with Lowenfeld in London in 1941 with the first introduction of the World Technique to the Institute for Therapeutic Pedagogy in Stockholm (Bowyer, 1970). The Erica Method parallels the tools and methods of Lowenfeld and is used for diagnostic and therapeutic applications.

Charlotte Buhler, noted child development researcher at the University of Vienna, also adapted the World Technique to her research and clinical needs. Taken with the ability of the World Technique to portray the workings of the child's mind, Buhler (1951) worked to standardize the technique for use as a diagnostic test in the study of children's cognitive and developmental processes. With Lowenfeld's original support and encouragement, Buhler observed world making at the clinic in London. Buhler named her tool the *World Test*. With the use of a limited number of miniature figures, numbering between 160 and 300, the World Test is a diagnostic instrument which is conducted on a table top, rather than in sand, and is scored using a standardized rating scale designed to discern clinical (pathological) from normal (non-pathological) worlds. When Lowenfeld and Buhler later met in 1950 to discuss their work, Lowenfeld found Buhler's World Test to be quite at cross-purposes to her work with the World Technique (Bowyer, 1970; Lowenfeld, 1950a, 1950b).

Buhler influenced the work of two French clinicians, de Beaumont and Arthus, who, after seeing a demonstration of the world material by Buhler in Holland in the 1940's, returned to France to develop what they called the *Village Test*, another modification of the World Technique adapted for clinical assessment (Arthus, 1949; Bowyer, 1970). The Village Test equipment and interpretation was then standardized by Pierre Mabille (1950).

Coincidental with the work of Lowenfeld and Buhler was the development of the Dramatic Productions Test (DPT) by Erik Homberger (1937), later known as Erik Erikson. Although unaware of the World Technique or the World Test, Erikson used miniature figures in a defined space to attempt to better understand human behavior. Erikson utilized the DPT in two well documented studies: one of college students at Harvard, and the other as part of a twenty-year longitudinal developmental study at the University of California at Berkeley (Erikson, 1951). Asking the participants to *—make a dramatic scene*, in the Harvard study, Erikson surmised that what appeared in their miniature configurations on the table top were scenes representative of trauma from childhood. Erikson concluded that the DPT configurations were continuations of where the participants had left off in their childhood attempts to overcome the trauma through the active repetition of play. In the developmental study Erikson saw similar themes of early trauma in addition to scenes of family conflict, themes of illness or somatic concerns and psychosexual conflicts.

Another adaptation of Lowenfeld's World Technique to assessment and diagnosis was that of Austrian clinicians Hedda Bolgar and Lisolette Fischer, who were interested in developing a non-verbal projective instrument to assist in clinical diagnosis. Familiar with the work of both Lowenfeld and Buhler, they developed the *Little World Test* in the mid 1930's (Bolgar & Fischer, 1940). The Little World Test consists of 232 standardized colorful wood or metal miniatures of a simple or schematic design and is conducted on an octagonal table surface. The test is scored in six categories, choice, quantity, form, content, behavior and verbalization and is used to distinguish clinical from normal profiles (Bowyer, 1970).

Scottish psychologist and academician, Laura Ruth Bowyer (aka Pickford) made an avid study of the World Technique. With Margaret Lowenfeld's encouragement she wrote a comprehensive survey of the history and uses of the World Technique and made significant contributions to work with the World Technique (Bowyer, 1970). Among other contributions to her work in the Lowenfeld tradition, Bowyer developed scoring categories to better analyze worlds and deduced developmental norms for children and adults from clinical and normal populations.

Another adaptation of Lowenfeld's World Technique to diagnostic purposes was made by L.N.J. Kamp at the University of Utrecht in the Netherlands. Kamp, had employed the World Technique to formulate a developmental scale when working in the public schools in Topeka, Kansas in the 1940's. Working with E.S. Kessler of Georgetown University, Kamp devised scoring procedures to determine developmental norms as indicated in world productions (Kamp & Kessler, 1970).

Dutch educator, P.C. Ojemann drew upon the work of Kamp and that of educator, Maria J. Krabbe (1991) to develop her *Wereldspel* table top village construction test for the diagnosis of what she called *image thinking* as a learning style for the early detection of learning difficulties in school children (Ojemann, Personal communication, November 1992, Groningen, Holland).

Another formidable figure in the development of the therapeutic use of miniatures in sand was Dora Maria Kalff. A neighbor and friend of Emma and Carl Jung in Switzerland, Kalff was encouraged by Jung to pursue a psychological career (Mitchell & Friedman, 1994; Kalff, 2003). Having observed Kalff's abilities with children, Jung suggested that Kalff direct her attention to this unexplored area in Jungian psychology. This posed many logistical difficulties for Kalff. Traditional Jungian analysis is unsuited to children, as they have not yet evolved the cognitive skills or developmental capacities that predispose them to a verbal analysis. Kalff began her study in 1949 at the Jung Institute in Kusnaacht, Switzerland, and in 1954 attended a lecture presented by Margaret Lowenfeld on the World Technique. Kalff was intrigued and impressed with the possibility of using the World Technique as a symbolic tool with children. With Jung's encouragement, Kalff went to London to study the World Technique with Margaret Lowenfeld upon completing her analytical training in 1956 (Weinrib, 1983/2004).

Recognizing the archetypal content and symbolic process of the worlds, Kalff adapted the World Technique to Jungian theory and named her technique *sandplay* therapy, to distinguish it from Lowenfeld's World Technique.

Whereas Margaret Lowenfeld (1979/1993) customarily interpreted the Worlds for the children before the end of treatment, Dora Kalff (1980/2003) recognized that a delayed interpretation was important, because it allowed the client the opportunity to undergo transformation at the deepest levels of the psyche. Rooted in the fundamental Jungian concept that the psyche has an inherent tendency to move toward wholeness, Kalff saw that the therapist's silent, but knowing attendance to the sandplay process activated these potentials in the client. Whereas Lowenfeld regarded the World Technique as a means for the communication and expression of children's thoughts and emotions and as a vehicle for the release of conflicts and tension resulting from discrepancies between their inner and outer realities, Kalff saw the immediacy of the reordering of the psyche occurring in the creation of the sandplay, itself. With her Jungian background and deeply intuitive nature, Kalff recognized that a process of archetypal symbolic transformation occurred through a series of sandplays and felt that it was a perfect vehicle for the Jungian treatment of children.

Kalff and Lowenfeld communicated about their differing approaches to the sand tray and agreed in the late 1950's to the difference in names to distinguish the two approaches (Mitchell & Friedman, 1994). Sandplay therapy has since grown in popularity as a valued therapeutic medium among Jungian analysts and Jungian oriented therapists. As occurred with the World Technique, sandplay has also come into favor for use with adult clients as well as children.

References

Allen, R.E. (2007) Human ecology economics: A new framework for sustainability. NY: Routledge.

Amatruda , K. & Helm-Simpson, P. (1997). *Sandplay the sacred healing: A guide to symbolic process.* Novato, CA: Trance Sand Dance Press.

Ammann, R. (1991). *Healing and transformation in sandplay: Creative processes become visible.* La Salle, IL: Open Court.

Arthus, H. (1949). *Le Village: Test d'activite creatice.* Paris: Presses Universitaires de France.

Bahti, M. & Bahti, T. (1997). *Southwestern Indian ceremonials..* Las Vegas, NV: K.C. Publications.

Baldrian, F. (1995). Taoism (C. Le Blanc, Trans.). In M. Eliade (Ed.), *The encyclopedia of religion*, Vol. 14 (pp.288-305). New York: Macmillan Publishing Company.

Baum, L. F. (2003). *The wonderful wizard of oz.* New York: Modern Library.

Baum, N. (2002). People with Schizophrenia. In N. Baum & B. Weinberg (Eds.), *In the hands of creation: Sandplay images of birth and rebirth.* Toronto: Muki Baum Association.

Bolgar, H. & Fischer, L.K. (1940). The toy test: A psychodiagnostic method. *Psychological Bulletin*, 37. 17-18.

Bowyer, R. (1956). *The importance of sand in the World Technique: An experiment. A normative study of sand tray worlds.* Paper read at British Psychological Society Annual General Meeting, Manchester, England.

Bowyer, R. (1970). *The Lowenfeld world technique: Studies in personality.* London: Pergamon Press.

Bradway, K. & McCoard, B. (1997). *Sandplay: Silent workshop of the psyche.* New York: Routledge.

Brill, A.A. (1966). *The basic writings of Sigmund Freud.* New York: The Modern Library.

Bryant, B. (1993). *The wheel of time sand mandala: Visual scripture of Tibetan Buddhism.* San Francisco: Harper Collins.

Buhler, C. (1941). Symbolic action in children. *Transactions of the New York Academy of Science*, 17. 63-65.

Buhler, C. (1951a). The world test: Manual of directions. *Journal of Child Psychiatry*, 2. 24-35.

Buhler, C (1951b). The world test, a projective technique. *The Journal of Child Psychiatry*, 2:1. 4-23.

Buhler, C., Kelly (Lumry), G. & Carrol, S. (1951). World-test standardization studies. *The Journal of Child Psychiatry*, 2. 76.

Buhler, C (1952). National differences in world test projection patterns. *Journal of Projective Techniques*, 16:1. 42-55.

Burke, V.J. (1996). Sandtray characteristics of school children by gender, ages seven through eleven. *Masters Abstracts International*, 35-01.

Cirlot, J.E. (1971). *A dictionary of symbols*. New York: Philosophical Library.

Cohn, D.P. (2000). Gender differences among children during the struggle stage of sand tray therapy. *Dissertation Abstracts International*, 61(5-B), 2749.

Collins, S. (1995). Buddhist Concepts. In M. Eliade (Ed.), *The encyclopedia of religion*, Vol. 13 (pp.443-6). New York: Macmillan Publishing Company.

Cory, G.A. & Gardner, R. (Eds.) (2002). The evolutionary neuroethology of Paul MacLean: Convergences and frontiers. Westport, CT: Praeger.

Davidson, H.R. E. (1964). *Gods and myths of northern Europe*. Baltimore, MD: Penguin Books.

Dillard, A. (1999). *For the time being*. New York: Alfred A. Knoph.

De Groot, J. J. M. (1964). *The Religious System of China Vol. 6*. Taipei. (Original work published 1910)

de Vries, A. (1984). *Dictionary of symbols and imagery*. Amsterdam, The Netherlands: Elsevier Science Publishers B.V.

Donelan, J. (2000). What makes sandplay unique? Sandplay therapists' views on how sandplay relates to verbal techniques and the beneficial effects of using these modalities concurrently. *Dissertation Abstracts International*, 60 (9-B): 4884.

Eastwood, P. S. (2002). *Nine windows to wholeness: Exploring numbers in sandplay therapy*. Honolulu, Hi: Sanity Press.

Ebrey, P.B. (Ed.). (1993). *Chinese civilization: A sourcebook* (2nd ed.). New York: The Free Press.

Edgerton, F. (1944). *The Bhagavad Gita*. New York: Harper Torchbooks.

Edinger, E.F. (1972). *Ego & archetype: Individuation and the religious function of the psyche*. Boston: Shambhala.

Edinger, E.F. (1991). *Anatomy of the psyche: Alchemical symbolism in psychotherapy.* La Salle, IL: Open Court. (Original work published 1985)

Eliade, M. (1959). *The sacred and the profane. The nature of religion.* (W. Trask, Trans.). London: Harcourt Brace Jovanovich.

Eliade, M. (1974). *Shamanism: Archaic techniques of ecstasy.* (W.R. Trask, Trans.) Princeton, NJ: Princeton University Press. (Original work published 1964)

Eliade, M. (1979). *The forge and the crucible: The origins and structures of alchemy, 2d ed.* (S. Corrin, Trans.) Chicago: University of Chicago Press.

Eliade, M. (1991). *Images and symbols: Studies in religious symbolism.* (P. Mairet, Trans.). Princeton, NJ: Princeton University Press. (Original work published 1952)

Eliade, M. (1996). *Patterns in comparative religions.* Lincoln, NE: University of Nebraska Press. (Original work published 1958)

Erikson, E.H. (1951). Sex differences in the play configurations of pre-adolescents. *American Journal of Orthopsychiatry,* 21. 667-92.

Erikson, E.H. (1963). *Childhood and society.* New York: W.W. Norton & Company, Inc. (Original work published 1950)

Erikson, E.H. (1980). *Identity and the life cycle.* New York: W.W. Norton & Company. (Original work published 1959)

Flavell, J.H. (1963), *The developmental psychology of Jean Piaget.* New York: D. Van Nostrand Company.

Frazer, J.G. (2002). *The golden bough.* Indypublish.Com. (Original work published 1922)

Freud, S. (1933). Collected papers. *London: Hogarth Press.*

Freud, S. (1966). *The basic writings of Sigmund Freud: The interpretation of dreams* (A.A. Brill, Trans., Ed.). New York: Modern Library. (Original work published 1913)

Gilligan, C. (1993). *In a different voice: psychological theory and women's development.* Cambridge: Harvard University Press.

Gimbutas, M. (1963). *The Balts.:Ancient peoples and places, vol. 33.* Praeger, London.

Glendenning, C. (1994). *"My name is Chellis & I'm in recovery from western civilization."* Boston: Shambala Publications, Inc..

Goswami, A., Reed, R.E. & Goswami, M. (1993). *The self-aware universe: How consciousness creates the material world..* New York: Tarcher/Putnam.

Gould, S.J. (1977). *Ontogeny and phylogeny.* Cambridge: Harvard University Press.

Graves, R. (1994). *The white goddess.* New York: Farrar, Straus and Giroux.

Griffin-Pierce, T. (1995). *The encyclopedia of native America..* Viking: New York.

Grimm (1972). *The complete Grimm's fairy tales.* New York: Pantheon Books.

Grof, S. (1976). *Realms of the human unconscious.* New York: Dutton Paperback.

Grubbs, G. (1991). *A categorical and comparative analysis of the sandplay process of abused and non abused children.* Doctoral dissertation: California Graduate School of Family Psychology.

Grubbs, G. (2005). *The sandplay categorical checklist (SCC) for sandplay analysis.* Woodinville, WA: Rubedo Publications.

Haeffner, M. (1994). *Dictionary of alchemy: From Maria Prophetissa to Isaac Newton.* San Francisco: Acquarian.

Hamilton, E. (1942). *Mythology.* Boston: Little, Brown and Company.

Harman, W. (1988). *Global mind change: The new age revolution in the way we think.* New York: Warner Books.

Harding, G. (1972). *Spieldiagnostik.* (Trans into German: Bohm, E.) Weinheim: Beltz Verlag. (Original work published 1969)

Hearn, M. (1973). *The annotated Wizard of Oz: The wonderful wizard of oz by L. Frank Baum.* Clarkson, Potter, Inc.: New York.

Herbart, J.F. (1901). *Outlines of educational doctrine.* New York: Macmillan.

Homberger, E. (1937). Dramatic productions test. (Part of larger article, Configurations in play: Clinical notes). *Psychoanalytic Quarterly,* 6. 139-214.

Hveberg, H. (1962). *Of gods and giants: Norse mythology.* P.S. Iversen, Trans.). Oslo: Johan Grundt Tanum Forlag.

I ching: Book of changes (1971). (R. Wilhelm & C.F. Baynes, Trans.). Princeton, NJ: Princeton University Press. (Original Bollingen Foundation publication 1950)

Janet, P. (1903). *Les obsessions et la psychasthenie.* Paris.

Jones, L.E. (1982). The development of structure in the world of expression: A cognitive-developmental analysis of children's "sand worlds". *Dissertation Abstracts International,* 43-09B.

Jung, C.G. (1976). *Symbols of transformation: An analysis of the prelude to a case of schizophrenia.* (R.C.F. Hull, Trans.). Princeton, NJ: Princeton University Press. (Original work published 1956)

Jung, C.G. (1977). *Psychology and alchemy.* (R.F.C. Hull, Trans.)

Princeton: Princeton University Press.
(Original work published 1953)

Jung, C.G. (1977). *Psychological types.* (R.C.F. Hull Revision of H.G. Baynes, Trans.). Princeton, NJ: Princeton University Press. (Original work published 1971)

Jung, C.G. (1977) *Two essays on analytical psychology.* (R.C.F. Hull, Trans.). Princeton, NJ: Princeton University Press. (Original work published 1953)

Jung, C.G. (1980). *The archetypes and the collective unconscious.* (R.C.F. Hull, Trans.). Princeton, NJ: Princeton University Press. (Original work published 1959)

Jung, C.G. (1981). *The development of personality* . (R.F.C. Hull, Trans.). Princeton, NJ: Princeton University Press. (Original work published 1954)

Jung, C.G. (1981). *The structure and dynamics of the psyche.* (R.C.F. Hull, Trans.). Princeton, NJ: Princeton University Press. (Original work published 1960)

Jung, C.G. (1983). *Alchemical studies.* (R.F.C. Hull, Trans.) Princeton, NJ: Princeton University Press. (Original work published 1967)

Kalff, D.M. (2003). *Sandplay: A psychotherapeutic approach to the psyche.* Cloverdale, CA: Temenos Press. (Original work published 1980)

Kalff, D.M. (1988). Sandplay in Switzerland. (Seminar notes).. Zurich: University of California at Santa Cruz.

Kalff, M. (1993). Twenty points to be considered in the interpretation of a sandplay. *Journal of Sandplay Therapy,* 2:2. 17-35.

Kamp, L.N.J. & Kessler, E.S. (1970). The world test: Developmental aspects of a play technique. *Journal of Child Psychology and Psychiatry,* 11. 81-108.

Kawai, H. (1988). *The Japanese psyche: Major motifs in the fairy tales of Japan.* Dallas, TX: Spring Publications, Inc.

Kiepenheuer, K. (1990). *Crossing the bridge: A Jungian approach to adolescence* . (K.R. Schneider, Trans.). La Salle, IL: Open Court.

Klein, M. (1932). *Psychoanalysis of children.* New York: Norton.

Krabbe, M.J. (1991). *The image thinker at school.* Amsterdam: Stichting Beelddenken.

Leach, M. and Fried, J. (Eds.). (1972). *Funk & Wagnalls standard dictionary of folklore mythology and legend.* San Francisco: Harper & Row, Publishers.

Levinson, D.J. (1978). *The seasons of a man's life.* New York: Ballantine Books.

Lowenfeld, M. (1939). The world pictures of children: A method of recording and studying them. *British Journal of Medical Psychology,* 18:1. 65-101.

Lowenfeld, M. (1946). Discussion on the value of play therapy in child psychiatry. *Proceedings of the Royal Society of Medicine,* 39. 439-42.

Lowenfeld, M. (Ed.) (1948). *On the psychotherapy of children. A report of a conference held at the Institute of Child Psychology, London, August, 1948, on the theory and technique of direct objective therapy.* London: The Institute of Child Psychology.

Lowenfeld, M. (1950a). Combined approach to the study of treatment of disturbed children. *American Journal of Psychotherapy,* 4. 627-42.

Lowenfeld, M. (1950b). The nature and use of the Lowenfeld world technique in work with children and adults. *The Journal of Psychology,* 30. 325-31.

Lowenfeld, M. (1993). *Understanding children's sandplay: Lowenfeld's world technique.* Great Britain: Antony Rowe Ltd.. (Originally published as *The world technique,* George Allen & Unwin Ltd., 1979)

Lucas, G. (Writer/Director). (1977). *Star wars* [Motion picture]. United States: Lucasfilm. (Released by 20th Century Fox)

Lumry, G.K. (1951). A study of world test characteristics as a basis for discrimination between various clinical categories. *The Journal of Child Psychiatry,* 2. 24-35.

Mabille, P. (1950). *La technique du test du village.* Paris: Presses Universitaires de France. (Reprinted: Dufour, 1970.)

Mahler, M.S., Pine, F. & Bergman, A. (1975). *The psychological birth of the human infant: Symbiosis and individuation.* New York: Basic Books, Inc.

Major, J.S. (1995). Yin-Yang Wu-Hsing. In M. Eliade (Ed.), *The encyclopedia of religion,* Vol. 15 (p. 515). New York: Macmillan Publishing Company.

Markell, M.J. (2002). *Sand, water, silence: The embodiment of spirit, explorations in matter and psyche.* London: Jessica Kingsley Publishers.

Meador, B.D.S. (1994). *Uncursing the dark: Treasures from the underworld.* Wilmette, IL: Chiron Publications.

Metzner, R. (1994) *The well of remembrance: Rediscovering the earth wisdom myths of northern Europe.* Boston: Shambhala.

Miller, J.B. (1984). *The development of women's sense of self.* Work in Progress: The Stone Center, No. 12. Wellesley: Wellesley College.

Miller, J.B. (1986). *Toward a new psychology of women.* Boston: Beacon Press.

Miller, J.B. (1991). *The construction of anger in women and men.* In J. Jordan, et al, *Women's growth in connection* (pp. 181-196). New York: The Guilford Press.

Mitchell, A.G. (1993). *Hindu gods and goddesses.* New Delhi: UBS Publishers' Distributors Ltd.

Mitchell, R.R. & Friedman, H.S. (1994). *Sandplay: Past, present and future.* New York: Routledge.

Montague, A. (1981). *Growing young.* New York: McGraw-Hill Book Company.

Morena, G.D. (2001. *The wisdom of oz.* Berkeley, CA: Frog, Ltd.

Nestler, E.J., Hyman, S.E. & Malenka, R.C. (2001). *Molecular neuropharmacology: A foundation for clinical neuroscience.* New York: McGraw-Hill Companies, Inc.

Neumann, E. (1971). *The origins and history of consciousness* (R.F.C. Hull, Trans.). Princeton, NJ: Princeton University Press.

Neumann, E. (1972). *The great mother: An analysis of the archetype* (R. Manheim, Trans.). Princeton, NJ: Princeton University Press. (Original work published 1955)

Neumann, E. (1973). *Amor and psyche: The psychic development of the feminine, a commentary on the tale by Apuleius* (R. Manheim, Trans.). Princeton, NJ: Princeton University Press. (Original work published 1953)

Neumann, E. (1973). *The child: Structure and dynamics of the nascent personality* (R. Manheim, Trans.). New York: Harper & Row.

Newberg, A. & D'Aquili, E. (2001). *Why God won't go away: Brain science & the biology of belief.* New York: Ballantine Books.

Nicholson, M.J. (1997). *Mountain gloom and mountain glory: The development of the aesthetics of the infinite.* Seattle: University of Washington Press (Original work published 1959).

OED *Oxford English Dictionary* (2nd ed.). New York: Oxford University Press Inc.

Pennington, Y.V. (1996). The sandtray assessment of development: A refinement of Bowyer's research into Lewin's theory of development: A preliminary investigation of the instrument (Kurt Lewin). *Dissertation Abstracts International*, 57-04B.

Perry, B.D. (2001). The neuroarcheology of childhood maltreatment: The neurodevelopmetnal costs of adverse childhood events. *The cost of maltreatment: Who pays? We all do*, 15-37. (K. Franey, R. Geffner & R. Falconer, Eds.) San Diego, CA: Family Violence and Sexual Assault Institute.

Perry, B.D. (2002). Childhood experience and the expression of genetic potential: What childhood neglect tells us about nature and nurture. *Brain and Mind*, 3, 79-100.

Pestalozzi, J.H. (1895). *Leonard and Gerard*. Boston: Heath.

Piaget, J. (1975). *The child's conception of the world*. Totowa, NJ: Littlefield, Adams & Co. (Original work published 1929)

Piaget, J. (1976). *Judgment and reasoning in the child*. Totowa, NJ: Littlefield, Adams & Co. (Original work published 1928)

Piaget, J. (1970). Piaget's theory. In P.H. Mussen (Ed.), *Carmichael's manual of child psychology* (Vol. I, 3rd ed.). New York: Wiley.

Qur'an. (1996). (Abdullah Yusuf Ali, Trans.). Maryland: Amana Publications.

Rao, T.A.G. (1985). *Elements of Hindu iconography* (Vols. 1-2). Delhi: Motilal Banarsidass (Original work published 1914).

Reyna, R. (1993). *Dictionary of Oriental philosophy*. New Delhi: Munshiram Manoharlal Publishers Pvt. Ltd.

Reynolds, D.W. (1998). *Star Wars: The visual dictionary: The ultimate guide to Star Wars characters and creatures*. New York: DK Publishing.

Ryce-Menuhin, J. (1992). *Jungian sandplay: The wonderful therapy*. New York: Routledge.

Siegel, D.J. (1999). *The developing mind: How relationships and the brain interact to shape who we are*. New York: The Guilford Press.

Smith. H. (1992). *Forgotten truth: the common vision of the world's religions*. San Francisco: Harper San Francisco.

Smitter, M. (2002, December). *Sand*. Retrieved 1/10/03, from http://www.seafriends.org.nz/oceano/sand.htm

Stein, M. (1982). The aims and goal of Jungian analysis. In M. Stein (Ed.), *Jungian analysis* (pp. 27-44). Boulder, Co: Shambala.

Steinhardt, L. (2000). *Foundation and form in Jungian sandplay*. London: Jessica Kingsley Publishers.

Stern, D.N. (1985). *The interpersonal world of the infant: A view from psychoanalysis and developmental psychology*.

New York: Basic Books, Inc.
Storm, H. (1972). *Seven arrows.* New York: Harper and Row.
Sturluson, S. (1984). *The prose edda: Tales from Norse mythology* (J. I. Young, Trans.). Berkeley, CA: University of California Press. (Original work published 1954)
Thomas, D.H., Miller, J., White, R., Nabokov, P. & Deloria, P.J. (1993). *The native Americans: An illustrated history.* Atlanta: Turner Publishing, Inc.
Turner, B. (1994). Symbolic process and the role of the therapist in sandplay. *Journal of Sandplay Therapy,* 3 (2), 84-95.
Turner, B. (1996a). *The witch: some considerations for female development.* Unpublished manuscript, California Institute of Integral Studies, San Francisco.
Turner, B. (1996b). *The witch.* Unpublished manuscript.
Turner, B. (1998). An evaluation of the effectiveness of training in Subjective Immersion Analysis as an analytic tool in Jungian sandplay therapy. *Dissertation Abstracts International,* 9904979.
Turner, B. (Ed.) (2004). *H.G. Wells Floor Games: A father's account of play and its legacy of healing.* Cloverdale, CA: Temenos Press.
Turner, G. (1979). *Indians of North America.* Blandford Press: Great Britain.
Walker, E.H. (2000). *The physics of consciousness.* Cambridge, MA: Perseus Publishing.
Weinrib, E.L. (2004). *Images of the self: The sandplay therapy process.* Cloverdale: Temenos Press. (Original work published 1983)
Wells, H.G. (1911). *Floor games.* London: Frank Palmer.
Werner, H. (1973). *Comparative psychology of mental development.* New York, International Universities Press, Inc. (Original work published 1940)
Wickes, F. (1966). *The inner world of childhood.* New York: Spectrum. (Original work published 1927)
Winnicott, D.W. (1992). *Through paediatrics to psycho-analysis: Collected papers.* New York: Brunner/Mazel. (Original work published 1958)
Woodman, M. & Dickson, E. (1996). *Dancing in the flames: The dark goddess in the transformation of consciousness.* Boston: Shambhala.
Zimmer, H. (1971). *The philosophies of India.* (J. Campbell, Ed.) Princeton, NJ: Princeton University Press.

INDEX

A

B

C

D

E

F

G

H

I

J

K

L

M

N

O

S

U

V

Y

Z